State of the Art Brain Tumor Diagnostics, Imaging, and Therapeutics

Guest Editor

MENG LAW, MD

NEUROIMAGING CLINICS OF NORTH AMERICA

www.neuroimaging.theclinics.com

Consulting Editor
SURESH K. MUKHERJI, MD

August 2010 • Volume 20 • Number 3

SAUNDERS an imprint of ELSEVIER, Inc.

W.B. SAUNDERS COMPANY
A Division of Elsevier Inc.

1600 John F. Kennedy Boulevard • Suite 1800 • Philadelphia, Pennsylvania 19103-2899

http://www.theclinics.com

NEUROIMAGING CLINICS OF NORTH AMERICA Volume 20, Number 3
August 2010 ISSN 1052-5149, ISBN 13: 978-1-4377-1838-6

Editor: Joanne Husovski
Developmental Editor: Donald Mumford

Neuroimaging Clinics of North America (ISSN 1052-5149) is published quarterly by Elsevier Inc., 360 Park Avenue South, New York, NY 10010-1710. Months of issue are February, May, August, and November. Business and editorial offices: 1600 John F. Kennedy Blvd., Suite 1800, Philadelphia, PA 19103-2899. Business and editorial offices: 6277 Sea Harbor Drive, Orlando, FL 32887-4800. Periodicals postage paid at New York, NY, and additional mailing offices. Subscription prices are USD 293 per year for US individuals, USD 415 per year for US institutions, USD 150 per year for US students and residents, USD 339 per year for Canadian individuals, USD 520 per year for Canadian institutions, USD 431 per year for international individuals, USD 520 per year for international institutions and USD 215 per year for Canadian and foreign students and residents. To receive student/resident rate, orders must be accompanied by name of affiliated institution, date of term, and the *signature* of program/residency coordinator on institution letterhead. Orders will be billed at individual rate until proof of status is received. Foreign air speed delivery is included in all *Clinics* subscription prices. All prices are subject to change without notice. POSTMASTER: Send address changes to *Neuroimaging Clinics of North America*, Elsevier Health Sciences Division, Subscription Customer Service, 3251 Riverport Lane, Maryland Heights, MO 63043. Telephone: 1-800-654-2452 (U.S. and Canada); 314-447-8871 (outside U.S. and Canada). Fax: 314-447-8029. E-mail: journalscustomerservice-usa@elsevier.com (for print support); journalsonlinesupport-usa@elsevier.com (for online support).

Reprints. For copies of 100 or more of articles in this publication, please contact the Commercial Reprints Department, Elsevier Inc., 360 Park Avenue South, New York, NY 10010-1710. Tel.: 212-633-3812; Fax: 212-462-1935; E-mail: reprints@elsevier.com.

Neuroimaging Clinics of North America is covered by *Excerpta Medical/EMBASE,* the RSNA Index of Imaging Literature, *MEDLINE/PubMed (Index Medicus),* MEDLINE/MEDLARS, SciSearch, Research Alert, and Neuroscience Citation Index.

Printed and bound in the United Kingdom
Transferred to Digital Print 2011

Neuroimaging Clinics of North America

FORTHCOMING ISSUES	RECENT ISSUES

THE CLINICS ARE NOW AVAILABLE ONLINE!

Access your subscription at:
www.theclinics.com

Contributors

CONSULTING EDITOR

SURESH K. MUKHERJI, MD
Professor and Chief of Neuroradiology and Head and Neck Radiology; Professor of Radiology, Otolaryngology Head and Neck Surgery and Radiation Oncology, University of Michigan Health System, Ann Arbor, Michigan

GUEST EDITOR

MENG LAW, MD, FRACR
Professor of Radiology and Neurological Surgery, Director of Neuroradiology, Department of Radiology, Keck University of Southern California School of Medicine, USC Medical Center, Los Angeles, California

AUTHORS

KENNETH ALDAPE, MD
Department of Pathology, The University of Texas M.D. Anderson Cancer Center, Houston, Texas

PETER B. BARKER, DPhil
Professor, Russell H. Morgan Department of Radiology and Radiological Science, Johns Hopkins University School of Medicine; Kennedy Krieger Institute, Baltimore, Maryland

CAMERON BRENNAN, MD
Brain Tumor Center, Memorial Sloan-Kettering Cancer Center; Department of Neurosurgery, Weill Medical College of Cornell University; Department of Neurosurgery, Memorial Sloan-Kettering Cancer Center; Human Oncology and Pathogenesis Program, Memorial Sloan-Kettering Cancer Center, New York, New York

NICOLE BRENNAN, BA
Department of Radiology, Memorial Sloan-Kettering Cancer Center, New York, New York

MICHAEL D. CHAN, MD
Department of Radiation Oncology, Wake Forest University Health Sciences, Winston-Salem, North Carolina

SUSAN M. CHANG, MD
Department of Neurologic Surgery, University of California, San Francisco, San Francisco, California

RIVKA R. COLEN, MD
Fellow in Radiology, Department of Radiology, Brigham and Women's Hospital, Harvard Medical School, Boston, Massachusetts

CLARE H. CUNLIFFE, MD
Assistant Professor and Medical Investigator, Office of the Medical Investigator, University of New Mexico, Albuquerque, New Mexico

INGEBORG FISCHER, MD
Department of Pathology, The University of Texas M.D. Anderson Cancer Center, Houston, Texas; Departement Neuropathologie, Universitaetsspital Zurich, Schmelzbergstrasse, Zurich, Switzerland

MARY E. FOWKES, MD, PhD
Assistant Professor, Division of Neuropathology, Department of Pathology, Mount Sinai Hospital, New York, New York

JUSTIN F. FRASER, MD
Department of Neurosurgery, Weill Medical
College of Cornell University, New York, New York

KETAN B. GHAGHADA, PhD
Assistant Professor, School of Health Information
Sciences, The University of Texas Health Science
Center at Houston, Houston, Texas

AJAY GUPTA, MD
Neuroradiology Service, Department of Radiology,
Memorial Sloan-Kettering Cancer Center,
New York, New York

CATHERINE R. HAWLEY, BS
Vanderbilt University School of Medicine,
Nashville, Tennessee

ANDREI I. HOLODNY, MD
Chief of Neuroradiology Service, Department of
Radiology, Memorial Sloan-Kettering Cancer
Center; Professor of Radiology, Department of
Radiology, New York Presbyterian Hospital/Weill
Cornell Medical College; Brain Tumor Center,
Memorial Sloan-Kettering Cancer Center,
New York, New York

JASON M. HOOVER, MD
Department of Neurologic Surgery, Mayo Clinic,
Rochester, Minnesota

ALENA HORSKÁ, PhD
Assistant Professor, Russell H. Morgan
Department of Radiology and Radiological
Science, Johns Hopkins University School of
Medicine, Baltimore, Maryland

ALAN JACKSON, PhD, FRCP, FRCR, FBIR
Professor, School of Cancer and Imaging
Sciences, Wolfson Molecular Imaging Centre,
The University of Manchester, Manchester,
United Kingdom

FERENC A. JOLESZ, MD
B. Leonard Holman Professor of Radiology,
Department of Radiology, Brigham and Women's
Hospital, Harvard Medical School, Boston,
Massachusetts

GLENN LESSER, MD
Department of Internal Medicine (Hematology and
Oncology), Wake Forest University Health
Sciences, Winston-Salem, North Carolina

**SAMANTHA JANE MILLS, MB ChB, MRCP,
FRCR**
Professor, School of Cancer and Imaging
Sciences, Wolfson Molecular Imaging Centre,
The University of Manchester, Manchester,
United Kingdom

AARON M. MOHS, PhD
Emory-Georgia Tech Center for Cancer
Nanotechnology Excellence Distinguished Fellow,
Department of Biomedical Engineering, Emory
University and Georgia Institute of Technology,
Atlanta, Georgia

SRINIVASAN MUKUNDAN Jr, MD, PhD
Section Head of Neuroradiology, Department of
Radiology, Brigham and Women's Hospital;
Associate Professor of Radiology, Harvard
Medical School, Boston, Massachusetts

YOAV PARAG, MD
Division of Neuroradiology, Department of
Radiology, Mount Sinai Hospital, New York,
New York

IAN F. PARNEY, MD, PhD
Department of Neurologic Surgery, Mayo Clinic,
Rochester, Minnesota

NEIL PATEL, BS
University of Illinois College of Medicine, Urbana,
Illinois

JAMES M. PROVENZALE, MD
Professor, Departments of Radiology and
Oncology, Emory University School of Medicine;
Professor, Department of Biomedical Engineering,
Georgia Institute of Technology, Atlanta, Georgia;
Professor, Department of Radiology, Duke
University Medical Center, Durham, North Carolina

EUDOCIA C. QUANT, MD
Instructor in Neurology Harvard Medical School,
Division of Cancer Neurology, Department of
Neurology, Brigham and Women's Hospital;
Center for Neuro-Oncology, Dana-Farber/Brigham
and Women's Cancer Center, Boston,
Massachusetts

AKASH SHAH, MD
Neuroradiology Service, Department of Radiology,
Memorial Sloan-Kettering Cancer Center,
New York, New York

EDWARD G. SHAW, MD
Department of Radiation Oncology, Wake Forest
University Health Sciences, Winston-Salem,
North Carolina

**STAVROS MICHAEL STIVAROS, MB ChB,
FRCR**
Professor, School of Cancer and Imaging
Sciences, Wolfson Molecular Imaging Centre, The
University of Manchester, Manchester,
United Kingdom

STEPHEN B. TATTER, MD, PhD
Department of Neurosurgery, Wake Forest
University Health Sciences, Winston-Salem,
North Carolina

GERARD THOMPSON, MB ChB, MRCS
Professor, School of Cancer and Imaging
Sciences, Wolfson Molecular Imaging Centre,

The University of Manchester, Manchester,
United Kingdom

PATRICK Y. WEN, MD
Professor of Neurology, Harvard Medical School,
Division of Cancer Neurology, Department of
Neurology, Brigham and Women's Hospital;
Center for Neuro-Oncology, Dana-Farber/Brigham
and Women's Cancer Center, Boston,
Massachusetts

ROBERT J. YOUNG, MD
Director of 3T Neuroimaging, Neuroradiology
Service, Department of Radiology, Memorial
Sloan-Kettering Cancer Center; Assistant
Professor of Radiology, Department of Radiology,
New York Presbyterian Hospital/Weill Cornell
Medical College; Brain Tumor Center, Memorial
Sloan-Kettering Cancer Center, New York,
New York

Contents

> To keep up with advances in central nervous system (CNS) tumor diagnosis and discovery of new entities, the classification of these tumors requires periodic review and revision. Since the initial 1979 publication from the World Health Organization (WHO) of Histological Typing of Tumours of the Central Nervous System, 3 further editions have been published, cataloging the advances in CNS tumor classification and diagnosis over the past 3 decades. In this article, we discuss select new additions to the current classification, including new diagnostic tools, differential diagnoses, and management implications.

> Diffuse gliomas in adults continue to have a dismal prognosis with the current standard therapeutic methods, including maximal surgical resection, radiation, and chemotherapy. The pathogenesis of adult glioma is complex, involving the loss of function of tumor suppressor genes and activation of oncogenes, which are involved in a network of interconnected signaling pathways. Through activation of these pathways, characteristics of malignant gliomas, including uncontrolled proliferation and growth, invasion, and angiogenesis, are driven. Evolving therapeutic approaches are focused on specifically targeting these genetic lesions. This content gives an overview of the current knowledge about the pathogenesis of adult diffuse gliomas, emphasizing new targeted treatment approaches.

> In the past decade, numerous advances in the understanding of brain tumor physiology, tumor imaging, and tumor therapy have been attained. In some cases, these advances have resulted from refinements of pre-existing technologies (eg, improvements of contrast-enhanced magnetic resonance imaging). In other instances, advances have resulted from development of novel technologies. The development of nanomedicine (ie, applications of nanotechnology to the field of medicine) is an example of the latter. In this review, the authors explain the principles that underlay nanoparticle design and function as well as the means by which nanoparticles can be used for imaging and therapy of brain tumors.

The utility of magnetic resonance spectroscopy (MRS) in diagnosis and evaluation of treatment response to human brain tumors has been widely documented. The role of MRS in tumor classification, tumors versus nonneoplastic lesions, prediction of survival, treatment planning, monitoring of therapy, and post-therapy evaluation is discussed. This article delineates the need for standardization and further study in order for MRS to become widely used as a routine clinical tool.

The advanced imaging techniques outlined in this article are only slowly establishing their place in surgical practice. Even a low risk of false information is unacceptable in neurosurgery, thus decision-making is necessarily conservative. As more validation studies and greater experience accrue, surgeons are becoming more comfortable weighing the quality of information from functional imaging studies. Advanced imaging information is highly complementary to established surgical "good practice" such as anatomic planning, awake craniotomy, and electrocortical stimulation; its greatest impact is perhaps on how neurosurgery is planned and discussed before the patient is ever brought to the operating room. Access to functional magnetic resonance (MR) imaging, diffusion tractography, and intraoperative MR imaging can influence neurosurgical decisions before, during, and after surgery. However, the widespread adoption of these techniques in neurosurgical practice remains limited by the lack of standardized methods, the need for validation across institutions, and the unclear cost-effectiveness particularly for intraoperative MR imaging. Before advanced imaging results can be used therapeutically, it is incumbent on the neurosurgeon and neuroradiologist to develop a working understanding of each technique's strengths and weaknesses, positive and negative predictive values, and modes of failure. This content presents several imaging methods that are increasingly used in neurosurgical planning. As these techniques are progressively applied to surgery, radiologists, medical physicists, neuroscientists, and engineers will be necessary partners with the treating neurosurgeon to bridge the gap between the experimental and the therapeutic.

The use of biomarkers of microvascular structure and function from perfusion and permeability imaging is now well established in neuro-oncological research. There remain significant challenges to be overcome before these techniques and related biomarkers can find general clinical acceptance. Core to this is the standardization of acquisition and processing protocols for robust use across multiple clinical sites. The potential clinical benefits of these approaches are already becoming clear, particularly in the setting of novel antiangiogenic therapies. With an increasing body of evidence in the scientific literature, and with a steadily falling barrier to entry, the coming decade should see rapid developments in imaging biomarkers, and facilitate their transition into routine clinical practice.

Magnetic resonance image-guided focused ultrasound surgery (MRgFUS) has surfaced as a viable noninvasive image-guided therapeutic method that integrates focused ultrasound (FUS), the therapeutic component, with magnetic resonance imaging (MRI), the image guidance module, into a real-time therapy delivery system with closed-loop control of energy delivery. The main applications for MRgFUS of the brain are thermal ablations for brain tumors and functional neurosurgery, and nonthermal, nonablative uses for disruption of the blood brain barrier (BBB) or blood clot and hematoma dissolution by liquification. The disruption of the BBB by FUS can be used for targeted delivery of chemotherapy and other therapeutic agents. MRI is used preoperatively for target definition and treatment planning, intraoperatively for procedure monitoring and control, and postoperatively for validating treatment success. Although challenges still remain, this integrated noninvasive therapy delivery system is anticipated to change current treatment paradigms in neurosurgery and the clinical neurosciences.

Treatment of glioblastoma multiforme remains a major challenge despite advances in standard therapy, including surgery, radiation, and chemotherapy. The field of nanomedicine is expected to have a major impact on the treatment and management of brain tumors. Over the past decade, significant efforts have been made in using nanoparticles for diagnosis and treatment of brain tumors. One class of nanoparticles, liposomes, have received considerable attention for use as nanocarriers for delivery of therapeutics and contrast agents. The purpose of this article is to present the advances in the design and functional characteristics of liposomes for applications in brain tumor imaging.

The eloquent brain can be identified using functional MR (fMR) imaging for the gray matter and diffusion tensor (DT) imaging for the white matter. fMR imaging and DT imaging are especially important for patients with tumors near the important motor and language centers of the brain, where the normal anatomic references may be distorted by the tumor and associated edema. This article explains fMR imaging and DT imaging techniques and illustrates their clinical applications and limitations.

Radiation therapy remains a critical therapeutic modality in the treatment of adult brain tumors. However, its use continues to evolve depending on the histologic findings of the brain tumor. In high-grade gliomas, current trials focus on the addition of systemic agents and optimization of target delineation to improve the therapeutic ratio of radiotherapy. In low-grade gliomas, the life expectancy is much greater, and the possibility of late effects of radiotherapy have shaped contemporary trials to attempt to identify groups that benefit from radiotherapy versus the ones that may defer radiotherapy until tumor progression. With primary central nervous system lymphoma, the advent of high-dose methotrexate-based chemotherapy and the risk of severe early neurocognitive toxicity have brought the role of radiotherapy into question. With meningioma, the use of normal tissue-sparing techniques such as radiosurgery has allowed for the successful treatment of patients who are eminently curable and with a life expectancy that is generally no different than that of

Clinical Trials in Brain Tumor Surgery

Jason M. Hoover, Susan M. Chang, and Ian F. Parney

The prognosis for patients diagnosed with primary central nervous system tumors, such as gliomas, remains generally poor. Improved treatment (standard therapies and novel strategies) is needed. Glioma surgery is a key part of standard treatment and has established roles in providing tissue for diagnosis and in tumor debulking. Several techniques to increase safe surgical resection have been investigated. In addition, novel surgical modalities introducing therapeutic agents locally are increasingly common. This article reviews recent glioma surgery clinical trials, focusing on outcome studies, novel surgical techniques, and local therapeutic agent delivery.

Novel Medical Therapeutics in Glioblastomas, Including Targeted Molecular Therapies, Current and Future Clinical Trials

Eudocia C. Quant and Patrick Y. Wen

The prognosis for glioblastoma is poor despite optimal therapy with surgery, radiation, and chemotherapy. New therapies that improve survival and quality of life are needed. Research has increased our understanding of the molecular pathways important for gliomagenesis and disease progression. Novel agents have been developed against these targets, including receptor tyrosine kinases, intracellular signaling molecules, epigenetic abnormalities, and tumor vasculature and microenvironment. This article reviews novel therapies for glioblastoma, with an emphasis on targeted agents.

Foreword

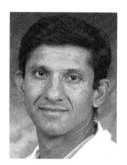

Suresh K. Mukherji, MD
Consulting Editor

I am convinced that the future of radiology is biologic imaging. With advancements such as routine submillimeter imaging capabilities with CT & MR, dynamic 3-D rotational neuroangiography, 4-D ultrasound, and stereotactic mammography, one wonders if the limits of anatomic imaging have been reached.

The concept of biologic imaging defines the ability to directly image and assess various physiologic and metabolic processes at the cellular and subcellular levels. My definition of biologic imaging includes recent advances in radiotracer chemistry, nanotechnology, perfusion imaging (CT and MR imaging), diffusion imaging, MR spectroscopy, functional MR imaging, and recently introduced material density imaging.

As this new frontier is crossed, with greater acceptance of these physiologic and metabolic techniques by referring physicians, what "keeps me up at night" is whether or not biologic imaging will continue to be performed by radiologists.

Our field is entering an era of subspecialization heralded by the new American Board of Radiology certifying examination and the maintenance of certification process. In order to continue to maintain our pivotal role in these new imaging frontiers, future radiologists need to become familiar with tumor biology, treatment options, and physiologic response to prevent us from being marginalized from the biologic imaging techniques they initially developed.

In this issue of *Neuroimaging Clinics of North America*, Dr Meng Law has done an incredible job introducing the current and future challenges of the role of biologic imaging techniques in brain tumor imaging. He has skillfully separated this issue into 3 distinct sections: diagnostics, treatment planning, and therapeutics. He has brought together internationally recognized thought leaders in advanced imaging techniques (spectroscopy, perfusion, diffusion tensor, functional MR imaging, nanotechnology, novel gadolinium/liposomal contrast agents, and MR imaging–guided focused ultrasound surgery), neuro-oncology, radiation oncology, and neurosurgery.

I want to personally thank Dr Law for his tireless efforts in producing such an outstanding contribution. This state-of-the-art publication will be a classic reference for all individuals participating in the field of neuro-oncology.

As you can probably tell, Meng and I have known each other for many years. He and I have held several high-level scientific discussions on the golf course. Meng is a gifted individual who is recognized as an international authority on the applications of advanced MR techniques for diagnosis and treatment monitoring of brain tumors. My only concern is related to his mathematical skills. I am somewhat confused how Meng continues to insist, "18 holes" multiplied by "7 strokes per hole" equals "72." Maybe Dr Law will be willing to edit a future issue of *Neuroimaging Clinics of North America* on his definition of "New Math Techniques and Iterative Reconstruction"!

Suresh K. Mukherji, MD
University of Michigan Health System
1500 East Medical Center Drive
Ann Arbor, Michigan 48109-5030, USA

E-mail address:
mukherji@med.umich.edu

Neuroimag Clin N Am 20 (2010) xiii
doi:10.1016/j.nic.2010.04.010
1052-5149/10/$ – see front matter

Preface

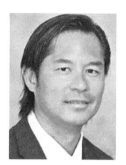

Meng Law, MD, FRACR
Guest Editor

When Suresh Mukherji asked if I could serve as guest editor for *Neuroimaging Clinics of North America*, I was grateful and honored because it provided an excellent opportunity to contribute a truly unique offering on the "State of Art of Brain Tumor Diagnostics, Imaging, and Therapeutics." Then I realized Suresh also had an ulterior motive, which was to hamper my efforts in improving my golf game so he could one day be competitive on the golf course! Suresh has been a friend and colleague for many years. He has provided guidance on just about every facet of neuroradiology, and golf. Needless to say, I owe many of my professional successes and almost all of my failures on the golf course to this advice.

Nevertheless, I certainly did not want to eschew this unique opportunity, which has allowed me to bring together some true experts not only in brain tumor imaging but also in diagnostic pathology and therapeutics. I believe that to completely understand the pathophysiology behind the advanced biologic imaging techniques and nanotechnology, we must first understand the pathology and molecular biology in brain tumors. Just as important, to be a good diagnostician and fully understand the direction brain tumor diagnostics and imaging is taking, knowledge of current radiation oncology, neuro-oncology, and neurosurgical therapies and clinical trials is critical.

The final product is, I hope, an educational and eye-opening snapshot of current brain tumor diagnostics and therapeutics. This work is divided into three sections: diagnostics, therapy planning and imaging, and therapeutics. The diagnostics section discusses the new World Health Organization (WHO) classification of brain tumors as well as novel molecular tools available for the characterization of tumor subtypes and biology. In the therapy planning and imaging section, along with the advanced imaging techniques of spectroscopy, perfusion, diffusion tensor, and functional MR imaging in presurgical and therapy evaluation, I have included contributions on the applications of nanotechnology, novel gadolinium/liposomal contrast agents, and MR imaging–guided focused ultrasound surgery. In the therapeutics section, there are three superb contributions on the state of the art of radiation oncology, neurosurgery, and neuro-oncology.

Pathology has always been critical to the understanding of radiology. In the first article, I have asked my colleagues from Mount Sinai Medical Center, headed by Mary Fowkes, to provide an update on pathology and molecular biology in brain tumors. Six new entities described in the WHO classification of central nervous system tumors and new developments that have been reported in the literature since 2007 are described. In particular, pertinent clinical, radiologic, and pathologic features that may aid in differential diagnosis from more familiar, well-established tumors have been emphasized, which could potentially have an impact on future management of these tumors. Inge Fisher and Ken Aldape provide a summary of the genetic and molecular biology in gliomas as well as the current molecular tools available in clinical practice. Because multiple molecular mechanisms and pathways are implicated in gliomagenesis and progression, multitarget therapies are likely to be required for successful

Neuroimag Clin N Am 20 (2010) xv–xviii
doi:10.1016/j.nic.2010.05.002

neuroimaging.theclinics.com

therapy, a recurrent theme in this edition of *Neuro-imaging Clinics of North America*.

In the main section on therapy planning and imaging, the first contribution is from Aaron Mohs and Jim Provenzale. Pro's expertise in neuroradiology and nanotechnology has resulted in an educated summary of current nanotechnology and its applications in brain tumor imaging. Having studied spectroscopy as a clinician, I have come to appreciate the clinical usefulness of magnetic resonance spectroscopy. To really appreciate its subtleties, however, I have always had to defer to true spectroscopists. Peter Barker and Alena Horska not only provide perspective on the clinical application of magnetic resonance spectroscopy in brain tumors but also clearly echo my sentiments on current advanced imaging tools, which are that robust and automated procedures are needed to collect data, analyze data, and display results in a timely fashion. Standardization across sites and different vendors of acquisition and analysis techniques are also important as, ultimately, are computer-aided detection techniques so that these tools can be used in a busy clinical setting. Alan Jackson and his colleagues provide an overview of perfusion imaging and, again, Alan states that barriers remain to the standardization of imaging biomarkers for use across multiple clinical sites. Some microvascular imaging biomarkers, notably cerebral blood volume, are already amenable to widespread implementation and standardization.

Presurgical planning is critical to providing optimum postoperative outcome, and advances in functional MR imaging and diffusion tensor imaging have allowed mapping eloquent cortical and white matter tracts. My colleagues at Memorial Sloan-Kettering Cancer Center are internationally recognized practitioners and leaders in presurgical mapping. Their contribution includes the potential pitfalls facing novices who are unfamiliar with cortical reorganization, atypical brain dominance, brain plasticity, and vascular decoupling, which can result in inconsistencies in mapping cortical and subcortical structures. This is further reinforced in a review by Robert Young, Nicole Brennan, Justin Fraser, and Cameron Brennan, which again emphasizes these pitfalls and also the challenges facing intraoperative electrophysiologic mapping. They also provide an interesting perspective on the economics and-complexity of operating intraoperative MR imaging systems and the current value of this technology.

This section also discusses some groundbreaking work being done at the Brigham and Women's Hospital that will likely revolutionize current treatment paradigms of brain tumors and other central nervous system disorders. Srini Mukundan and his colleagues have worked for many years on liposomal and novel gadolinium contrast agents. For most of those with little experience in this field, Srini describes nanoparticle platforms available for use as contrast agents, the design and functional properties of liposomes, and the development of MR imaging–based liposomal contrast agents and their usefulness in brain tumors. Ferenc Jolesz and Rivka Colen describe MR image–guided focused ultrasound surgery in the treatment of benign and malignant brain tumors, vascular malformations, and ischemic or hemorrhagic stroke as well as the nonablative targeted delivery of therapeutic drugs, genes, and antibodies. The integration of MR imaging guidance with advanced phased array ultrasound technology has allowed this new therapeutic modality to emerge as a viable noninvasive alternative to current surgical and minimally invasive treatments.

Therapeutics is critical in altering patient outcome and, as Suresh mentions in his foreword, the underlying molecular biology is now bringing imaging and therapeutics closer together. It is likely that personalized therapy targeted to a particular tumor or patient will stem from understanding the underlying molecular biology. Ed Shaw, a world-renowned radiation oncologist, and his colleagues provide an excellent review of the current approaches, challenging dilemmas in radiaton oncology, and the role of clinical trials in addressing these dilemmas. These contemporary trials are trying to optimize the therapeutic ratio between therapeutic gains versus treatment toxicity. The table summarizing the clinical trials for each of the different neoplasms is an invaluable resource.

Jason Hoover, Susan Chang, and Ian Parney review recent glioma surgery clinical trials focusing on outcome studies, novel surgical techniques, and local therapeutic agent delivery. Their contribution is a review of surgical techniques not only for the surgeons but also for anyone involved in the management of brain tumors, including neuro-oncologists and neuroradiologists. Finally, Eudocia Quant and Patrick Wen provide a phenomenal summary of clinical trials and the state of the art in neuro-oncology. Tables 1 to 3 summarize the current agents and ongoing trials beautifully in article by Quant and Wen. Malignant transformation in gliomas is the result of sequential accumulation of genetic aberrations and deregulation of growth factor signaling pathways. Even though the complexity of the molecular abnormalities in glioblastoma multiformes and the redundancy of the signaling pathways make it unlikely that single agents will achieve great success, there has been significant interest in this approach. Ultimately, like most diseases resistant to monotherapy (eg, tuberculosis and AIDS), it is likely that polytherapy will be most effective on multiple signaling pathways and ultimately more successful in the treatment of malignant glioma. Other issues in this review are the radiographic controversies and challenges faced with the current response criteria. Pseudophenomena, such as pseudoprogression in response to temozolomide/radiation therapy and pseudoresponse in response to antiangiogenic agents, have resulted in new radiographic response criteria for high-grade gliomas that are being developed by the international Response Assessment in Neuro-Oncology Working Group.

My hope is that this issue serves as a reference for neuroradiologists, neuro-oncologists, radiation oncologists, and neurosurgeons as well as providing some thought provoking reading for anyone interested in where molecular nanotechnology and liposomal technology are headed. I would like to thank Joanne Husovski for her efforts and support in putting this edition together. Last and by no means least I want to personally thank Suresh again for allowing me this opportunity.

Meng Law, MD, FRACR
Department of Radiology
Keck USC School of Medicine
USC Medical Center, 1520 San Pablo Street
Suite L 1600, Los Angeles, CA 90033, USA

E-mail address:
meng.law@usc.edu

DEDICATION

To my parents, Lawrence and Sue Law, for always instilling integrity, respect, and hard work in all aspects of my life.

State-of-the-Art Pathology: New WHO Classification, Implications, and New Developments

Clare H. Cunliffe, MD[a],*, Ingeborg Fischer, MD[b],
Yoav Parag, MD[c], Mary E. Fowkes, MD, PhD[d]

KEYWORDS

- Pathology • Brain tumor • WHO Classification
- New developments • New entities

To keep up with advances in central nervous system (CNS) tumor diagnosis and discovery of new entities, the classification of these tumors requires periodic review and revision. Since the initial 1979 publication from the World Health Organization (WHO) of *Histological Typing of Tumours of the Central Nervous System,* 3 further editions have been published, cataloging the advances in CNS tumor classification and diagnosis over the past 3 decades. The second edition, published in 1993, incorporated advances in tumor classification resulting from the use of immunohistochemical techniques in diagnosis. Subsequently, the third edition, published in 2000, elaborated on the use of genetic techniques as an aid to tumor diagnosis, as well as describing associated clinical and radiologic findings and prognostic factors. The current 2007 edition includes several new entities, variants, and patterns of differentiation, and expands on the use of molecular techniques in diagnosis and prognostication. In this article, we discuss select new additions to the current classification, including new diagnostic tools, differential diagnoses, and management implications.

ANGIOCENTRIC GLIOMA, WHO GRADE 1

Angiocentric glioma is a low-grade indolent cortically based tumor of the cerebrum usually presenting in children with a history of seizures.[1–6] The tumor was first recognized in as a new entity in 2005.[1,2] The name originates from the presence of perivascular tumor cells, which are mostly bipolar, and are arranged in a circumferential, longitudinal, or perpendicular orientation to blood vessels.[1,2]

A total of 26 cases had been described at the time of publication of the 2007 WHO *Classification of Tumours of the Central Nervous System*, with a mean age of 17 years.[7] However, all but 2 of the 26 presented with seizures in childhood.[1–3] Five cases, all 13 years of age or younger,[4–6] have been described since. One additional cortical tumor in a 5-year-old presenting with headaches has been reported, with features described as

[a] Office of the Medical Investigator, University of New Mexico, 700 Camino de Salud NE, Albuquerque, NM 87106, USA
[b] Department Neuropathologie, Universitaetsspital Zurich, Schmelzbergstrasse 12, 8091 Zurich, Switzerland
[c] Division of Neuroradiology, Department of Radiology, Mount Sinai Hospital, 1, Gustave L. Levy Place, New York, NY 10029, USA
[d] Division of Neuropathology, Department of Pathology, Mount Sinai Hospital, 1, Gustave L. Levy Place, New York, NY 10029, USA
* Corresponding author.
E-mail address: clare@drcunliffe.com

Neuroimag Clin N Am 20 (2010) 259–271
doi:10.1016/j.nic.2010.04.001
1052-5149/10/$ – see front matter © 2010 Published by Elsevier Inc.

ependymoma or angiocentric glioma.[8] Most of the patients had a preceding history of either refractory epilepsy or childhood seizures,[1–6] but one case presented with headache, loss of visual acuity, and no seizure history.[5]

Radiographically, the tumor appears as an ill-defined cortical lesion that is hyperintense on T2-weighted magnetic resonance images, and noncontrast enhancing on T1-weighed images, with superficial extension into the associated subjacent white matter.[1,2,4,5] Diffusion tensor imaging tractography has revealed tumor displacement of fibers.[6] One case has been reported to contain microcalcifications not detected radiographically.[2] The presence of a T2/FLAIR (fluid attenuated inversion recovery) "stalk-like" extension of the cortical tumor extending to the ventricle was described in a case series by Lellouch-Tubiana and colleagues.[2]

Histologically, the tumor is composed of a monomorphic population of cells, most with bipolar or fusiform cell processes, infiltrating the cortex as a single cell population with associated entrapped cortical neurons[1] or as masses of fusiform cells.[1,2] In less cellular areas, the tumor cells can have a circumferential and longitudinal orientation to blood vessels including capillaries (Fig. 1A).[1] In more densely cellular areas, the tumor cells are more radially oriented, forming perivascular pseudorosettes[1,4] and nodules of compact tumor cells.[1] The tumor is also reported to have subpial spread, with the tumor cells oriented perpendicular to the pial surface.[1] The cells are variably glial fibrillary acidic protein (GFAP) and EMA immunopositive and typically vimentin immunopositive (see Fig. 1B, C).[1–4] When positive, EMA usually has a dotlike immunopositive staining pattern similar to ependymomas,[1,3] but unlike ependymomas, angiocentric glioma tumor cells are CD99 immunonegative.[1] The tumor is variably immunopositive for neuronal markers, such as synaptophysin, NeuN, and chromogranin.[1,2,4]

Electron microscopy of some cases has revealed focal microlumina with associated microvilli and "zipper-like" intracellular junctions,[1,3] suggesting an ependymal phenotype. Preusser and colleagues[3] postulate an origin from radial glia, the basis for this theory being the radial orientation of tumor cells within the cortex, and the immunopositivity of the tumor for GFAP, vimentin, and S100. Chromosomal comparative genomic hybridization analysis of tumor DNA has revealed a loss of chromosomal bands 6q24-q25 and gain of chromosomal band 11p11.2.[3]

In one patient, placement of depth electrodes within the tumor revealed ictal activity centered

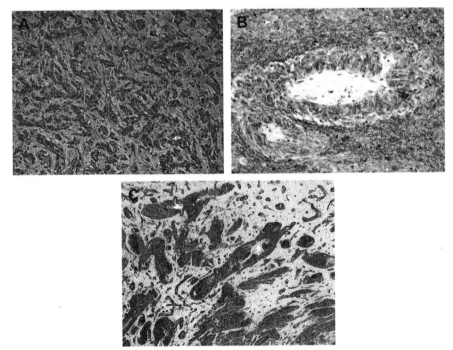

Fig. 1. Angiocentric gliomas: 13-year-old child with medically refractory epilepsy. (A) Circumferential and longitudinal arrangement of perivascular tumor cells around small blood vessels (hematoxylin-eosin, original magnification ×200). The perivascular radial orientation of tumor cells is highlighted by immunostains for (B) GFAP (original magnification ×400) and (C) vimentin (original magnification ×40).

within the tumor before spread to the surrounding cortex, suggesting the utility of tumor depth electrodes to define tumor extent before surgery.[6] Although typically a low-grade tumor, at least one reported case progressed following subtotal resection, with recurrent seizures and death 62 months after initial resection.[1] In contrast, a second case had small polymorphous areas histologically, but showed no evidence of recurrence after 9 months of follow-up.[4] Each of these cases had an elevated MIB-1(Ki-67) labeling index, 10% and 8% respectively. Following gross total or subtotal resection, most patients have been seizure free without progression.[1,3–5]

ATYPICAL CHOROID PLEXUS PAPILLOMA, WHO GRADE 2

Most intraventricular choroid plexus tumors (CPT) are benign and designated choroid plexus papilloma (CPP) with a current WHO classification of Grade 1.[9] CPPs have a low rate of recurrence and do not require adjuvant therapy following gross total resection.[10,11] Much less common are choroid plexus carcinomas (CPC), which exhibit clear features of malignancy.[11,12] However, brain invasion is not the sole criteria for malignancy.[13] Diagnosis of CPC requires the presence of 4 of the 5 following atypical histologic features: high mitotic activity, increased cellularity, nuclear pleomorphism, sheeting of tumor cells, and necrosis.[11,12] CPCs are classified as WHO Grade 3 tumors.[9] A new intermediate category is described in the current WHO classification: atypical choroid plexus papilloma (APP), WHO Grade 2,[9] which has an uncertain clinical prognosis. Childhood CPTs most commonly occur in the lateral ventricles, whereas adult CPTs most commonly occur in the posterior fossa.[14] CPTs account for 0.4% to 1.0% of adult intracranial tumors, but 4.0% of pediatric intracranial tumors.[14] APPs have been found to occur at a significantly younger age (median age of 0.7 years) than either CPPs or CPCs (both with a median age of 2.3 years).[15] The main feature distinguishing APP from CPP is an elevated mitotic activity defined as equal to or greater than 2 per 10 high-powered fields.[12] Mitotic count is the only *histologic* feature independently associated with tumor recurrence, while achievement of gross total resection is the main *clinical* feature impacting the likelihood of tumor recurrence.[12] Malignant progression in choroid plexus papillomas is rare, but there is at least one report of an APP occurring as a recurrence after a 15-year dormant period following resection of a CPP.[13,16] A recent study of 106 patients with choroid plexus tumors

revealed a 5-year event-free survival of 92%, 83%, and 28% for CPP, APP, and CPC respectively.[15] APPs have a risk of metastasizing almost equal to CPCs, whereas CPPs metastasize at a rate of 5%.[15] The clinical symptoms of choroid plexus tumors include headache, nausea, vomiting, altered visual acuity, and papilledema, commonly attributable to the presence of hydrocephalus.[14,17,18]

Generally, magnetic resonance imaging (MRI) is considered the best choice for diagnosis of CPTs, the tumors appearing as homogeneous or heterogeneous, hyperdense or hyperintense masses that are contrast enhancing (**Fig. 2**A, B).[18,19]

Histologically, APPs are composed of fibrovascular papillary structures having a simple layer of cuboidal or columnar epithelial cells with slight nuclear atypia, sometimes in a pseudo-columnar architecture.[11,12,14] The thin fibrovascular papillary fronds tend to maintain their normal papillary architecture, but present with at least one atypical feature, most commonly elevated mitotic activity[11,12,14] (see **Fig. 2**C, D). Immunohistochemically, the tumor cells are typically immunopositive for cytokeratin, GFAP, S100, and TTR, but immunonegative for carcinoembryonic antigen (CEA).[13] Immunohistochemical staining for p53 and MIB-1 may be helpful in determining the tumor grade. Both CPPs and APPs are typically immunonegative for p53 (0% and 9.5% respectively), whereas CPCs are typically immunopositive (47.1%).[13,15] Immunohistochemical stains for MIB-1 reveal an increasing labeling index with increasing grade (1.3, 9.1, and 20.3 for CPPs, APPs, and CPCs respectively) (see **Fig. 2**E).

Genetic analysis of APPs has revealed variable cytogenetic and genomic abnormalities, including normal chromosomal karyotype.[20] Most studies have demonstrated normal or hyperdiploid karyotypes for CPCs.[20]

The histologic grade of CPTs is important because CPPs tend not to recur or need treatment with adjuvant therapy, although long-term follow-up is still recommended. In contrast, although APPs have a higher rate of incomplete resection and metastasis than CPPs, they appear to respond favorably to chemotherapy with complete, partial, or stable remission in most cases.[15]

PAPILLARY GLIONEURONAL TUMOR, WHO GRADE 1

The entity "papillary glioneuronal tumor" (PGNT) was first defined by Komori and colleagues,[21] who described a mixed glial and neuronal tumor with indolent behavior and good prognosis, which

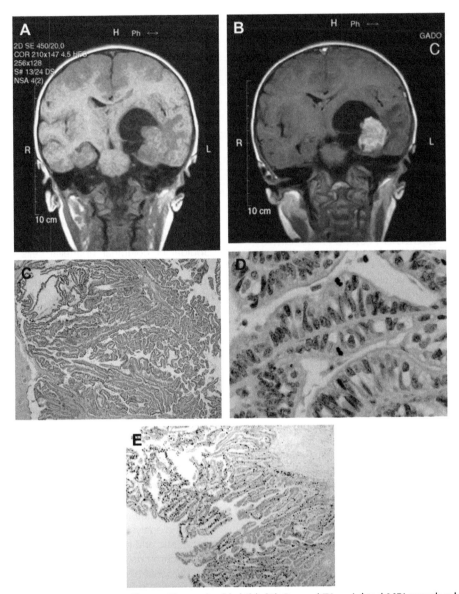

Fig. 2. Atypical choroid plexus papilloma: 15-month-old child. (*A*) Coronal T1-weighted MRI reveals a heterogeneous, hyperintense tumor within the temporal horn of the left lateral ventricle. (*B*) Coronal post-contrast T1-weighted MRI reveals the tumor to be contrast enhancing. (*C*) The tumor is composed of an arborizing network of papillary fronds with an overlying single layer of epithelial cells (hematoxylin-eosin, original magnification ×20). (*D*) Pseudostratified cuboidal to columnar epithelial cells. Two mitotic figures are seen at the center of the field (hematoxylin-eosin, original magnification ×400). (*E*) The MIB-1 labeling index is elevated, at 10% to 20% (MIB-1 immunostain, original magnification ×40).

is characterized as WHO grade 1. The tumor has been reported in patients from 7 to 75 years of age, but most tumors present in young adults.[21–23] PGNTs typically present as cerebral lesions with both cystic and solid areas[21,23–26] and can be large,[25,27] reportedly up to 9 cm. The tumors have a greater than 7-year progression-free survival following gross total resection.[28] PGNTs

typically do not have atypical features such as high mitotic activity, necrosis, and vascular hyperplasia/endothelial hyperplasia.[21,25,29,30] However, PGNTs with elevated proliferation rates and aggressive behavior have been reported.[23,31] Two recently reported cases of aggressive PGNTs had an initial MIB-1 labeling index of 1% and 4% respectively, and rapidly recurred despite gross total resection. Another reported case had an elevated labeling index of 10%, and had mini-gemistocytic cells; this tumor rapidly progressed despite partial resection and adjuvant radio-chemotherapy. However, a case reported by Vaquero and Coca in 2006[31] had an elevated MIB-1 labeling index of 15% and was symptom-free 5 years after radical surgery and radiotherapy, indicating that high proliferation rate alone does not always predict aggressive behavior. PGNTs are associated with focal hemorrhage and there is at least one reported case of progressive super-ficial siderosis attributable to chronic subarach-noid hemorrhage.[32,33]

Clinically, PGNTs commonly present with mild neurologic symptoms such as headache and vision changes,[21,22,31,34] but the tumors can also present with nausea and vomiting, seizures, or hemiparesis.[24,25,29] Asymptomatic cases discov-ered incidentally have also been reported.[27]

Radiographically, the tumors are most com-monly found to have large uniloculated or multilo-culated cysts with an associated mural nodule.[21,23–26,35] On MRI, the tumors are typically hypointense on T1, hyperintense on T2, and usually show enhancement of the mural nodule and sometimes enhancement of the cyst wall (Fig. 3A–C).[21,22,34,35] Typically, PGNTs have little associated edema or mass effect.[35]

Histologically, the tumors are composed of compact areas of pseudopapillary-appearing thick hyalinized blood vessels lined by 1 or 2 cell layers of small astrocytic tumor cells with round uniform nuclei (see Fig. 3D).[21,22] These astrocytic cells are immunopositive for GFAP and S100.[21,22,25,26] Surrounding the astrocytic cells are oligodendro-cytic cells with round nuclei and scant to indistinct cytoplasm that are immunopositive for Olig2, a nonspecific marker for oligodendrocyte differen-tiation.[36,37] The cells within the spaces between the pseudopapillary vessels are composed of var-iably small and medium-sized neuronal tumor cells and, when present, large ganglion tumor cells. These small, medium, and large neuronal cells are each immunopositive for neuronal markers such as synaptophysin, NeuN, neurofilament (NF), and neuron specific enolase (NSE).[21,25] Most PGNTs have no necrosis, few if any areas of vascular proliferation, a low MIB-1 proliferation index (<1%), and most of the cases have been p53 im-munonegative.[25,27,29,30,35,36] Rosenthal fibers, eosinophilic granular bodies, hemosiderin, and calcifications are commonly present at the periphery of the tumors.[27,30]

Electron microscopy has confirmed the pres-ence of microfilaments within glial processes, and microtubules within immature neurons.[23]

One report of chromosomal analysis of a PGNT identified genetic alteration of chromosome 7 alone, with breakpoints at 7p22.[38] No deletions of chromosomes 1p or 19q have been reported.[28]

Although PGNTs tend to have good prognosis with no need for adjuvant therapy following gross total resection, reports of atypical and aggressive PGNTs suggest the need for ongoing careful re-porting of atypical features for future therapeutic implications.

ROSETTE-FORMING GLIONEURONAL TUMOR OF THE FOURTH VENTRICLE, WHO GRADE 1

This tumor is a mixed glial-neuronal neoplasm affecting predominantly young adults, and centered on the region of the fourth ventricle. The tumor was originally described as a distinct entity by Komori and colleagues[39–41] in 2002 in a series of 11 posterior fossa tumors. Before this, a tumor with the same histologic appearance was described as dysembryoplastic neuroepithe-lial tumor of the cerebellum by Kuchelmeister and colleagues[42] in 1995. At the time of the current WHO guide going to press, 17 cases had been reported.[43] Since then, a further 12 cases have been described.[41,44–47] One of these cases had the characteristic histomorphology, but was located in the optic chiasm and left optic nerve of a patient with neurofibromatosis type 1.[47]

Rosette-forming glioneuronal tumor of the fourth ventricle (RGNT) occurs over an age range of 12 to 59 years, with a possible slight female predilec-tion.[43] Patients typically present with headaches and ataxia as a result of obstructive hydroceph-alus,[40,43] and may occasionally experience neck pain.[43] RGNT has a midline location, involving the fourth ventricle and/or aqueduct. At the periphery, the tumor may also involve the cerebellar vermis, adjacent brain stem, thalamus, or pineal gland.[43,48] The tumor may be multicentric.[28]

Upon MRI, the tumor is relatively circumscribed and is mostly solid with heterogeneous areas, the solid portions of the tumor being iso- to hypoin-tense on T1-weighted imaging and hyperintense on T2 imaging.[40,43,48] It may be partially cystic or multiloculated, and dense calcifications have been seen in some examples.[48] Multicentric, flaccid curvilinear or ring enhancement appears to be characteristic for RGNT.[48] In contrast, the ring enhancement that can be seen in pilocytic astrocytomas is usually solitary. Radiologically, distinction of RGNT from medulloblastoma (which can also have a similar location) can be achieved because medulloblastomas have high density on computed tomography (CT) and diffusion

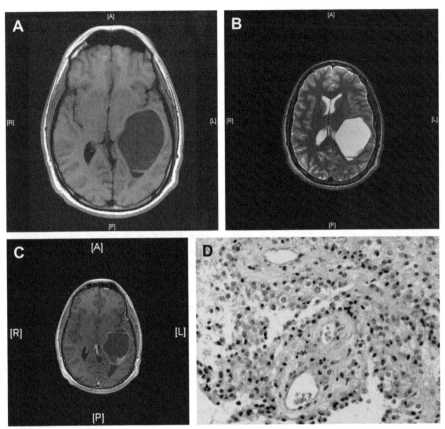

Fig. 3. Papillary glioneuronal tumor: 21-year-old man with a large multiloculated cystic mass within the left temporal lobe. (A) The mass is hypointense on axial T1-weighted MRI. (B) Axial T2-weighted MRI further demonstrates the cystic nature of the lesion and the lateral mural nodule. (C) Axial postcontrast T1-weighted MRI reveals rim enhancement of the tumor, with associated mass effect and midline shift. (D) Pseudopapillary architecture comprising central blood vessels surrounded by 1 to 2 layers of pseudostratified cells with pale cytoplasm. The inner cell layer has hyperchromatic nuclei (hematoxylin-eosin, original magnification ×200).

restriction on MRI, reflecting the high cellularity of this tumor.[48]

Histologically, the biphasic nature of RGNT is reflected in its distinct glial and neurocytic components (Fig. 4A). The tumor has an overall low cellularity.[43] The glial component closely resembles pilocytic astrocytoma, composed of elongated "piloid" glial cells within a variably compact to loose fibrillary background, sometimes with microcystic areas (see Fig. 4B). Also like pilocystic astrocytoma, there may admixed Rosenthal fibers, eosinophilic granular bodies (EGBs), microcalcifications, and hemosiderin deposits. Similarly, thick-walled hyalinized vessels and glomeruloid vascular structures may be present.[28,40,43] Therefore, recognition of the accompanying neurocytic component is important to avoid confusion with pilocytic astrocytoma. The "neurocytic" portions of the tumor contain cells with round nuclei and finely speckled chromatin, arranged in perivascular pseudorosettes and small neurocytic rosettes surrounding a central core of neuropil (see Fig. 4C).[28] There may be an interspersed mucinous matrix with microcysts.[43] Occasional ganglion cells may be seen.[40,43] As may be expected, the neuropil matrix is immunopositive for synaptophysin, as are the neurocytic cells (see Fig. 4D). There is similar labeling of these cells for MAP-2 and NSE. The glial component is labeled by immunostains for GFAP and S100 protein.[28] Depending on plane of section, the neurocytic component can histologically resemble dysembryoplastic neuroepithelial tumor (DNT), with perivascular columns of tumor cells suspended within a mucoid matrix.[28]

Distinction of this tumor from pilocytic astrocytoma and DNT depends on recognition of the biphasic nature of the tumor and also correlation with the clinico-radiologic presentation. Typically, pilocytic astrocytomas are seen in a younger age

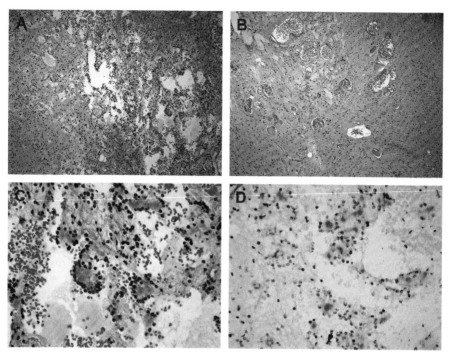

Fig. 4. Rosette-forming glioneuronal tumor of the fourth ventricle. (*A*) The biphasic nature of the tumor is demonstrated, with the rosette-forming neurocytic component to the right, and the glial component to the left of the image (hematoxylin-eosin, original magnification ×100). (*B*) Glial component with features resembling pilocytic astrocytoma (hematoxylin-eosin, original magnification ×100). (*C*) Neurocytic component, with rosettes containing fine neuropil cores (hematoxylin-eosin, original magnification ×400). (*D*) The neuropil cores are highlighted by an immunostain for synaptic vesicle protein (SV2 immunostain, original magnification ×400).

group and are most commonly seen in the cerebellum and brain stem; imaging commonly revealing a cystic neoplasm with a mural nodule.[40] DNT is usually supratentorial, intracortical, and multinodular, with a predilection for the temporal lobe and occurring in young patients with a history of seizures.[28,43]

The RGNT has low MIB-1 proliferation indices, less than 3%, reflecting its slow-growing, indolent nature.[43] Mitotic activity and necrosis are not normally present.[40]

It is thought that RGNT arises from pluripotential cells in remnants of germinal matrix within the subependymal plate along the aqueduct and fourth ventricle, potentially explaining its midline cerebellar location.[43–45]

Survival following excision of the tumors is good;[43] however, radical excision is commonly associated with considerable morbidity, frequently with multiple cranial nerves affected, particularly cranial nerves 6 and 7.[46] Disabling postoperative deficits have been described in about half the cases.[43] Therefore, correct diagnosis of this tumor is important to avoid overaggressive surgical management and the ensuing neurologic deficits.[45]

PAPILLARY TUMOR OF THE PINEAL REGION, WHO GRADE 2–3

Although papillary tumors of pineal origin were first described by Trojanowski and colleagues[49] in 1981 and Vaquero and colleagues in 1990,[50] the entity papillary tumor of the pineal region (PTPR) was first coined by Jouvet and colleagues in 2003.[51] Tumors of the pineal region constitute less than 1% of all intracranial tumors,[50] and papillary tumors of the pineal gland are rare. The behavior of these tumors is unclear, with a high risk for local recurrence and rare potential craniospinal dissemination, hence a WHO designation of grade 2–3.[52,53]

The age distribution of the tumor is 5 to 66 years of age,[54,55] but most occur in older patients than patients with choroid plexus tumors.[55] PTPR is associated with an overall 5-year survival of 73%,[51] but recurrence occurs in 70% of cases with cerebrospinal fluid (CSF) dissemination in 7% of cases.[54] The overall prognosis is largely dependent on complete resection. The tumor cells are thought to originate from cytokeratin-positive specialized ependymal cells with abundant secretory granules of the specialized ependyma of the subcommissural organ (SCO).[51]

Clinically, PTPR tends to present with headache[56] and vision disturbances. However, the tumor has also presented with generalized seizures as the first clinical symptom.[57] The tumors typically produce obstructive triventricular hydrocephalus[52,57–59] at the aqueduct[57,59] and radiographically appear as well-circumscribed lesions with cystic and solid components at the pineal region[52,54,58–61] ranging in size from 23 to 50 mm.[54,57] However, at least one case of a simultaneous multicentric tumor of the pineal and suprasellar region has been reported.[60]

On CT, the tumor is usually hypodense, but enhances with contrast.[56] The tumor is variably hyperintense on T1-weighted MRI[58,60,61] with cystic areas demonstrated on T2-weighted MRI (Fig. 5A). Tumors are commonly heterogeneous throughout or homogeneous within solid areas on T1-weighted images with contrast enhancement (see Fig. 5B).[52,57,58,61] Fat-saturated T1-weighted MRI imaging can help to exclude benign lesions such as teratoma, dermoid cyst, or lipomas[61] and angiography can help differentiate vascular malformations and aneurysms.[61] Tracer uptake into the lesion can be seen with ^{111}In-DTPA-pentetreotide scans[60] or [^{18}F] fluorodeoxyglucose uptake on positron emission tomography.[62] The correct diagnosis of this tumor cannot be made by radiology alone,[53] and instead requires tissue for histologic diagnosis.

The tumor may be found to adhere to the aqueduct but has not been found to invade the adjacent thalamus.[57] Hemorrhage, fresh and old, has infrequently been reported within the tumor.[57]

Histologically, PTPR has focal ependymal-like features with both loose and solid papillary growth, epithelial-like cells arranged in true rosettes,[54,57] and also around blood vessels forming perivascular pseudorosettes[54,55] (see Fig. 5C). The tumor cells have moderate amounts of eosinophilic cytoplasm with round-to-oval nuclei, prominent nucleoli,[53] and reported nuclear grooves.[63] The tumor cells are not uncommonly vacuolated[55,57] with signet-ring cells[53] (see Fig. 5D). Focal necrosis is common[51,54,55] but, despite the aggressive nature of the tumor, mitotic figures are mostly reported to be rare.[57,59,60,64] However, some tumors with moderate mitotic activity have been described.[53] MIB-1 immunohistochemical staining has revealed a variable labeling index of less than 5% to greater than 10%.[54]

Immunohistochemically, they are similar to choroid plexus tumors with immunopositivity for cytokeratin and immunonegativity for GFAP.[54] The tumor cells are consistently immunopositive for NSE and cytokeratins CK18 and KL1 (100%)[52,54,55,65]; mostly immunopositive for MAP-2 and vimentin[52,54,55,65]; immunonegative for NF, TPH, AFP, melan A, NeuN, PLAP, and CK20[52,54,65]; mostly immunonegative for GFAP, TTR, and Kir7.1[52,54,55]; and variably immunopositive or immunonegative for synaptophysin, EMA, Chromogranin A, and S100 (see Fig. 5E).[54,55,57,65]

PTPR are associated with several chromosome alterations, including loss in chromosomes 10 and 22q, and gain in chromosomes 4, 8, 9, and 12.[55] Tumor cells were also found to have high mRNA gene expression of SPDEF, KRT18, and mRNAs of genes encoding proteins expressed in SCO cells.[66]

Early diagnosis with aggressive surgical resection, aiming for gross total resection, is the only significant factor in overall survival and recurrence.[54] However, because many patients experience local recurrence, most are treated with either adjuvant radiotherapy[54] alone or in combination with chemotherapy, despite frequent poor response.[60] Spinal cord dissemination is rare,[54] but one reported case without surgery developed subsequent CSF dissemination,[54] and one other case had CSF dissemination at the time of diagnosis.[60] The benefit of adjuvant chemotherapy and radiotherapy is still unclear.

PITUICYTOMA, WHO GRADE 1

The pituicytoma is a rare, low-grade glial neoplasm of the sella turcica and suprasellar region, occurring around the pituitary stalk and posterior pituitary.[67–69] Although the diagnosis of pituicytoma had previously been applied loosely, to include granular oncocytomas and pilocytic astrocytomas, the current diagnostic criteria restricts this diagnosis to tumors thought to originate from cells within the neurohypophysis and infundibulum.[67–71] However, pituicytomas have also been postulated to arise from folliculostellate cells of the adenohypophysis (anterior pituitary), which are thought to be involved in hormonal regulation of the neurohypophysis by cytokines and growth hormones.[72] To date, fewer than 30 cases of pituicytoma have been documented.[7] So far, all reported cases have occurred in adults, with a preponderance of male patients.[71] There has been one report of a pituicytoma in a 66-year-old with a parathyroid adenoma and follicular carcinoma.[68] A case of multiple endocrine neoplasia type 2 associated with a granular cell tumor has been reported but, as stated previously, this tumor is no longer considered in the same category as pituicytoma.[68,73] Hemorrhage into

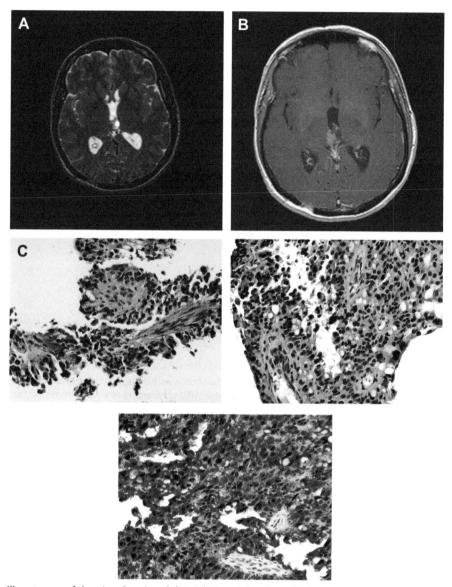

Fig. 5. Papillary tumor of the pineal region. (*A*) Axial T2-weighted MRI highlights the solid and cystic components of the pineal tumor. (*B*) Axial postcontrast T1-weighted MRI demonstrating contrast enhancement of the solid portion of the tumor. (*C*) Perivascular pseudorosettes in a papillary architecture (hematoxylin-eosin, original magnification ×200). (*D*) Tumor with signet cells (hematoxylin-eosin, original magnification ×200). (*E*) Tumor cells are S100-immunopositive (S100 immunostain with red chromagen, original magnification ×200).

a pituicytoma and the overlying third ventricle has been reported, with resulting severe headache.[74] Similar to the incidental finding of pituitary adenomas and carcinoma metastatic in pituitaries from autopsy specimens, a pituicytoma has been identified during autopsy.[75]

Clinically, pituicytomas tend to have visual disturbances and associated field cuts,[69,76,77] hypoprolactinemia with associated amenorrhea and decreased libido,[71] panhypopituitarism,[77] as well as normal pituitary and thyroid function.[69] Despite the location of pituicytomas adjacent to the optic system and the associated visual changes experienced by patients with this tumor, there have been no reports of invasion into the optic system or hypothalamus.[78]

Radiographically, pituicytomas are usually well-circumscribed, noninfiltrating tumors that are isointense on T1-weighted MRI images and either hyperintense or isointense on T2-weighted MRI images.[67,69] Pituicytomas are usually homogeneously contrast enhancing[67,69] (**Fig. 6**A) and one

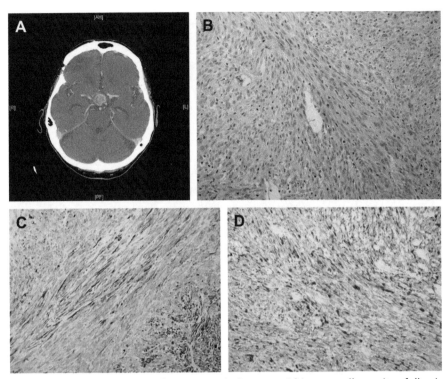

Fig. 6. Pituicytoma: 81-year-old woman with recurrent pituicytoma within suprasellar region, following an initial resection 9 years earlier. (*A*) Coronal CT, soft tissue window with contrast, reveals a 19-mm contrast-enhancing mass involving the sellar and suprasellar compartments. (*B*) Spindled cells in fascicles, with mild cytologic atypia (hematoxylin-eosin, original magnification ×100). The tumor cells are diffusely immunopositive for (*C*) vimentin (original magnification ×100), and (*D*) GFAP (original magnification ×100).

tumor has been reported to have rapid early-phase enhancement with contrast.[79] Although pituicytomas are usually solid, at least one case of a cystic pituicytoma has been reported.[67] In one case, angiography of a pituicytoma reportedly found multiple feeding blood vessels, including feeder vessels from both internal carotid arteries and the right posterior communicating artery.[80]

Histologically, the tumors are typically composed of spindled cells in a storiform and interlocking fascicular architecture.[68] The tumor cells commonly have little to no nuclear pleomorphism, and no necrosis or vascular/endothelial hyperplasia (see **Fig. 6**B).[69,74,76,79,80] Rosenthal fibers and bipolar cells are often absent.[69,70,74,76] Although eosinophilic granular bodies are also usually absent,[69,70] they have been seen on occasion.[75] Herring bodies are infrequently reported or absent.[70] Tumor cells are usually immunopositive for S100 and vimentin (see **Fig. 6**C), variably immunopositive for GFAP (see **Fig. 6**D), and immunonegative for synaptophysin and NF.[67,69] Tumor cells have been reported to be immunopositive for CD44 and CD56, and immunonegative for EMA, Keratin (CAM5.2), desmin, CEA, and

p53.[69] Most cases of pituicytoma have a low MIB-1 labeling index (0.5% to 2.0%).[67] Unlike granular cell tumors, there is no PAS positivity within the tumor cells of pituicytoma.[81] Reticulin staining usually produces only perivascular staining, with no staining around individual tumor cells.[67]

Electron microscopy has revealed tumor cells without interdigitating cell membranes,[77] which are commonly found to contain cytoplasmic intermediate filaments and abundant mitochondria.[67,76,82]

Pituicytomas are slow-growing neoplasms, and appear to be essentially cured after complete excision. In a study of 9 patients, the 6 who underwent complete excision of their tumors experienced no recurrences during a range of follow-up periods up to 99 months.[67] However, subtotally resected tumors have a tendency to recur,[72,80,82] albeit over a period of months to years.[71] So far, there are no reports of malignant transformation or craniospinal dissemination.[71] Complications following surgery are infrequent, and have included diabetes insipidus, which may be transient, and hypopituitarism.[81]

SUMMARY

We have reviewed 6 new entities that were described in the current WHO *Classification of Central Nervous System Tumors*, including associated new developments that have been reported in the literature since 2007. In particular, we emphasized pertinent clinical, radiologic, and pathologic features that may aid in differential diagnosis from more familiar, well-established tumors. The histogenesis and genetic alterations within these entities were also touched upon, representing ongoing areas of research that could potentially have an impact on future management of these tumors.

REFERENCES

1. Wang M, Tihan T, Rojiani AM, et al. Monomorphous angiocentric glioma: a distinctive epileptogenic neoplasm with features of infiltrating astrocytoma and ependymoma. J Neuropathol Exp Neurol 2005;64(10):875–81.
2. Lellouch-Tubiana A, Boddaert N, Bourgeois M, et al. Angiocentric neuroepithelial tumor (ANET): a new epilepsy-related clinicopathological entity with distinctive MRI. Brain Pathol 2005;15(4):281–6.
3. Preusser M, Hoischen A, Novak K, et al. Angiocentric glioma: report of clinico-pathologic and genetic findings in 8 cases. Am J Surg Pathol 2007;31(11):1709–18.
4. Sugita Y, Ono T, Ohshima K, et al. Brain surface spindle cell glioma in a patient with medically intractable partial epilepsy: a variant of monomorphous angiocentric glioma? Neuropathology 2008;28(5):516–20.
5. Shakur SF, McGirt MJ, Johnson MW, et al. Angiocentric glioma: a case series. J Neurosurg Pediatr 2009;3(3):197–202.
6. Fulton SP, Clarke DF, Wheless JW, et al. Angiocentric glioma-induced seizures in a 2-year-old child. J Child Neurol 2009;24(7):852–6.
7. Louis DN, Ohgaki H, Wiestler OD, et al. The 2007 WHO classification of tumours of the central nervous system. Acta Neuropathol 2007;114(2):97–109.
8. Lum DJ, Halliday W, Watson M, et al. Cortical ependymoma or monomorphous angiocentric glioma? Neuropathology 2008;28(1):81–6.
9. Rousseau A, Mokhtari K, Duyckaerts C. The 2007 WHO classification of tumors of the central nervous system—what has changed? Curr Opin Neurol 2008;21(6):720–7.
10. McEvoy AW, Harding BN, Phipps KP, et al. Management of choroid plexus tumours in children: 20 years experience at a single neurosurgical centre. Pediatr Neurosurg 2000;32(4):192–9.
11. Jeibmann A, Wrede B, Peters O, et al. Malignant progression in choroid plexus papillomas. J Neurosurg 2007;107(Suppl 3):199–202.
12. Jeibmann A, Hasselblatt M, Gerss J, et al. Prognostic implications of atypical histologic features in choroid plexus papilloma. J Neuropathol Exp Neurol 2006;65(11):1069–73.
13. Shintaku M, Nitta T, Matsubayashi K, et al. Ossifying choroid plexus papilloma recurring with features of atypical papilloma. Neuropathology 2008;28(2):160–4.
14. Uff CE, Galloway M, Bradford R. Metastatic atypical choroid plexus papilloma: a case report. J Neurooncol 2007;82(1):69–74.
15. Wrede B, Hasselblatt M, Peters O, et al. Atypical choroid plexus papilloma: clinical experience in the CPT-SIOP-2000 study. J Neurooncol 2009;95(3):383–92.
16. Tanaka K, Sasayama T, Nishihara M, et al. Rapid regrowth of an atypical choroid plexus papilloma located in the cerebellopontine angle. J Clin Neurosci 2009;16(1):121–4.
17. Irsutti M, Thorn-Kany M, Arrue P, et al. Suprasellar seeding of a benign choroid plexus papilloma of the fourth ventricle with local recurrence. Neuroradiology 2000;42(9):657–61.
18. Tena-Suck ML, Lopez-Gomez M, Salinas-Lara C, et al. Psammomatous choroid plexus papilloma: three cases with atypical characteristics. Surg Neurol 2006;65(6):604–10.
19. Li S, Savolaine ER. Imaging of atypical choroid plexus papillomas. Clin Imaging 1996;20(2):85–90.
20. Brassesco MS, Valera ET, Becker AP, et al. Grade II atypical choroid plexus papilloma with normal karyotype. Childs Nerv Syst 2009;25(12):1623–6.
21. Komori T, Scheithauer BW, Anthony DC, et al. Papillary glioneuronal tumor: a new variant of mixed neuronal-glial neoplasm. Am J Surg Pathol 1998;22(10):1171–83.
22. Tsukayama C, Arakawa Y. A papillary glioneuronal tumor arising in an elderly woman: a case report. Brain Tumor Pathol 2002;19(1):35–9.
23. Javahery RJ, Davidson L, Fangusaro J, et al. Aggressive variant of a papillary glioneuronal tumor. Report of 2 cases. J Neurosurg Pediatr 2009;3(1):46–52.
24. Borges G, Bonilha L, Menezes AS, et al. Long-term follow-up in a patient with papillary glioneuronal tumor. Arq Neuropsiquiatr 2004;62(3B):869–72.
25. Vajtai I, Kappeler A, Lukes A, et al. Papillary glioneuronal tumor. Pathol Res Pract 2006;202(2):107–12.
26. Chen L, Piao YS, Xu QZ, et al. Papillary glioneuronal tumor: a clinicopathological and immunohistochemical study of two cases. Neuropathology 2006;26(3):243–8.
27. Dim DC, Lingamfelter DC, Taboada EM, et al. Papillary glioneuronal tumor: a case report and review of the literature. Hum Pathol 2006;37(7):914–8.

28. Edgar MA, Rosenblum MK. Mixed glioneuronal tumors: recently described entities. Arch Pathol Lab Med 2007;131(2):228–33.

29. Celli P, Caroli E, Giangaspero F, et al. Papillary glioneuronal tumor. Case report and literature review. J Neurooncol 2006;80(2):185–9.

30. Williams SR, Joos BW, Parker JC, et al. Papillary glioneuronal tumor: a case report and review of the literature. Ann Clin Lab Sci 2008;38(3):287–92.

31. Vaquero J, Coca S. Atypical papillary glioneuronal tumor. J Neurooncol 2007;83(3):319–23.

32. Konya D, Peker S, Ozgen S, et al. Superficial siderosis due to papillary glioneuronal tumor. J Clin Neurosci 2006;13(9):950–2.

33. Buccoliero AM, Giordano F, Mussa F, et al. Papillary glioneuronal tumor radiologically mimicking a cavernous hemangioma with hemorrhagic onset. Neuropathology 2006;26(3):206–11.

34. Stosic-Opincal T, Peric V, Gavrilovic S, et al. Papillary glioneuronal tumor. AJR Am J Roentgenol 2005;185(1):265–7.

35. Prayson RA. Papillary glioneuronal tumor. Arch Pathol Lab Med 2000;124(12):1820–3.

36. Gelpi E, Preusser M, Czech T, et al. Papillary glioneuronal tumor. Neuropathology 2007;27(5):468–73.

37. Ishizawa T, Komori T, Shibahara J, et al. Papillary glioneuronal tumor with minigemistocytic components and increased proliferative activity. Hum Pathol 2006;37(5):627–30.

38. Faria C, Miguens J, Antunes JL, et al. Genetic alterations in a papillary glioneuronal tumor. J Neurosurg Pediatr 2008;1(1):99–102.

39. Komori T, Scheithauer BW, Hirose T. A rosette-forming glioneuronal tumor of the fourth ventricle: infratentorial form of dysembryoplastic neuroepithelial tumor? Am J Surg Pathol 2002;26(5):582–91.

40. Allende DS, Prayson RA. The expanding family of glioneuronal tumors. Adv Anat Pathol 2009;16(1):33–9.

41. Pimentel J, Resende M, Vaz A, et al. Rosette-forming glioneuronal tumor: pathology case report. Neurosurgery 2008;62(5):E1162–3 [discussion: E1163].

42. Kuchelmeister K, Demirel T, Schlorer E, et al. Dysembryoplastic neuroepithelial tumour of the cerebellum. Acta Neuropathol 1995;89(4):385–90.

43. Hainfellner JA, Scheithauer BW, Giangaspero F, et al. Rosette-forming glioneuronal tumour of the fourth ventricle. In: Louis DN, Ohgaki H, Wiestler OD, et al, editors, In: WHO classification of tumors of the central nervous system, vol. 1. Lyon (France): IARC Press; 2007. p. 115–6.

44. Vajtai I, Arnold M, Kappeler A, et al. Rosette-forming glioneuronal tumor of the fourth ventricle: report of two cases with a differential diagnostic overview. Pathol Res Pract 2007;203(8):613–9.

45. Marhold F, Preusser M, Dietrich W, et al. Clinicoradiological features of rosette-forming glioneuronal tumor (RGNT) of the fourth ventricle: report of four cases and literature review. J Neurooncol 2008;90(3):301–8.

46. Tan CC, Gonzales M, Veitch A. Clinical implications of the infratentorial rosette-forming glioneuronal tumor: case report. Neurosurgery 2008;63(1):E175–6 [discussion: E176].

47. Scheithauer BW, Silva AI, Ketterling RP, et al. Rosette-forming glioneuronal tumor: report of a chiasmal-optic nerve example in neurofibromatosis type 1: special pathology report. Neurosurgery 2009;64(4):E771–2 [discussion: E772].

48. Amemiya S, Shibahara J, Aoki S, et al. Recently established entities of central nervous system tumors: review of radiological findings. J Comput Assist Tomogr 2008;32(2):279–85.

49. Trojanowski JQ, Tascos NA, Rorke LB. Malignant pineocytoma with prominent papillary features. Cancer 1982;50(9):1789–93.

50. Vaquero J, Coca S, Martinez R, et al. Papillary pineocytoma. Case report. J Neurosurg 1990;73(1):135–7.

51. Jouvet A, Fauchon F, Liberski P, et al. Papillary tumor of the pineal region. Am J Surg Pathol 2003;27(4):505–12.

52. Buffenoir K, Rigoard P, Wager M, et al. Papillary tumor of the pineal region in a child: case report and review of the literature. Childs Nerv Syst 2008;24(3):379–84.

53. Dagnew E, Langford LA, Lang FF, et al. Papillary tumors of the pineal region: case report. Neurosurgery 2007;60(5):E953–5 [discussion: E953–5].

54. Fevre-Montange M, Hasselblatt M, Figarella-Branger D, et al. Prognosis and histopathologic features in papillary tumors of the pineal region: a retrospective multicenter study of 31 cases. J Neuropathol Exp Neurol 2006;65(10):1004–11.

55. Hasselblatt M, Blumcke I, Jeibmann A, et al. Immunohistochemical profile and chromosomal imbalances in papillary tumours of the pineal region. Neuropathol Appl Neurobiol 2006;32(3):278–83.

56. Roncaroli F, Scheithauer BW. Papillary tumor of the pineal region and spindle cell oncocytoma of the pituitary: new tumor entities in the 2007 WHO Classification. Brain Pathol 2007;17(3):314–8.

57. Kuchelmeister K, Hugens-Penzel M, Jodicke A, et al. Papillary tumour of the pineal region: histodiagnostic considerations. Neuropathol Appl Neurobiol 2006;32(2):203–8.

58. Cerase A, Vallone IM, Di Pietro G, et al. Neuroradiological follow-up of the growth of papillary tumor of the pineal region: a case report. J Neurooncol 2009;95(3):433–5.

59. Boco T, Aalaei S, Musacchio M, et al. Papillary tumor of the pineal region. Neuropathology 2008;28(1):87–92.

60. Sato TS, Kirby PA, Buatti JM, et al. Papillary tumor of the pineal region: report of a rapidly progressive

tumor with possible multicentric origin. Pediatr Radiol 2009;39(2):188–90.

61. Chang AH, Fuller GN, Debnam JM, et al. MR imaging of papillary tumor of the pineal region. AJNR Am J Neuroradiol 2008;29(1):187–9.

62. Inoue T, Kumabe T, Kanamori M, et al. Papillary tumor of the pineal region: a case report. Brain Tumor Pathol 2008;25(2):85–90.

63. Varikatt W, Dexter M, Mahajan H, et al. Usefulness of smears in intra-operative diagnosis of newly described entities of CNS. Neuropathology Jun 25 2009. [Epub ahead of print].

64. Shibahara J, Todo T, Morita A, et al. Papillary neuroepithelial tumor of the pineal region. A case report. Acta Neuropathol 2004;108(4):337–40.

65. Santarius T, Joseph JA, Tsang KT, et al. Papillary tumour of the pineal region. Br J Neurosurg 2008; 22(1):116–20.

66. Fevre-Montange M, Champier J, Szathmari A, et al. Microarray analysis reveals differential gene expression patterns in tumors of the pineal region. J Neuropathol Exp Neurol 2006;65(7):675–84.

67. Brat DJ, Scheithauer BW, Staugaitis SM, et al. Pituicytoma: a distinctive low-grade glioma of the neurohypophysis. Am J Surg Pathol 2000;24(3):362–8.

68. Schultz AB, Brat DJ, Oyesiku NM, et al. Intrasellar pituicytoma in a patient with other endocrine neoplasms. Arch Pathol Lab Med 2001;125(4): 527–30.

69. Katsuta T, Inoue T, Nakagaki H, et al. Distinctions between pituicytoma and ordinary pilocytic astrocytoma. Case report. J Neurosurg 2003;98(2):404–6.

70. Uesaka T, Miyazono M, Nishio S, et al. Astrocytoma of the pituitary gland (pituicytoma): case report. Neuroradiology 2002;44(2):123–5.

71. Brat DJ, Scheithauer BW, Fuller GN, et al. Newly codified glial neoplasms of the 2007 WHO Classification of Tumours of the Central Nervous System: angiocentric

glioma, pilomyxoid astrocytoma and pituicytoma. Brain Pathol 2007;17(3):319–24.

72. Ulm AJ, Yachnis AT, Brat DJ, et al. Pituicytoma: report of two cases and clues regarding histogenesis. Neurosurgery 2004;54(3):753–7 [discussion: 757–8].

73. Cusick JF, Ho KC, Hagen TC, et al. Granular-cell pituicytoma associated with multiple endocrine neoplasia type. J Neurosurg 1982;56(4):594–6.

74. Benveniste RJ, Purohit D, Byun H. Pituicytoma presenting with spontaneous hemorrhage. Pituitary 2006;9(1):53–8.

75. Takei H, Goodman JC, Tanaka S, et al. Pituicytoma incidentally found at autopsy. Pathol Int 2005; 55(11):745–9.

76. Hurley TR, D'Angelo CM, Clasen RA, et al. Magnetic resonance imaging and pathological analysis of a pituicytoma: case report. Neurosurgery 1994; 35(2):314–7 [discussion: 317].

77. Roncaroli F, Scheithauer BW, Cenacchi G, et al. 'Spindle cell oncocytoma' of the adenohypophysis: a tumor of folliculostellate cells? Am J Surg Pathol 2002;26(8):1048–55.

78. Nakasu Y, Nakasu S, Saito A, et al. Pituicytoma. Two case reports. Neurol Med Chir (Tokyo) 2006;46(3): 152–6.

79. Thiryayi WA, Gnanalingham KK, Reid H, et al. Pituicytoma: a misdiagnosed benign tumour of the posterior pituitary. Br J Neurosurg 2007;21(1):47–8.

80. Gibbs WN, Monuki ES, Linskey ME, et al. Pituicytoma: diagnostic features on selective carotid angiography and MR imaging. AJNR Am J Neuroradiol 2006;27(8):1639–42.

81. Wolfe SQ, Bruce J, Morcos JJ. Pituicytoma: case report. Neurosurgery 2008;63(1):E173–4 [discussion: E174].

82. Kowalski RJ, Prayson RA, Mayberg MR. Pituicytoma. Ann Diagn Pathol 2004;8(5):290–4.

Molecular Tools: Biology, Prognosis, and Therapeutic Triage

Ingeborg Fischer, MD[a,b], Kenneth Aldape, MD[a,*]

KEYWORDS

- Glioma • Malignant tumor • Targeted therapy
- Molecular • Genetic

GLIOMA CLASSIFICATION

The current World Health Organization (WHO) classification recognizes astrocytic, oligodendroglial, and mixed oligoastrocytic gliomas, largely based on morphology. Tumor classification and grade remain an important prognostic factor: survival rates for WHO grade II oligodendroglioma are approximately 80% at 5 years and 65% for fibrillary astrocytoma at 5 years.[1] In anaplastic (WHO grade III) tumors, the median survival time is 3.5 years for oligodendroglial and 1.7 years for astrocytic tumors.[2] Glioblastoma (WHO grade IV) is associated with a dismal prognosis, with a median survival of approximately 1 year.

GENETIC AND MOLECULAR CHARACTERISTICS

Diffusely infiltrating gliomas of different lineage and grade not only are morphologically different but also have some distinct genetic characteristics (Fig. 1). With malignant progression, genetic alterations accumulate: for example, TP53 mutations and overexpression of platelet-derived growth factor (PDGF) ligands and receptors (PDGFRs) in low-grade astrocytomas are followed by accumulation of genetic alterations of cell-cycle regulatory pathways, including deletion or mutations of cyclin-dependent kinase (CDK) inhibitor, p16INK4A/CDKN2A, or the retinoblastoma susceptibility locus 1, with the progression to anaplastic astrocytoma followed by amplification or overexpression of CDK4 and loss of heterozygosity (LOH) of chromosome 10q in malignant progression of secondary glioblastomas (Fig. 2).[3–6]

It has been suggested that secondary glioblastomas in some instances acquire genotypic and phenotypic characteristics of primitive neuroectodermal tumors.[7] In contrast, primary glioblastomas are characterized by frequent amplification of epidermal growth factor receptor (EGFR) and infrequent TP53 mutations.[2,8]

In oligodendrogliomas, the molecular-genetic hallmark is deletion of the chromosomal arms 1p and 19q, which is present in up to 80% of cases. It is often due to an unbalanced translocation t(1;19)(q10;p10).[9]

The 1p/19q deletion is of prognostic and predictive significance in diffuse glioma, especially high-grade tumors. A landmark study of 35 anaplastic oligodendroglioma tumor samples demonstrated that those patients whose tumors exhibited 1p/19q loss had a therapeutic response and longer survival times than patients whose tumors lacked this change.[10] Since that time, it has been suggested that oligodendrogliomas are inherently more responsive to treatment as compared with other diffuse gliomas.[11,12] Although combined 1p/19q loss was initially suggested as a predictive marker for response to alkylating chemotherapy, subsequent studies indicate that it is more generally

[a] Department of Pathology, Unit 085, The University of Texas M.D. Anderson Cancer Center, 1515 Holcombe Boulevard, Houston, TX 77030, USA
[b] Department of Neuropathology, University Hospital Zurich, Switzerland
* Corresponding author.
E-mail address: kaldape@mdanderson.org

Neuroimag Clin N Am 20 (2010) 273–282
doi:10.1016/j.nic.2010.05.004
1052-5149/10/$ – see front matter © 2010 Published by Elsevier Inc.

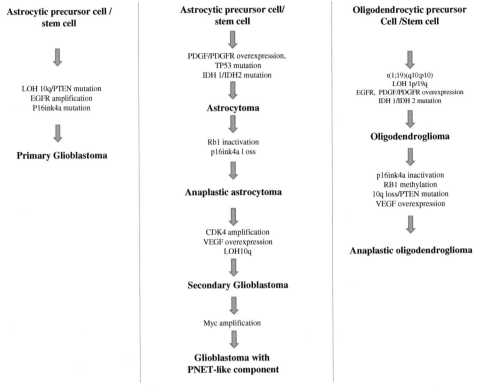

Fig. 1. Glioma development and progression. Tumors originate from neural stem cells or glial precursor cells transformed through genetic alterations, which accumulate during malignant progression. p16ink4a, CDKN2A (cyclin-dependent kinase inhibitor 2A).

associated with improved response to genotoxic agents in general, including radiotherapy.[13–15] Nonetheless, the assessment of 1p/19q status in oligodendroglial tumors is currently a widely performed molecular-genetic test in neuro-oncologic practice.[13] Although 1p/19q status seems to influence treatment decisions in some settings, opinions vary on the treatment implications based on the results of 1p/19q status in these tumors.[16] Putative tumor suppressor genes have not been identified on these chromosomal arms; therefore, the link between molecular pathogenesis of

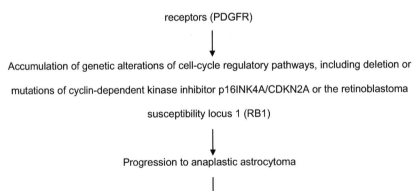

TP53 mutations and overexpression of platelet derived growth factor (PDGF) ligands and receptors (PDGFR)

Accumulation of genetic alterations of cell-cycle regulatory pathways, including deletion or mutations of cyclin-dependent kinase inhibitor p16INK4A/CDKN2A or the retinoblastoma susceptibility locus 1 (RB1)

Progression to anaplastic astrocytoma

Amplification or overexpression of cyclin-dependent kinase 4 (CDK4) and loss of heterozygosity (LOH) of chromosome 10q in malignant progression of secondary glioblastomas

Fig. 2. Flowchart depicting malignant progression of low-grade astrocytomas in terms of genetic alterations.

oligodendrogliomas and the therapeutic implication is still missing in this case. Other mechanisms of tumor development and progression appear similar to those seen in astrocytic tumors, including deregulation of cell cycle proteins[6] and their inhibitors, loss of phosphatase and tensin homolog deleted on chromosome 10 (PTEN),[17] and up-regulation of angiogenic factors[18] with the progression to anaplastic oligodendroglioma.

The molecular and genetic alterations underlying the tumorigenesis and progression of mixed oligoastrocytomas resemble those of astrocytic or oligodendroglial tumors. Tumors that have 1p/19q deletions do not have TP53 mutations and vice versa, indicating that even if morphologically ambiguous, oligoastrocytomas genetically resemble pure oligodendrogliomas or astrocytoma. Although recognized by the WHO, the use of the mixed oligoastrocytoma diagnosis remains suboptimal due to its ambiguity and difficult with respect to reproducible classification among neuropathologists.[11] A challenge for the future is to identify molecular signatures to more precisely define the clinical behavior of these morphologically ambiguous tumors in individual cases.

Most recently, a common genetic mutation for low-grade gliomas of astrocytic and oligodendroglial lineage has been described, which can also be found in secondary glioblastomas arising from a lower-grade glioma: mutations in the isocitrate-dehydrogenase 1 and 2 genes were found in 90% of diffuse astrocytomas and 85% of secondary glioblastomas analyzed. In oligodendrogliomas, isocitrate dehydrogenase (IDH) mutations were found in 84% of grade II and 94% of grade III lesions. In contrast, only 5% of primary glioblastomas carry an IDH mutation according to this study.[19] A summary of novel treatments aimed at the components of the malignant phenotype is given in **Fig. 3**.

TREATMENT TARGETS
Growth Factor Signaling Pathways—Receptor Tyrosine Kinase Inhibition

Mitogenic growth signals enable tumor cells to move from a quiescent state into a proliferative state. They are transmitted into the cell by transmembrane receptors that bind diffusible growth factors, extracellular matrix (ECM) components, and cell-to-cell adhesion/interaction molecules. Glioma cells (over)express growth factors and corresponding receptors, for example PDGF, PDGFRs, transforming growth factor (TGF)-β, and EGFR, allowing for paracrine and autocrine growth stimulation.[20,21] In addition, growth-stimulating signaling independentlof ligand binding

can occur in tyrosine kinase receptors due to a mutation (for example, EGFR variant type III [EGFRvIII], discussed later).

PDGF/PDGFRs

Coexpression of PDGF and PDGFRs exists in gliomas of all grades and is held to be an early oncogenic event, even though expression directly increases with glioma grade.[22] PDGF promotes not only growth but also angiogenesis through an autocrine loop.[22,23] Imatinib mesylate (Gleevec, Novartis, East Hanover, NJ, USA), a kinase inhibitor of PDGFRs, c-Kit and bcr-abl, has demonstrated progression-free survival (PFS) at 6 years of 32% in patients who had immunohistochemical expression of PDGFRs.[24] Thus, detection of the target protein may be helpful in predicting response to Gleevec.[25]

EGFR

EGFR is the most frequently amplified gene in glioblastoma.[4,5,26] EGFR amplification is associated with EGFR overexpression.[27,28] EGFRvIII is a truncated variant of EGFR found in 20% to 50% of glioblastomas with EGFR amplification. It results in a deletion in exons 2–7 of the EGFR mRNA, thereby removing the extracellular ligand-binding domain of the receptor.[29] Thus, EGFRvIII is constitutively activated, signaling through the phosphatidylinositol-3 kinase (PI3K), RAS, and mitogen-activated protein (MAP)-kinase (MAPK) pathways, independently of its ligand. The increased activity of EGFR promotes tumor growth through many different mechanisms, promoting survival, invasion, and angiogenesis.[30] In accordance with these effects, EGFRvIII positivity in glioblastoma multiforme (GBM) has been linked to a more aggressive clinical phenotype with shorter overall survival times.[31] Because EGFRvIII is a tumor-specific change on normal cells, it is a promising therapeutic target.[32]

EGFR-targeted therapies include the monoclonal antibodies to EGFR (cetuximab [Erbitux, Bristol-Myers Squibb, New York, NY, USA]) and EGFR kinase inhibitors, gefitinib (Iressa [ZD1839], AstraZenaca, Wilmington, DE, USA) and erlotinib (Tarceva [OSI-774], Genentech, South San Francisco, CA, USA). In glioblastomas, clinical response to treatment with cetuximab has been reported in several cases.[33] Phase I and II clinical trials are ongoing. Gefitinib and erlotinib resulted in radiographic response, but no survival benefit in clinical trials for malignant gliomas. Attempts at correlation of treatment response with molecular characteristics of gliomas produced notable result in retrospective evaluation of tumor tissues

Novel Treatment approaches in gliomas	
1. Inhibition of growth signals	
PDGFR	imatinib mesylate (*Gleevec*)
EGFR	cetuximab (*Erbitux*), geftinib (*Iressa*), erlotinib (*Tarceva*)
TGF-β	AP-12009
Ras	Tipifarnib *(Zarnestra)*, lonafarnib (*Sarasar*)
mTOR	Sirolimus *(Rapamune)*, temsirolimus *(Torisel)*, everolimus (*Certican*)
2. Reconstituting cell cycle brakes	
proteasome	bortezomib *(Velcade)*
P53	Gene therapy
3. Anti-angiogenesis	
VEGF	bevacizumab *(Avastin)*
VEGFR	Vatalanib /PTK787, cediranib/AZD2171
4. Anti-Invasion	
Integrins	Cillengitide/EMD121974
Matrix Metalloproteases	marimastat

Fig. 3. Therapeutic approaches targeting individual or multiple aspects of the malignant phenotype.

from patients enrolled in clinical trials. Coexpression of normal PTEN and mutant EGFRvIII and combined low levels of AKT and overexpression of EGFR have been identified as predictors of radiographic response.[34–36]

TGF-β

TGF-β is a polypeptide growth factor that binds to its serine-threonine kinase receptor, TGF-βR. TGF-βR phosphorylates the Smad transcription factors, which regulate the transcription of TGF-β responsive genes. In normal cells, TGF-β promotes apoptosis and differentiation and blocks cell proliferation. In neoplastic cells, inactivation of TGF-β through mutation of the receptor or downstream Smad proteins results in uncontrolled proliferation. Gliomas coexpress TGF-β and its receptors in an autocrine loop. The expression levels of TGF-β increase with tumor grade. The TGF-β receptors are, however, not mutated in high-grade gliomas, suggesting a downstream signaling disruption.[37,38] TGF-β also promotes invasion by inducing the expression of matrix metalloproteinase (MMP)-2.[39] In epithelial tumors, TGF-β is associated with tumor progression and metastatic phenotype by inducing transdifferentiation, termed the epithelial-to-mesenchymal transition.[40,41] Recent findings indicating an analogous transition in malignant glioma[42] raise the possibility that TGF-β may play a role in this process. Therapeutic exploitation of the TGF-β pathway has been attempted with antisense oligonucleotide, AP12009, which has been tested in clinical trials on malignant gliomas with modest success.[43] One protein of the TGF-β superfamily,

MIC-1/GDF15, may be useful as a prognostic biomarker in glioblastoma patients: the level of MIC-1/GDF15 protein in the CSF determined by ELISA revealed a shorter survival in patients with elevated levels.[44]

Ras-Raf-MEK-MAPK

The MAPK pathway is activated through integrins or receptor tyrosine kinase (RTK) receptors, which bind growth factors, such as TGF-β. RTK activation results in receptor dimerization and downstream activation of Ras and phosphorylation of MAPK by MEK (mitogen-activated protein kinase kinase), which in turn phosphorylates nuclear transcription factors that induce the expression of genes promoting cell cycle progression, for example, cyclin D1. Although Ras is often activated in gliomas, it does not usually carry any mutations. Rather, Ras activity in gliomas is determined by inappropriate RTK or integrin activation.[45,46] The rate-limiting step of maturation of Ras is farnesylation. Farnesyltransferase inhibitors, however, including tipifarnib (Zarnestra [R115777], Johnson & Johnson, Brunswick, NJ, USA) and lonafarnib (Sarasar [SCH66336], Schering-Plough, Kenilworth, NJ, USA), have led to mixed results: although there was some efficacy in recurrent GBM, the treatment of residual disease yielded stable disease as the best response in a phase II clinical trial.[47,48]

PI3K/PTEN/AKT/mTOR

The PI3K pathway is an important mediator of cell growth and proliferation. Its activation is frequent and associated with poor prognosis in glioma patients.[49] In many cases, loss of PTEN, a major tumor suppressor that is inactivated in up to 50% of high-grade gliomas by mutations or epigenetic mechanisms, results in uncontrolled PI3K signaling and AKT activation.[50,51] Downstream from Akt, the serine/threonine kinase, mammalian target of rapamycin (mTOR), regulates protein translation involving initiation factor 4E-binding protein-1 and the ribosomal S6 kinase. Approaches to blocking this signaling cascade include the mTOR inhibitors, rapamycin (sirolimus [Rapamune], Pfizer, New York, NY, USA) and its synthesized analogs, temsirolimus (Torisel, Wyeth) and everolimus (Certican [RAD001], Novartis), which have been evaluated in clinical trials.[52,53] In a phase II clinical trial of temsirolimus on 65 GBM patients, a radiographic response to treatment was observed in 36% of patients.[53]

PROLIFERATION: RECONSTITUTION OF BRAKES ON THE TUMOR CELL CYCLE
Rb Pathway

A central effector of the antiproliferative signaling is the retinoblastoma protein (pRb). It blocks proliferation by sequestering the transcription factor, E2F, which is necessary for the progression from the G1 into S phase. Disruption of the pRb pathway liberates E2Fs and thus allows cell proliferation. The retinoblastoma pathway can be disrupted in different ways. Functional pRb may be lost through mutation of its gene, which occurs in 25% of high-grade gliomas. The pRb can be inactivated by cyclin D1 and CDK4 and CDK6 complexes through hyperphosphorylation.[54] Amplification of the CDK4 and CDK6 genes also result in functional inactivation of RB in high-grade gliomas.[55,56] In addition, RB activity is lost through the inactivation of a critical negative regulator of CDK4 and CDK6, p16^{Ink4a}.[57]

Disruptions of the pRb pathway are frequent in high-grade gliomas and tend to involve only one component of the pathway in any given tumor.[58]

Because cyclins and CDK inhibitors are subject to proteosomal degradation, the cell cycle regulation can be modified through proteasome inhibitors, such as bortezomib (Velcade, Millenium Pharmaceuticals, Cambridge, MA, USA). This proteasome inhibitor induces expression of p21 and p27 decreases levels of CDK2, CDK4, and E2F4, and leads to apoptosis in vitro glioma cell lines.[59] A phase I clinical trial of bortezomib in combination with temozolomide and radiotherapy showed safety and tolerability for patients with newly diagnosed and recurrent malignant gliomas.[60]

p53 Pathway

The p53 protein plays a role in cell cycle control, DNA damage response, cell death and differentiation. Its regulatory function in the cell cycle consists of a control function at the G1 to S phase transition point, which is effected through its downstream transcriptional target CDNK1A, which encodes the protein for the CDK2 inhibitor, p21. The proapoptotic effect of p53 is mediated by its up-regulation of proapoptotic proteins, such as BAX.

Molecular therapeutic approaches directed at loss of p53 function in gliomas attempt to restore p53 function, mainly through delivery of the p53 gene.[61] In a phase I clinical trial of adenovirus-mediated gene transfer for recurrent gliomas, treatment was well tolerated by patients, PFS was 13 weeks, and overall survival was 43 weeks.[62] A limitation of this treatment approach, as observed with gene therapy approaches in general, has been poor diffusion of the vector into the affected brain tissue.

FORMATION OF NEW BLOOD VESSELS: ANTIANGIOGENIC TREATMENT

Angiogenesis, the new formation of blood vessels from pre-existing ones, is a key step in malignant progression of gliomas.[63,64] Angiogenesis is controlled through many angiogenic and antiangiogenic factors. High-grade gliomas have the ability to tip the angiogenic-antiangiogenic balance and induce vascular proliferation through a multitude of mediating substances, including vascular endothelial growth factor (VEGF), acidic and basic fibroblast growth factor, hepatocyte growth factor, and stromal cell–derived factor 1.[23,65] Of these, VEGF is perhaps the best studied.

The expression of VEGF is in part mediated by the transcription factor, HIF-1, which is itself activated through hypoxia or up-regulated expression of intracellular signaling pathways induced by growth factors, such as EGF and PDGF-A.[65] Its inhibition has found its way into clinical application in the form of several agents, of which bevacizumab (Avastin, Genentech) is the most well known. This is a humanized neutralizing monoclonal antibody to VEGF, which demonstrated a 63% radiographic response to treatment in a phase 2 clinical trial in malignant gliomas in combination with irinotecan. The 6-month PFS in this study was 38% and the 6-month overall survival probability was 72%.[66,67]

In patients with recurrent malignant gliomas, antitumor activity of bevacizumab used as a single agent has been demonstrated.[68] For patients with progression during a bevacizumab-containing regimen, however, alternative therapeutic strategies should be considered, because a retrospective analysis by Quant and others demonstrated lack of response to a second bevacizumab-containing regimen.[69] A different strategy to inhibit VEGF-mediated angiogenesis is to block the tyrosine kinase activity of the VEGF receptors.[70] These tyrosine kinase-inhibitors often have intrinsic activity against more than one receptor and are thus referred to as "multi-RTK inhibitors." The advantage lies in the ability to block multiple signaling pathways active in the tumor. The pan-VEGF receptor inhibitor, AZD2171, has been reported to radiographically normalize tumor vasculature in glioblastoma patients and decrease edema.[71] The multireceptor-tyrosine kinase inhibitors, sunitinib and PTK787, for example, block VEGFR, PDGFRs, and c-Kit signaling.[72,73] Sorafenib unites activity against VEGFR, PDGFRs, Raf, and c-Kit. Vatalanib was well tolerated by patients with recurrent high-grade glioma in combination with imatinib and hydroxyurea.[73]

INVASION

An important hallmark of gliomas is their invasiveness. They diffusely infiltrate the surrounding brain tissue, making a complete surgical resection impossible to achieve. In it currently unclear whether or not the diffuse infiltration along white matter tracts seen in low-grade gliomas is the same process as the more destructive matrix remodeling and invasion exhibited by GBM, but at least for these high-grade tumors, it is felt that tumor cells must be able to attach to the ECM, break down ECM components, and move by extension of membrane protrusion and reorganization of the cytoskeleton. The ECM serves can be viewed as a scaffold that also engages in signaling processes with invading glioma cells. In the brain parenchyma, the main constituent proteins are hyaluron and glycosaminoglycan and in the perviascular space, where glioma cells migrate preferentially, fibronectin, laminin, collagen, and vitronectin.[74] Tumor cells form attachments to these components, which is necessary for migration. The most important group of adhesion molecules is the integrin family of transmembrane proteins that mediate attachment to ECM components. The expression of integrin proteins has been shown to correlate with migration and invasion in gliomas.[75] Furthermore, integrins are important for migration of endothelial cells, thus fostering angiogenesis. Cilengitide (EMD121974, EMD Pharmaceuticals, Durham, NC, USA), an inhibitor of αvβ3 and αvβ5

integrins, suppresses brain tumor growth through induction of apoptosis in vascular endothelial and brain tumor cells by blocking their interaction with the matrix proteins vitronectin and tenascin.[75,76] This drug has yielded a 6-month PFS of 15% and a median overall survival of 9.9 months in a phase II clinical trial for treatment of recurrent glioblastoma.[77]

Because the ECM is also a physiologic barrier to cell migration, glioma cells can break down the ECM by secreting proteases, such as MMPs and urokinase plasminogen activator.[78] The expression of MMPs and urokinase plasminogen activator increases with glioma grade and is inversely correlated with prognosis.[79–81] Blockage of MMPs can be achieved by inhibitors, such as marimastat, which has been tested in clinical trials on patients with anaplastic gliomas. It was found no more efficacious, however, than treatment with single-agent temozolomide.[82]

EGFR signaling also contributes to invasion. Glioblastomas with constitutively active EGFRvIII receptors are more invasive in vitro than those with wild-type EGFR.[30] Downstream signaling molecules, most prominently phosphorylated Akt,[83,84] are also implicated in invasion, demonstrating that the PI3K-Akt pathway is not only instrumental to growth and inhibition of apoptosis but also for tumor invasion.

MOLECULAR MARKERS IN CURRENT CLINICAL APPLICATION

To date, assessment of 1p/19q status by polymerase chain reaction or fluorescence in situ hybridization is the only established molecular marker in neuro-oncologic practice (discussed previously). A second candidate biomarker in the phase of validation is the methylation status of the promoter of the O6-methylguanine-DNA-methyltransferase (MGMT) gene, which has been correlated with the response to temozolomide in a landmark European Organisation for Research and Treatment of Cancer study.[85,86] This gene encodes for a DNA repair enzyme, which confers resistance to alkylating chemotherapeutic agents as temozolomide. The transcription of this gene is silenced through promoter methylation in approximately 50% of glioblastomas, rendering the tumor more sensitive to treatment. A current multicenter trial of cilengitide (Cilengitide, Temozolomide, and Radiation Therapy in Treating Patients with Newly Diagnosed Glioblastoma and Methylated Gene Promoter Status [CENTRIC]; study number EMD 121974-011) for treatment of newly diagnosed glioblastoma specifically enrolls patients with a methylated MGMT-promoter.

MOLECULAR SUBTYPES IDENTIFIED VIA HIGH-THROUGHPUT SCREENS

Several studies have described molecular subtyping of gliomas based on high-throughout screens, mainly through expression microarrays.[42,87–90] Although the specifics of the subclassification schemes vary, a common thread is the finding of a subclass of tumors, which has been termed "mesenchymal" (due to overexpression of genes associated with mesenchyme) as well as a "proneural" subclass (due to overexpression of genes associated with neural development). Mesenchymal tumors tend to be overwhelmingly grade IV/GBM, whereas proneural tumors include grade II-III infiltrating gliomas as well as some GBMs. Proneural tumors tend to be from younger patients and display a less aggressive clinical behavior. More recently data from The Cancer Genome Atlas described a classification scheme that included mesenchymal and proneural subclasses as well as two additional subclasses.[90] Part of the difference in the specifics of classification schemes relate to the statistical algorithms used to generate the subclasses, and there is currently a lack of consensus as to optimal methods for doing so.

Further work from The Cancer Genome Atlas incorporating data from CpG island methylation screens identified a subset of GBMs that show concordant methylation of a cassette of genes. This finding was termed, *the CpG island methylator phenotype (CIMP)*, similar to what has been described in other tumor types, including colorectal tumors. CIMP-positive tumors represented 5% to 10% of GBMs, showed improved prognosis, and were overwhelmingly in the proneural subgroup. Examination of grade II-III gliomas showed that a high proportion of these tumors were CIMP positive. Finally, a positive correlation of CIMP status with mutations in IDH1 was demonstrated.[91] Currently, the functional relationship, if any, between DNA methylation and IDH1 mutation is unknown, but these two markers identify a subtype of glioma with improved outcome.

SUMMARY AND FUTURE PERSPECTIVE

With the rapid development of molecular tools to identify the biologic basis for glioma development and progression, much knowledge has been accumulated in the past years that will be translated into daily clinical practice by therapy targeting determinants of the malignant phenotype. Because the mechanisms and pathways implicated in gliomagenesis and progression are interconnected, multitarget therapies may be more successful in prolonging survival times than single-agent chemotherapy. Molecular-genetic analysis will perhaps reveal clinically important subgroups. Future clinical trials should incorporate biomarker-based analyses that would allow the identification of drugs that may be more or less effective against specific molecular subgroups. Information gained from such trials could lead to the possibility of tailoring future treatments according to the genetic profile of the tumor, and improving overall patient outcomes.

REFERENCES

1. Okamoto Y, Di Patre PL, Burkhard C, et al. Population-based study on incidence, survival rates, and genetic alterations of low-grade diffuse astrocytomas and oligodendrogliomas. Acta Neuropathol 2004;108(1):49–56.
2. Ohgaki H, Kleihues P. Population-based studies on incidence, survival rates, and genetic alterations in astrocytic and oligodendroglial gliomas. J Neuropathol Exp Neurol 2005;64(6):479–89.
3. Ohgaki H. Genetic pathways to glioblastomas. Neuropathology 2005;25(1):1–7.
4. Ohgaki H, Dessen P, Jourde B, et al. Genetic pathways to glioblastoma: a population-based study. Cancer Res 2004;64(19):6892–9.
5. Ohgaki H, Kleihues P. Genetic pathways to primary and secondary glioblastoma. Am J Pathol 2007;170(5):1445–53.
6. Wolter M, Reifenberger J, Blaschke B, et al. Oligodendroglial tumors frequently demonstrate hypermethylation of the CDKN2A (MTS1, p16INK4a), p14ARF, and CDKN2B (MTS2, p15INK4b) tumor suppressor genes. J Neuropathol Exp Neurol 2001;60(12):1170–80.
7. Perry A, Miller R, Guirati M, et al. Malignant gliomas with neuroblastic (PNET-like) components (GBM-PNET): a clinicopathologic and genetic study of 28 cases. Neuro Oncol 2007;9(4):543.
8. Houillier C, Lejeune J, Benouaich-Amiel A, et al. Prognostic impact of molecular markers in a series of 220 primary glioblastomas. Cancer 2006;106(10):2218–23.
9. Griffin CA, Burger P, Morsberger L, et al. Identification of der(1;19)(q10;p10) in five oligodendrogliomas suggests mechanism of concurrent 1p and 19q loss. J Neuropathol Exp Neurol 2006;65(10):988–94.
10. Cairncross JG, Ueki K, Zlatescu MC, et al. Specific genetic predictors of chemotherapeutic response and survival in patients with anaplastic oligodendrogliomas. J Natl Cancer Inst 1998;90(19):1473–9.
11. Kros JM, Gorlia T, Kouwenhoven MC, et al. Panel review of anaplastic oligodendroglioma from European Organization For Research and Treatment of

Cancer Trial 26951: assessment of consensus in diagnosis, influence of 1p/19q loss, and correlations with outcome. J Neuropathol Exp Neurol 2007;66(6): 545–51.

12. van den Bent MJ. Anaplastic oligodendroglioma and oligoastrocytoma. Neurol Clin 2007;25(4):1089–99, ix–x.

13. Aldape K, Burger PC, Perry A. Clinicopathologic aspects of 1p/19q loss and the diagnosis of oligo-dendroglioma. Arch Pathol Lab Med 2007;131(2): 242–51.

14. Van Den Bent MJ. Guidelines for the treatment of oli-godendroglioma: an evidence-based medicine approach. Forum (Genova) 2003;13(1):18–31.

15. Weller M, Berger H, Hartmann C, et al. Combined 1p/19q loss in oligodendroglial tumors: predictive or prognostic biomarker? Clin Cancer Res 2007; 13(23):6933–7.

16. Abrey LE, Louis DN, Paleologos N, et al. Survey of treatment recommendations for anaplastic oligoden-droglioma. Neuro Oncol 2007;9(3):314–8.

17. Sasaki H, Zlatescu MC, Betensky RA, et al. PTEN is a target of chromosome 10q loss in anaplastic oli-godendrogliomas and PTEN alterations are associ-ated with poor prognosis. Am J Pathol 2001;159(1): 359–67.

18. Chan AS, Leung SY, Wong MP, et al. Expression of vascular endothelial growth factor and its receptors in the anaplastic progression of astrocytoma, oligo-dendroglioma, and ependymoma. Am J Surg Pathol 1998;22(7):816–26.

19. Yan H, Parsons DW, Jin G, et al. IDH1 and IDH2 mutations in gliomas. N Engl J Med 2009;360(8): 765–73.

20. Guha A, Dashner K, Black PM, et al. Expression of PDGF and PDGF receptors in human astrocytoma operation specimens supports the existence of an autocrine loop. Int J Cancer 1995;60(2):168–73.

21. Maher PA. Nuclear Translocation of fibroblast growth factor (FGF) receptors in response to FGF-2. J Cell Biol 1996;134(2):529–36.

22. Hermanson M, Funa K, Hartman M, et al. Platelet-derived growth factor and its receptors in human glioma tissue: expression of messenger RNA and protein suggests the presence of auto-crine and paracrine loops. Cancer Res 1992; 52(11):3213–9.

23. Dunn IF, Heese O, Black PM. Growth factors in glioma angiogenesis: FGFs, PDGF, EGF, and TGFs. J Neurooncol 2000;50(1–2):121–37.

24. Savage DG, Antman KH. Imatinib mesylate—a new oral targeted therapy. N Engl J Med 2002;346(9): 683–93.

25. Haberler C, Gelpi E, Marosi C, et al. Immunohisto-chemical analysis of platelet-derived growth factor receptor-alpha, -beta, c-kit, c-abl, and arg proteins in glioblastoma: possible implications for patient selection for imatinib mesylate therapy. J Neurooncol 2006;76(2):105–9.

26. von Deimling A, von Ammon K, Schoenfeld D, et al. Subsets of glioblastoma multiforme defined by molecular genetic analysis. Brain Pathol 1993;3(1): 19–26.

27. Fischer I, de la Cruz C, Rivera AL, et al. Utility of chromogenic in situ hybridization (CISH) for detec-tion of EGFR amplification in glioblastoma: compar-ison with fluorescence in situ hybridization (FISH). Diagn Mol Pathol 2008;17(4):227–30.

28. Tripp SR, Willmore-Payne C, Layfield LJ. Relation-ship between EGFR overexpression and gene amplification status in central nervous system gliomas. Anal Quant Cytol Histol 2005;27(2):71–8.

29. Ekstrand AJ, Longo N, Hamid ML, et al. Functional characterization of an EGF receptor with a truncated extracellular domain expressed in glioblastomas with EGFR gene amplification. Oncogene 1994; 9(8):2313–20.

30. Lal A, Glazer CA, Martinson HM, et al. Mutant epidermal growth factor receptor up-regulates molecular effectors of tumor invasion. Cancer Res 2002;62(12):3335–9.

31. Pelloski CE, Ballman KV, Furth AF, et al. Epidermal growth factor receptor variant III status defines clin-ically distinct subtypes of glioblastoma. J Clin Oncol 2007;25(16):2288–94.

32. Jungbluth AA, Stockert E, Huang HJ, et al. A monoclonal antibody recognizing human cancers with amplification/overexpression of the human epidermal growth factor receptor. Proc Natl Acad Sci U S A 2003;100(2):639–44.

33. Belda-Iniesta C, Carpeno Jde C, Saenz EC, et al. Long term responses with cetuximab therapy in glio-blastoma multiforme. Cancer Biol Ther 2006;5(8): 912–4.

34. Haas-Kogan DA, Prados MD, Lamborn KR, et al. Biomarkers to predict response to epidermal growth factor receptor inhibitors. Cell Cycle 2005;4(10): 1369–72.

35. Haas-Kogan DA, Prados MD, Tihan T, et al. Epidermal growth factor receptor, protein kinase B/Akt, and glioma response to erlotinib. J Natl Cancer Inst 2005;97(12):880–7.

36. Mellinghoff IK, Wang MY, Vivanco I, et al. Molecular determinants of the response of glioblastomas to EGFR kinase inhibitors. N Engl J Med 2005; 353(19):2012–24.

37. Platten M, Wick W, Weller M. Malignant glioma biology: role for TGF-beta in growth, motility, angio-genesis, and immune escape. Microsc Res Tech 2001;52(4):401–10.

38. Yamada N, Kato M, Yamashita H, et al. Enhanced expression of transforming growth factor-beta and its type-I and type-II receptors in human glioblas-toma. Int J Cancer 1995;62(4):386–92.

39. Wick W, Platten M, Weller M. Glioma cell invasion: regulation of metalloproteinase activity by TGF-beta. J Neurooncol 2001;53(2):177–85.

40. Lamouille S, Derynck R. Cell size and invasion in TGF-beta-induced epithelial to mesenchymal transition is regulated by activation of the mTOR pathway. J Cell Biol 2007;178(3):437–51.

41. Zavadil J, Bottinger EP. TGF-beta and epithelial-to-mesenchymal transitions. Oncogene 2005;24(37): 5764–74.

42. Phillips HS, Kharbanda S, Chen R, et al. Molecular subclasses of high-grade glioma predict prognosis, delineate a pattern of disease progression, and resemble stages in neurogenesis. Cancer Cell 2006;9(3):157–73.

43. Schlingensiepen KH, Schlingensiepen R, Steinbrecher A, et al. Targeted tumor therapy with the TGF-beta2 antisense compound AP 12009. Cytokine Growth Factor Rev 2006;17(1–2):129–39.

44. Shnaper S, Desbaillets I, Brown DA, et al. Elevated levels of MIC-1/GDF15 in the cerebro-spinal fluid (CSF) of patients are associated with glioblastoma and worse outcome. Int J Cancer 2009;125(11): 2624–30.

45. Jeuken JW, van der Maazen RW, Wesseling P. Molecular diagnostics as a tool to personalize treatment in adult glioma patients. Tech Canc Res Treat 2006;5(3):215–29.

46. Knobbe CB, Reifenberger J, Reifenberger G. Mutation analysis of the Ras pathway genes NRAS, HRAS, KRAS and BRAF in glioblastomas. Acta Neuropathol 2004;108(6):467–70.

47. Cloughesy TF, Wen PY, Robins HI, et al. Phase II trial of tipifarnib in patients with recurrent malignant glioma either receiving or not receiving enzyme-inducing antiepileptic drugs: a North American Brain Tumor Consortium Study. J Clin Oncol 2006;24(22): 3651–6.

48. Moyal EC, Laprie A, Delannes M, et al. Phase I trial of tipifarnib (R115777) concurrent with radiotherapy in patients with glioblastoma multiforme. Int J Radiat Oncol Biol Phys 2007;68(5):1396–401.

49. Chakravarti A, Zhai G, Suzuki Y, et al. The prognostic significance of phosphatidylinositol 3-kinase pathway activation in human gliomas. J Clin Oncol 2004;22(10):1926–33.

50. Knobbe CB, Merlo A, Reifenberger G. Pten signaling in gliomas. Neuro Oncol 2002;4(3): 196–211.

51. Knobbe CB, Reifenberger G. Genetic alterations and aberrant expression of genes related to the phosphatidyl-inositol-3'-kinase/protein kinase B (Akt) signal transduction pathway in glioblastomas. Brain Pathol 2003;13(4):507–18.

52. Fan QW, Knight ZA, Goldenberg DD, et al. A dual PI3 kinase/mTOR inhibitor reveals emergent efficacy in glioma. Cancer Cell 2006;9(5):341–9.

53. Galanis E, Buckner JC, Maurer MJ, et al. Phase II trial of temsirolimus (CCI-779) in recurrent glioblastoma multiforme: a North Central Cancer Treatment Group Study. J Clin Oncol 2005;23(23):5294–304.

54. Aktas H, Cai H, Cooper GM. Ras links growth factor signaling to the cell cycle machinery via regulation of cyclin D1 and the Cdk inhibitor p27KIP1. Mol Cell Biol 1997;17(7):3850–7.

55. Reifenberger G, Ichimura K, Reifenberger J, et al. Refined mapping of 12q13-q15 amplicons in human malignant gliomas suggests CDK4/SAS and MDM2 as independent amplification targets. Cancer Res 1996;56(22):5141–5.

56. Reifenberger G, Reifenberger J, Ichimura K, et al. Amplification of multiple genes from chromosomal region 12q13-14 in human malignant gliomas: preliminary mapping of the amplicons shows preferential involvement of CDK4, SAS, and MDM2. Cancer Res 1994;54(16):4299–303.

57. Serrano M, Hannon GJ, Beach D. A new regulatory motif in cell-cycle control causing specific inhibition of cyclin D/CDK4. Nature 1993;366(6456):704–7.

58. Ueki K, Ono Y, Henson JW, et al. CDKN2/p16 or RB alterations occur in the majority of glioblastomas and are inversely correlated. Cancer Res 1996;56(1): 150–3.

59. Yin D, Zhou H, Kumagai T, et al. Proteasome inhibitor PS-341 causes cell growth arrest and apoptosis in human glioblastoma multiforme (GBM). Oncogene 2005;24(3):344–54.

60. Kubicek GJ, Werner-Wasik M, Machtay M, et al. Phase I trial using proteasome inhibitor bortezomib and concurrent temozolomide and radiotherapy for central nervous system malignancies. Int J Radiat Oncol Biol Phys 2009;74(2):433–9.

61. Hupp TR, Lane DP, Ball KL. Strategies for manipulating the p53 pathway in the treatment of human cancer. Biochem J 2000;352(Pt 1):1–17.

62. Lang FF, Bruner JM, Fuller GN, et al. Phase I trial of adenovirus-mediated p53 gene therapy for recurrent glioma: biological and clinical results. J Clin Oncol 2003;21(13):2508–18.

63. Brat DJ, Castellano-Sanchez AA, Hunter SB, et al. Pseudopalisades in glioblastoma are hypoxic, express extracellular matrix proteases, and are formed by an actively migrating cell population. Cancer Res 2004;64(3):920–7.

64. Cheng SY, Huang HJ, Nagane M, et al. Suppression of glioblastoma angiogenicity and tumorigenicity by inhibition of endogenous expression of vascular endothelial growth factor. Proc Natl Acad Sci U S A 1996;93(16):8502–7.

65. Fischer I, Gagner JP, Law M, et al. Angiogenesis in gliomas: biology and molecular pathophysiology. Brain Pathol 2005;15(4):297–310.

66. Vredenburgh JJ, Desjardins A, Herndon JE 2nd, et al. Phase II trial of bevacizumab and irinotecan

in recurrent malignant glioma. Clin Cancer Res 2007;13(4):1253–9.

67. Vredenburgh JJ, Desjardins A, Herndon JE 2nd, et al. Bevacizumab plus irinotecan in recurrent glioblastoma multiforme. J Clin Oncol 2007;25(30): 4722–9.

68. Kreisl TN, Kim L, Moore K, et al. Phase II trial of single-agent bevacizumab followed by bevacizumab plus irinotecan at tumor progression in recurrent glioblastoma. J Clin Oncol 2009;27(5):740–5.

69. Quant EC, Norden AD, Drappatz J, et al. Role of a second chemotherapy in recurrent malignant glioma patients who progress on bevacizumab. Neuro Oncol 2009;11(5):550–5.

70. Kubo K, Shimizu T, Ohyama S, et al. Novel potent orally active selective VEGFR-2 tyrosine kinase inhibitors: synthesis, structure-activity relationships, and antitumor activities of N-phenyl-N'-{4-(4-quinolyloxy)phenyl}ureas. J Med Chem 2005;48(5):1359–66.

71. Batchelor TT, Sorensen AG, di Tomaso E, et al. AZD2171, a pan-VEGF receptor tyrosine kinase inhibitor, normalizes tumor vasculature and alleviates edema in glioblastoma patients. Cancer Cell 2007;11(1):83–95.

72. de Bouard S, Herlin P, Christensen JG, et al. Antiangiogenic and anti-invasive effects of sunitinib on experimental human glioblastoma. Neuro Oncol 2007;9(4):412–23.

73. Reardon DA, Egorin MJ, Desjardins A, et al. Phase I pharmacokinetic study of the vascular endothelial growth factor receptor tyrosine kinase inhibitor vatalanib (PTK787) plus imatinib and hydroxyurea for malignant glioma. Cancer 2009;115(10):2188–98.

74. Gladson CL. The extracellular matrix of gliomas: modulation of cell function. J Neuropathol Exp Neurol 1999;58(10):1029–40.

75. Tonn JC, Wunderlich S, Kerkau S, et al. Invasive behaviour of human gliomas is mediated by individually different integrin patterns. Anticancer Res 1998;18(4A):2599–605.

76. Taga T, Suzuki A, Gonzalez-Gomez I, et al. alpha v-Integrin antagonist EMD 121974 induces apoptosis in brain tumor cells growing on vitronectin and tenascin. Int J Cancer 2002;98(5):690–7.

77. Reardon DA, Fink KL, Mikkelsen T, et al. Randomized phase II study of cilengitide, an integrin-targeting arginine-glycine-aspartic acid peptide, in recurrent glioblastoma multiforme. J Clin Oncol 2008;26(34):5610–7.

78. Rao JS. Molecular mechanisms of glioma invasiveness: the role of proteases. Nat Rev Cancer 2003; 3(7):489–501.

79. Demuth T, Berens ME. Molecular mechanisms of glioma cell migration and invasion. J Neurooncol 2004;70(2):217–28.

80. Wang M, Wang T, Liu S, et al. The expression of matrix metalloproteinase-2 and -9 in human gliomas of different pathological grades. Brain Tumor Pathol 2003;20(2):65–72.

81. Yamamoto M, Sawaya R, Mohanam S, et al. Expression and localization of urokinase-type plasminogen activator in human astrocytomas in vivo. Cancer Res 1994;54(14):3656–61.

82. Groves MD, Puduvalli VK, Conrad CA, et al. Phase II trial of temozolomide plus marimastat for recurrent anaplastic gliomas: a relationship among efficacy, joint toxicity and anticonvulsant status. J Neurooncol 2006;80(1):83–90.

83. Joy AM, Beaudry CE, Tran NL, et al. Migrating glioma cells activate the PI3-K pathway and display decreased susceptibility to apoptosis. J Cell Sci 2003;116(Pt 21):4409–17.

84. Koul D, Shen R, Bergh S, et al. Inhibition of Akt survival pathway by a small-molecule inhibitor in human glioblastoma. Mol Cancer Ther 2006;5(3):637–44.

85. Hegi ME, Diserens AC, Godard S, et al. Clinical trial substantiates the predictive value of O-6-methylguanine-DNA methyltransferase promoter methylation in glioblastoma patients treated with temozolomide. Clin Cancer Res 2004;10(6): 1871–4.

86. Hegi ME, Diserens AC, Gorlia T, et al. MGMT gene silencing and benefit from temozolomide in glioblastoma. N Engl J Med 2005;352(10):997–1003.

87. Freije WA, Castro-Vargas FE, Fang Z, et al. Gene expression profiling of gliomas strongly predicts survival. Cancer Res 2004;64(18):6503–10.

88. Li A, Walling J, Ahn S, et al. Unsupervised analysis of transcriptomic profiles reveals six glioma subtypes. Cancer Res 2009;69(5):2091–9.

89. Nigro JM, Misra A, Zhang L, et al. Integrated array-comparative genomic hybridization and expression array profiles identify clinically relevant molecular subtypes of glioblastoma. Cancer Res 2005;65(5): 1678–86.

90. Verhaak RG, Hoadley KA, Purdom E, et al. Integrated genomic analysis identifies clinically relevant subtypes of glioblastoma characterized by abnormalities in PDGFRA, IDH1, EGFR, and NF1. Cancer Cell 2010;17(1):98–110.

91. Noushmehr H, Weisenberger DJ, Diefes K, et al. Identification of a Cpg island methylator phenotype that defines a distinct subgroup of Glioma. Cancer Cell 2010;17(5):510–22.

Applications of Nanotechnology to Imaging and Therapy of Brain Tumors

Aaron M. Mohs, PhD[a], James M. Provenzale, MD[a,b,c,d],*

KEYWORDS

• Nanomedicine • Brain tumor • Magnetic resonance imaging

Nanoparticles are colloidal particles in which one dimension of the particle is in the range of 10 to 100 nm. Nanoparticles have become a subject for current biomedical investigation because of their unique properties, which include strong optical properties for imaging, ability to be targeted against various molecular sites, and capacity to deliver a cargo of therapeutic drugs.[1–3] Although these properties have been explored in several areas of molecular and cellular imaging, applications in the neurosciences have been relatively underexplored. However, several novel imaging approaches and therapeutic advances for brain tumors are possible using nanotechnology. This article details types of nanoparticles and the means by which they may be used for imaging and therapy of brain tumors (Table 1).

NANOPARTICLES
Liposomes and Micelles

Liposomes are formed from concentric phospholipid bilayers in aqueous conditions that yield vesicular nanoparticles. The resulting structures have a hydrophilic, aqueous core surrounded by a hydrophobic lipid bilayer, very similar to living cells. Liposomes can vary in size from 100 nm (ie, the upper limit of the nanoscale) to 5 μm,

depending on the number of lipid bilayers present.[3] In the aqueous core, hydrophilic therapeutic drugs or imaging agents can be entrapped during the self-assembly process; similarly, hydrophobic substances such as drugs or imaging agents can be incorporated into the hydrophobic shell. Such incorporation of substances is highly beneficial. For instance, incorporation of drugs maximizes drug stability, promotes unimpeded transport to the intended target, and allows for controlled and extended drug release properties.[4] Targeting ligands can be placed on the surface of liposomes, which increases their capacity for delivery to specific tissues (eg, tumor environments). Because of their ease of preparation and biocompatibility, liposomes have found wide application for therapeutic agent or imaging agent delivery (Fig. 1).[5,6] In fact several US Food and Drug Administration (FDA)-approved liposome-based therapeutic agents are available on the market, including doxorubicin formulations for the treatment of Kaposi sarcoma, ovarian cancer, and multiple myeloma.[7] Other therapeutic applications of liposomes are in various stages of clinical trials.[8]

Micelles, like liposomes, are formed from the self-assembly in aqueous media of lipids or polymers that are amphiphilic (ie, have both

a Department of Biomedical Engineering, Emory University and Georgia Institute of Technology, 101 Woodruff Circle Northeast, Suite 2007, Atlanta, GA 30322, USA
b Department of Radiology, Emory University School of Medicine, Atlanta, GA 30322, USA
c Department of Oncology, Emory University School of Medicine, Atlanta, GA 30322, USA
d Department of Radiology, Duke University Medical Center, Durham, NC 27110, USA
* Corresponding author. Department of Radiology, Emory University School of Medicine, Atlanta, GA 30322.
E-mail address: prove001@mc.duke.edu

Neuroimag Clin N Am 20 (2010) 283–292
doi:10.1016/j.nic.2010.04.002

Table 1
Physical, chemical, optical properties and applications of nanoparticles

Particle Type	Composition	Shape	Size	Surface Coatings	Properties	Function	References
Liposome	Aqueous vesicle with lipid-bilayer	spherical	100 nm–5 μm	Polymeric	Aqueous vesicular center and surface, hydrophobic bilayer, self-assembly	Delivery of therapeutic payload or imaging agent	3
Micelle	self-assembled amphiphilic lipid/polymer	spherical	20 nm–200 nm	Hydrophilic component of amphiphile	Hydrophobic core, hydrophilic surface, self-assembly	Delivery of therapeutic payload or imaging agent	5
Iron Oxide	Fe_2O_3	Wide array, including sphere, rod, multifaceted	2–60 nm core, 10–100 nm after surface	Carboxylate, silicate, polymer	Paramagnetic metal, thermally active	Magnetic resonance imaging and therapy	11,49
Gold	Au(0), SERS reporter	Wide array, including sphere, rod, multifaceted	2 nm–250 nm	Carboxylate, silica, synthetic polymer, protein	Strong absorbance, plasmon resonance thermally active	Spectroscopy, imaging, therapy	17,20
Quantum Dots	Cd, Pd, Mg, Zn, S, Se, Te, In, P	Wide array including sphere, rod, multifaceted	2–19 nm core; 5–40 nm after coating	Small molecule, silica, polymeric ligand, amphiphilic polymer	Bright, stable, tunable fluorescence	Imaging, investigational tool	26,27

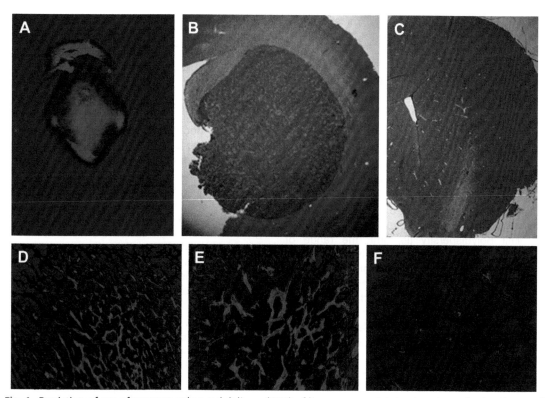

Fig. 1. Depiction of use of contrast-enhanced delivery (CED) of liposomes containing topotecan for treatment of brain tumors in a rat model. The intent of the experiment was to determine whether liposomal delivery of topotecan was more effective than intravenous administration. The tumor model was a U87MG intracranial xenograft. At 10 days after tumor implantation, fluorescent liposomes that were labeled with membrane-bound 1,1'-dioctadecyl-3, 3, 3', 3'-tetramethylindocarbocyanine-perchlorate (DiIC$_{18}$) were infused via CED. Rats were euthanized immediately after the infusions, and their brains were freshly frozen, cut with cryostat, and subjected to histologic examinations. After detecting the fluorescence using fluorescence microscopy, the same sections were stained with H & E. Fluorescence images were overlapped with H & E images (magnification × 12.5). (A) Fluorescence microscopy image of thin section of rat brain bearing tumor shows large accumulation of fluorescent liposomes within tumor. (B) Representative H & E image of U87MG xenograft on day 19 after implantation in rodent striatum. On day 10, this animal underwent CED with fluorescent liposomes that did not contain topotecan. The image shows a large, untreated tumor. (C) Representative H & E image of U87MG xenograft on day 19 after implantation in striatum in rat treated with liposomal topotecan. The image shows a fibrotic cavity containing small remnant of tumor. Thereafter, differences in tumor vasculature densities among various groups of animals were evaluated by immunohistological detection of laminin, a major protein in the basal lamina. Seven days after tumor implantation, rats were randomly divided into three groups and treated with CED infusion of either DiIC$_{18}$ liposomes (control), free topotecan (0.5 mg/mL), or liposomal topotecan (0.5 mg/mL topotecan). Seven days after treatment, rats were euthanized and subjected to immunohistological detection of laminin. (D). Immunohistological stain for laminin in control animal shows high degree of tumor vascularity. (E) Immunohistological stain for laminin in animal treated with free topotecan also shows high degree of vascularity. (F) Immunohistological stain for laminin in animal treated with liposomal topotecan shows very low degree of vascularity. (*Courtesy of* R. Saito, Department of *Neurologic* Surgery, Brain Tumor Research Center University of California, San Francisco, San Francisco, CA.)

hydrophobic and hydrophilic segments). Unlike liposomes, the amphiphilic molecules self-assemble into a structure having a hydrophobic core with a hydrophilic surface. Thus, in addition to size, the major difference between micelles and liposomes is that entrapment of a relatively hydrophobic drug occurs in the core of the nanoparticle. The major attribute of micelles is that they can make soluble therapeutic agents that are normally insoluble in aqueous or biologic environments (see **Table 1**). The hydrophilic shell provides a protective layer that allows more of the drug to be delivered to the target tissue than the administration of free drug itself.[9] Another attribute of micelle nanoparticles is that the chemical constituents used to make them can be engineered to respond to different environments, or be sensitive to stimuli, thus controlling drug release at the desired target site.[10]

Iron Oxide Nanoparticles

Iron oxide (IO) nanoparticles are increasingly being used for a number of imaging and therapeutic applications. These particles can be synthesized by various methods. Most commonly, they are formed by coprecipitation involving reactions with amphoteric surfactants to limit polydispersity (ie, limit the range of size, shape, and mass characteristics),[11] which renders the nanoparticles hydrophobic. Surface modifications are needed to prevent aggregation in aqueous media. The surface atoms of IO act as Lewis acids that can be stabilized by small molecules with multiple coordinating groups, such as citric acid.[12] Inorganic materials (eg, silica) also are used to stabilize IO nanoparticles and provide a means to covalently attach surface ligands for targeting.[13] Polymeric coatings are yet another means of stabilizing surfaces for IO nanoparticles. Natural polymers are among the most common means of stabilizing IO particles to increase blood circulation times and allow conjugation of targeting ligands; examples of such polymers include several dextran derivatives, chitosan, and synthetic polymers, most notably poly(ethylene glycol).[11]

Owing to their ferromagnetic core, IO particles have high relaxivity, which renders them suitable as a magnetic resonance contrast agents; some very small IO nanoparticles that are in the size range of 2 to 18 nm (termed ultrasmall paramagnetic IO, or USPIO) are used as magnetic resonance contrast agents. USPIO nanoparticles produce an increase in signal intensity on T1-weighted images comparable to the positive enhancement from gadolinium(III) complexes.[14] Because of their high transverse relaxivity, however, these nanoparticles also decrease magnetic resonance signal on T2*-weighted images, thereby allowing them to be used with either T1-weighted imaging sequences or T2-weighted sequences (**Figs. 2** and **3**).[15] IO nanoparticles are among the most advanced nanoparticles in terms of translation into clinical use. Paramagnetic IO nanoparticles have already received approval by the FDA for some magnetic resonance imaging (MRI) studies of the bowel and abdominal viscera.[16]

Gold Nanoparticles

Gold nanoparticles are nanoscale clusters of neutral gold atoms prepared from the reduction of gold salts in appropriate agents (eg, citric acid).[17] This method of synthesis affords high reaction yield, good control of size, and a narrow degree of polydispersity. Because gold nanoparticles are not stable in high salt buffer, they must undergo surface modification for biomedical applications. Sulfur atoms form especially strong bonds with gold atoms. Therefore, stabilizing ligands that have a thiol group (ie, a compound that contains a functional group composed of a sulfur–hydrogen bond), such as glutathione or poly(ethylene glycol)-thiol, readily react with gold nanoparticles in aqueous conditions to increase colloidal stability. The versatile surface chemistry of gold nanoparticles allows them to be coated with various biologic targeting ligands.[18,19]

Gold nanoparticles have a deep red color due to the broad surface plasmon resonance (SPR) band in the visible region (approximately 520 nm).[20] This absorbance band is paramount to many aspects of the research performed with gold nanoparticles. The SPR effect is important, because it is the basis for many colorimetric assays using gold nanoparticles and gives information about the adsorption of materials onto the nanoparticle surface. Work by Mirkin and colleagues has used gold nanoparticles to measure biomolecule concentrations at near trace levels.[21] Alternatively, gold nanoparticles can be used for sensitive detection assays using surface-enhanced Raman spectroscopy (SERS). SERS refers to the Raman scattering enhancement by adsorbing molecules to metal surfaces. The enhancement factor can be as large as 10^{14} to 10^{15}, which allows for single molecule detection.[22,23]

Gold nanoparticles can be considered biologically inert, which results in very high biocompatibility. In fact, colloidal gold suspensions have been approved for human use for a number of decades to treat rheumatoid arthritis. Therefore, a wealth of research exists investigating the potential of gold nanoparticles for further in vivo development (eg, for therapeutic delivery[17] and SERS spectroscopy).[24] In the latter example, SERS nanoparticles are of interest because there is almost no SERS background signal with near-infrared excitation. In addition, SERS nanoparticles have a specific molecular spectra (or signature) that aids in distinguishing the nanoparticle from background fluorescence.

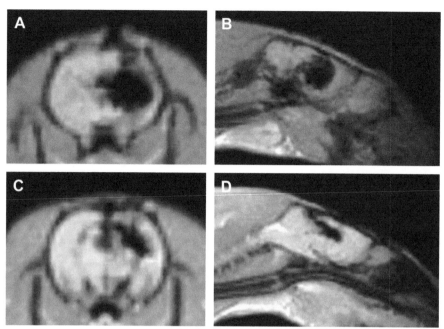

Fig. 2. In vivo magnetic resonance imaging of CED of iron oxide nanoparticles in rat brain tissue in two different animals. These images highlight the difference between efficient CED of nanoparticles and inefficient delivery. (*A*) Axial gradient echo magnetic resonance image showing accumulation of iron oxide nanoparticles within their intended target, the corpus striatum. Due to the susceptibility effects of the iron material generated by the gradient echo imaging technique, the nanoparticles appear as an area of diminished signal intensity. (*B*) Sagittal gradient echo magnetic resonance performed in the same animal as shown in **Fig. 2**A shows an area of diminished signal intensity in the corpus striatum due to the susceptibility effect produced by the iron oxide nanoparticles. (*C*) Axial gradient echo magnetic resonance image in a different animal than shown in **Figs. 2**A and B shows a linear region of diminished signal intensity, reflecting reflux of iron oxide nanoparticles along the path of the delivery catheter and into the ventricular system, (rather than delivery into the corpus striatum), indicating inefficient delivery. (*D*) Sagittal gradient-echo magnetic resonance image of the same animal shown in **Fig. 2**C again shows a linear accumulation of diminished signal intensity reflecting reflux of the iron oxide nanoparticles along the path of the delivery catheter. (*Courtesy of* Yael Mardor, PhD, The Advanced Technology Center, Sheba Medical Center, Tel-Hashomer, Israel.)

Finally, gold nanoparticles can be designed for absorption of light in the near-infrared portion of the light spectrum. Consequently, pulsed or continuous wave lasers have been used to selectively heat the gold nanoparticles that have been delivered to tumors for thermal ablation.[25]

Quantum Dots

Quantum dots are semiconductor nanocrystals for which the bandgap energy (ie, the minimum energy to excite an electron above the ground state) is size-dependent; this feature endows quantum dots with unique optical and electronic properties.[26,27] Quantum dots are composed of a metallic core and outer shell, which are necessary to provide the optical properties of a semiconductor. The cores commonly are comprised of cadmium sulfide, cadmium selenide, or cadmium

telluride.[28] To preserve the strong fluorescence emission of quantum dots, shells of wider bandgap energy (eg, zinc sulfide) are grown on the core; this shell provides electrical insulation and resistance to oxidation.[29] The size, chemical composition, and interaction between core and shell can be fine-tuned to produce highly specific optical properties, such as precisely defined emission wavelengths that allow the specific type of nanoparticle to be identified.[28] This feature allows different types of nanoparticles, each targeted against a different biomarker, to be used and discriminated from one another, which is a process termed multiplexed imaging. Quantum dots are commonly synthesized in high-temperature organic solvents that provide a surface of hydrophobic ligands. For use in biologically relevant environments, quantum dots are rendered water-soluble by several methods. Two such methods are (1) ligand exchange in a polar organic solvent

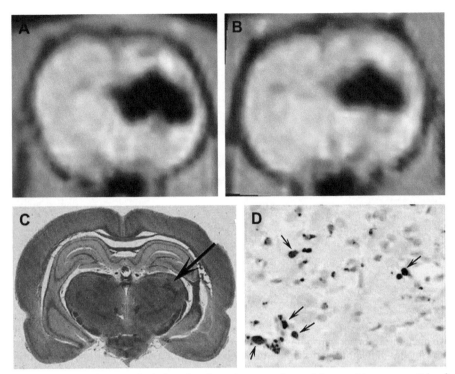

Fig. 3. Magnetic resonance images depicting the slow clearance time of iron oxide nanoparticles from brain. (*A*) Axial gradient-echo magnetic resonance images of a rat 1 day after CED of iron oxide nanoparticles shows region of diminished signal conforming to presence of nanoparticles. (*B*) Axial gradient-echo magnetic resonance images of same rat as shown in Fig. 3A performed 23 days after CED show retention of a large proportion of nanoparticles delivered weeks before. (*C*) Following extraction of brain tissue, slide of brain tissue using Prussian blue staining for iron shows iron staining at site of nanoparticle deposition (*arrow*). (*D*) Microscopic slide of brain tissue using Prussian blue staining shows residual nanoparticles either in or adjacent to the cells (*arrows*). (*Courtesy of* Yael Mardor, PhD, The Advanced Technology Center, Sheba Medical Center, Tel-Hashomer, Israel.)

followed by dialysis[30] and (2) micelle-like encapsulation of amphiphilic lipids or polymers.[31,32] For specific binding of quantum dots to different biologic targets (ie, biomarkers), quantum dots are often conjugated to targeting ligands in a final synthetic step.[33,34]

The optical properties of quantum dots are characterized by broad absorbance spectra and bright, stable fluorescence emission with a narrow emission spectra.[27] The broad absorption band allows for multiple excitation wavelengths to excite a single quantum dot and a single excitation source to excite many distinct colors of quantum dots (unlike organic dyes that have a relatively narrow absorbance band and can thus be excited solely by a single source). The narrow emission spectra of quantum dots are significant, because they allow different colors of quantum dots to be readily separated by physical filtering and computational techniques. Therefore, a single excitation source can illuminate many emission wavelengths (colors) of quantum dots. This property, combined with their brightness and enhanced photostability

(ie, continued brightness after exposure to excitation sources) renders quantum dots an ideal candidate for multiplexed imaging.[33] The increased photostability of quantum dots also makes them ideal candidates for live cell imaging; the prolonged exposure to an excitation source needed for imaging of living cells does not extinguish the bright signal emanating from quantum dots during an experiment.

Because quantum dots are composed of heavy metals, potential toxicity issues arise. If quantum dots are found to be toxic, their use in vivo will be greatly limited. Recent efforts from several groups have focused on developing biocompatible quantum dots. One approach is to minimize the length of exposure time in the body by development of quantum dots having a size small enough to guarantee rapid renal clearance; it is estimated that a size of less than 5 nm would be necessary.[35,36] A second, but equally challenging, approach to increase biocompatibility is to remove many of the heavy metals while retaining semiconductor optical properties. Several groups have worked on cadmium-free or cadmium-minimized quantum dots.[37,38]

APPLICATIONS OF NANOTECHNOLOGY IN THE IMAGING AND THERAPY OF BRAIN TUMORS
Targeted Delivery of Nanoparticles to Brain Tumors

Targeted delivery provides a means of providing more effective delivery of nanoparticles to brain tumors (whether for imaging or therapeutic purposes). Numerous methods have been developed for targeting, usually via application of antibodies (directed against tumor-related antigens) to the surface of nanoparticles. In addition to antibodies, examples of other tumor-targeting agents include peptides (eg, chlorotoxin), ferromagnetic agents, and cytokines.[39]

Nanoparticles for Drug Delivery

Another highly promising application of nanoparticles for treating brain tumors is delivery of chemotherapy. Advantages of nanoparticles in this setting include the potential for highly localized deposition of chemotherapy within the tumor as opposed to systemic delivery using standard chemotherapy formulations. For instance, even intravenous administration of such nanoparticles might provide a means of specific delivery of the agent if targeted nanoparticles solely or primarily were deposited within tumor. Nanoparticles offer several advantages along these lines (eg, the potential for incorporating relatively large amounts of chemotherapy into nanoparticles as well as for delivery of hydrophobic substances that might normally have very limited access to brain tumors because of the blood–brain barrier [BBB]).[40] By avoiding delivery of chemotherapy to nontarget organs outside the central nervous system (CNS), toxic effects might be minimized, and higher doses delivered to the tumor might be possible.

Impediments Posed by the BBB

Nanoparticle-based delivery of therapeutic agents offers a potential means to overcome the impediments provided by the BBB. The BBB serves to effectively exclude some small lipophilic molecules (depending on their physical properties), large lipophilic molecules (except for the few that are actively transported across the BBB), and most polar or ionized water-soluble molecules.[41] Additional barriers to transport exist in the form of membrane efflux pumps that actively transport molecules back into the vascular compartment (ie, the p-glycoprotein) and the pumps referred to

as the multidrug-resistance-associated protein (MRP) family.[41]

Two major means of delivering nanoparticle-mediated therapy are evident. The first, conventional, method is administration from a site outside the BBB (eg, oral or intravenous administration). Access across the BBB, however, is a formidable issue. As previously noted, a major issue faced in use of chemotherapy for treatment of brain tumors is inability of many agents to cross the BBB due to chemical composition and active processes that serve to transport molecules back into the intravascular compartment. Nonetheless, nanoparticles can be adapted to overcome the hurdles produced by the BBB. For instance, nanoparticles can be modulated to inhibit the p-glycoprotein drug efflux system and thus potentiate the effect of chemotherapy.[42] In addition, nanoparticles can be used to more effectively transport chemotherapy; sequestration of chemotherapeutic drugs within nanoparticles can slow the rate of drug degradation compared with freely circulating drug within the vascular compartment.[43]

Delivery of Chemotherapy-bearing Nanoparticles via Intravenous Infusion

Another application of superparamagnetic nanoparticles is targeted therapy of tumors. For such applications, various methods have been used to specifically target nanoparticles against brain tumor membrane receptors or proteins. As an example, investigators have developed nanoparticles that are targeted against membrane-bound matrix metalloproteinase-2 by coating the nanoparticles with chlorotoxin.[14] This modification of the nanoparticle allows tumors of neuroectodermal origin to be targeted. Such targeted nanoparticles reportedly have a very high rate of delivery to tumor compared with the same nanoparticles that lack the targeting mechanism of chlorotoxin.

Nanoparticles for Intraoperative Imaging

IO nanoparticles were among the first nanoscale imaging agents developed for brain tumor imaging. The introduction of these agents into the human clinical brain tumor environment has been rapid; they even have been successfully used for intraoperative imaging.[15] These nanoparticles are paramagnetic in nature and produce increased signal intensity on T1-weighted magnetic resonance images. They appear to accumulate in macrophages and reactive astrocytes within tumors and can be detected on MRI for a period of days after intravenous infusion. The accumulation within macrophages and astrocytes may allow for better delineation of tumor margins than allowable by imaging agents that solely depend upon leakage from the vascular pool (eg, conventional gadolinium-based contrast agents).[39] Initial studies using intraoperative MRI to guide resection of brain tumors in patients to whom such nanoparticles have been administered have proven promising.[15]

CED of Chemotherapy-bearing Nanoparticles

CED is a means to bypass the BBB by infusing materials directly into brain. By means of an indwelling catheter, therapeutic drug can be infused directly into native tumor, into tissues adjacent to native tumor, or into a postoperative cavity following partial resection of tumor. Following drug infusion, fluid pressure gradients induce drug distribution into interstitial spaces of the tumor.[44]

CED appears to be a promising method for delivering nanoparticles carrying chemotherapeutic drugs (see **Figs. 1–3**). Encapsulation of chemotherapy within nanoparticles, such as liposomes, allows for sustained release of the drug, enhances prolongation of drug half-life, and thus increases exposure of tumor cells to drug (see **Fig. 1**).[45] In a small animal model, pegylated liposomes containing chemotherapy have been used to successfully treat brain tumors (see **Fig. 1**).[46] Dual function nanoparticles containing both an MRI agent (eg, gadodiamide) and a chemotherapeutic agent also have been developed, which allow monitoring of drug distribution while also treating tumors. For instance, magnetic nanoparticles have been developed that can be used for CED delivery of drug while at the same time having MRI properties that allow transit of the nanoparticles (and, thereby, delivery of drug) to be monitored.[47] Studies using a liposome containing both gadodiamide and the chemotherapeutic agent topotecan additionally have been performed; these studies have shown increased drug delivery and increased median overall survival in rats bearing brain tumor xenografts.[48]

SUMMARY

This review has provided an introduction to some of the major forms of nanoparticles that have potential use for brain tumor imaging and therapy. The field of application of nanotechnology to medicine is a rapidly developing one. At this point in time, it appears highly likely that nanotechnology will play an important role in assessment and treatment of brain tumors, although the specific means by which this will be done remains to be determined.

REFERENCES

1. Ferrari M. Cancer nanotechnology: opportunities and challenges. Nat Rev Cancer 2005;5(3):161–71.
2. Alivisatos P. The use of nanocrystals in biological detection. Nat Biotechnol 2004;22(1):47–52.
3. Torchilin VP. Multifunctional nanocarriers. Adv Drug Deliv Rev 2006;58(14):1532–55.
4. Ruiz MA, Clares B, Morales ME, et al. Vesicular lipidic systems, liposomes, plo, and liposomes-plo: characterization by electronic transmission microscopy. Drug Dev Ind Pharm 2008;34(12):1269–76.
5. Torchilin VP. Peg-based micelles as carriers of contrast agents for different imaging modalities. Adv Drug Deliv Rev 2002;54(2):235–52.
6. Torchilin VP. Polymeric contrast agents for medical imaging. Curr Pharm Biotechnol 2000;1(2):183–215.
7. James ND, Coker RJ, Tomlinson D, et al. Liposomal doxorubicin (doxil): an effective new treatment for kaposi's sarcoma in aids. Clin Oncol (R Coll Radiol) 1994;6(5):294–6.
8. Torchilin VP. Recent advances with liposomes as pharmaceutical carriers. Nat Rev Drug Discov 2005;4(2):145–60.
9. Liu L, Venkatraman SS, Yang YY, et al. Polymeric micelles anchored with tat for delivery of antibiotics across the blood-brain barrier. Biopolymers 2008; 90(5):617–23.
10. Sethuraman VA, Lee MC, Bae YH. A biodegradable ph-sensitive micelle system for targeting acidic solid tumors. Pharm Res 2008;25(3):657–66.
11. Laurent S, Forge D, Port M, et al. Magnetic iron oxide nanoparticles: synthesis, stabilization, vectorization, physicochemical characterizations, and biological applications. Chem Rev 2008;108(6): 2064–110.
12. Sahoo Y, Goodarzi A, Swihart MT, et al. Aqueous ferrofluid of magnetite nanoparticles: fluorescence labeling and magnetophoretic control. J Phys Chem B 2005;109(9):3879–85.
13. Liu Q, Xu Z, Finch JA, et al. A novel two-step silica-coating process for engineering magnetic nanocomposites. Chem Mater 1998;10(12):3936–40.
14. Sun C, Veiseh O, Gunn J, et al. In vivo MRI detection of gliomas by chlorotoxin-conjugated superparamagnetic nanoprobes. Small 2008;4(3):372–9.
15. Neuwelt EA, Varallyay P, Bago AG, et al. Imaging of iron oxide nanoparticles by MR and light microscopy in patients with malignant brain tumours. Neuropathol Appl Neurobiol 2004;30(5):456–71.
16. Wang YX, Hussain SM, Krestin GP. Superparamagnetic iron oxide contrast agents: physicochemical characteristics and applications in MR imaging. Eur Radiol 2001;11(11):2319–31.
17. Ghosh P, Han G, De M, et al. Gold nanoparticles in delivery applications. Adv Drug Deliv Rev 2008; 60(11):1307–15.

18. Dixit V, Van den Bossche J, Sherman DM, et al. Synthesis and grafting of thioctic acid-peg-folate conjugates onto au nanoparticles for selective targeting of folate receptor-positive tumor cells. Bioconjug Chem 2006;17(3):603–9.

19. Paciotti GF, Myer L, Weinreich D, et al. Colloidal gold: a novel nanoparticle vector for tumor directed drug delivery. Drug Deliv 2004;11(3):169–83.

20. Daniel MC, Astruc D. Gold nanoparticles: assembly, supramolecular chemistry, quantum-size-related properties, and applications toward biology, catalysis, and nanotechnology. Chem Rev 2004;104(1):293–346.

21. Elghanian R, Storhoff JJ, Mucic RC, et al. Selective colorimetric detection of polynucleotides based on the distance-dependent optical properties of gold nanoparticles. Science 1997;277(5329):1078–81.

22. Nie S, Emory SR. Probing single molecules and single nanoparticles by surface-enhanced raman scattering. Science 1997;275(5303):1102–6.

23. Cao YC, Jin R, Mirkin CA. Nanoparticles with raman spectroscopic fingerprints for DNA and RNA detection. Science 2002;297(5586):1536–40.

24. Qian X, Peng XH, Ansari DO, et al. In vivo tumor targeting and spectroscopic detection with surface-enhanced raman nanoparticle tags. Nat Biotechnol 2008;26(1):83–90.

25. Huang X, El-Sayed IH, Qian W, et al. Cancer cell imaging and photothermal therapy in the near-infrared region by using gold nanorods. J Am Chem Soc 2006;128(6):2115–20.

26. Bruchez M Jr, Moronne M, Gin P, et al. Semiconductor nanocrystals as fluorescent biological labels. Science 1998;281(5385):2013–6.

27. Smith AM, Duan H, Mohs AM, et al. Bioconjugated quantum dots for in vivo molecular and cellular imaging. Adv Drug Deliv Rev 2008;60(11):1226–40.

28. Murray CB, Norris DJ, Bawendi MG. Synthesis and characterization of nearly monodisperse cde (e = sulfur, selenium, tellurium) semiconductor nanocrystallites. J Am Chem Soc 1993;115(19):8706–15.

29. Dabbousi BO, Rodriguez-Viejo J, Mikulec FV, et al. (CdSe)ZnS core–shell quantum dots: synthesis and characterization of a size series of highly luminescent nanocrystallites. J Phys Chem B 1997;101(46):9463–75.

30. Smith AM, Duan H, Rhyner MN, et al. A systematic examination of surface coatings on the optical and chemical properties of semiconductor quantum dots. Phys Chem Chem Phys 2006;8:3895–903.

31. Dubertret B, Skourides P, Norris DJ, et al. In vivo imaging of quantum dots encapsulated in phospholipid micelles. Science 2002;298(5599):1759–62.

32. Gao X, Cui Y, Levenson RM, et al. In vivo cancer targeting and imaging with semiconductor quantum dots. Nat Biotechnol 2004;22(8):969–76.

33. Xing Y, Chaudry Q, Shen C, et al. Bioconjugated quantum dots for multiplexed and quantitative immunohistochemistry. Nat Protoc 2007;2(5):1152–65.

34. Wu X, Liu H, Liu J, et al. Immunofluorescent labeling of cancer marker her2 and other cellular targets with semiconductor quantum dots. Nat Biotechnol 2003;21(1):41–6.

35. Choi HS, Liu W, Misra P, et al. Renal clearance of quantum dots. Nat Biotechnol 2007;25(10):1165–70.

36. Smith AM, Nie S. Minimizing the hydrodynamic size of quantum dots with multifunctional multidentate polymer ligands. J Am Chem Soc 2008;130(34):11278–9.

37. Pradhan N, Battaglia DM, Liu Y, et al. Efficient, stable, small, and water-soluble doped znse nanocrystal emitters as noncadmium biomedical labels. Nano Lett 2007;7(2):312–7.

38. Smith AM, Mohs AM, Nie S. Tuning the optical and electronic properties of colloidal nanocrystals by lattice strain. Nat Nanotechnol 2009;4(1):56–63.

39. Orringer DA, Koo YE, Chen T, et al. Small solutions for big problems: the application of nanoparticles to brain tumor diagnosis and therapy. Clin Pharmacol Ther 2009;85(5):531–4.

40. Gelperina S, Kisich K, Iseman MD, et al. The potential advantages of nanoparticle drug delivery systems in chemotherapy of tuberculosis. Am J Respir Crit Care Med 2005;172(12):1487–90.

41. Bart J, Groen HJ, Hendrikse NH, et al. The blood–brain barrier and oncology: new insights into function and modulation. Cancer Treat Rev 2000;26(6):449–62.

42. Chavanpatil MD, Khdair A, Gerard B, et al. Surfactant–polymer nanoparticles overcome p-glycoprotein-mediated drug efflux. Mol Pharm 2007;4(5):730–8.

43. Brioschi A, Zenga F, Zara GP, et al. Solid lipid nanoparticles: could they help to improve the efficacy of pharmacologic treatments for brain tumors? Neurol Res 2007;29(3):324–30.

44. Sampson JH, Raghavan R, Provenzale JM, et al. Induction of hyperintense signal on T2-weighted MR images correlates with infusion distribution from intracerebral convection-enhanced delivery of a tumor-targeted cytotoxin. AJR Am J Roentgenol 2007;188(3):703–9.

45. Moog R, Burger AM, Brandl M, et al. Change in pharmacokinetic and pharmacodynamic behavior of gemcitabine in human tumor xenografts upon entrapment in vesicular phospholipid gels. Cancer Chemother Pharmacol 2002;49(5):356–66.

46. Saito R, Krauze MT, Noble CO, et al. Convection-enhanced delivery of ls-tpt enables an effective, continuous, low-dose chemotherapy against malignant glioma xenograft model. Neuro Oncol 2006;8(3):205–14.

47. Perlstein B, Ram Z, Daniels D, et al. Convection-enhanced delivery of maghemite nanoparticles: Increased efficacy and MRI monitoring. Neuro Oncol 2008;10(2):153–61.

48. Grahn AY, Bankiewicz KS, Dugich-Djordjevic M, et al. Non-pegylated liposomes for convection-enhanced delivery of topotecan and gadodiamide in malignant glioma: initial experience. J Neurooncol 2009;95(2):185–97.

49. Peng XH, Qian X, Mao H, et al. Targeted magnetic iron oxide nanoparticles for tumor imaging and therapy. Int J Nanomedicine 2008;3(3):311–21.

Imaging of Brain Tumors: MR Spectroscopy and Metabolic Imaging

Alena Horská, PhD[a], Peter B. Barker, DPhil[a,b],*

KEYWORDS

- Brain tumors • Magnetic resonance spectroscopy
- Spectroscopic imaging • Metabolites

Localized proton magnetic resonance spectroscopy (MRS) of the human brain, first reported more than 20 years ago,[1–3] is a mature methodology that is used clinically in many medical centers worldwide for the evaluation of brain tumors.[4] Although there have been studies of human brain tumors using heteronuclei such as phosphorus (^{31}P) and sodium (^{11}Na),[5,6] by far the most spectroscopy studies use the proton (^{1}H) nucleus because of its high sensitivity and ease of implementation on commercial MR imaging scanners. This article will focus on proton MRS in human brain tumors.

There are two classes of spatial localization techniques for MRS. Single-voxel (SV) techniques record spectra from one region of the brain at a time (commonly used methods include the "point resolved spectroscopy sequence" [PRESS][7] and the "stimulated echo acquisition mode" [STEAM][8] sequences). Multivoxel techniques such as MRS imaging (MRSI)—also called "chemical shift imaging"[9]—simultaneously record spectra from multiple regions and thereby map out the spatial distribution of metabolites within the brain. MRSI is typically performed in 2- or 3-dimensions, but does not usually include full brain coverage. While SV-MRS and MRSI each have their own advantages and disadvantages (eg, in terms of spectral quality, scan time, spatial resolution, spatial coverage, and ease of use or interpretation), a key consideration for brain tumors is their metabolic inhomogeneity. For instance, the spectrum from the necrotic core of a high-grade brain tumor is quite different from a spectrum from the actively growing rim, whereas peritumoral edema is different from tumor invasion into surrounding brain tissue. For these reasons and others, high-resolution MRSI is often favored for evaluating brain tumor metabolism.[10]

Early in the development of human brain proton MRS, it was realized that brain tumors exhibited markedly different spectra from normal brain tissue.[4,11] It was found that nearly all brain tumors have decreased N-acetyl aspartate (NAA) signals, and often have increased levels of choline (Cho), leading to increased Cho/NAA ratios. The decrease in NAA is widely interpreted as the loss, dysfunction, or displacement of normal neuronal tissue because NAA is believed to be primarily of neuronal and axonal origin.[12] The Cho signal actually contains contributions from several different Cho-containing compounds, which are involved in membrane synthesis and degradation. It has been suggested that it is increased in brain tumors owing to increased membrane turnover. In vitro studies have indicated

Supported in part by National Institutes of Health grant P41 RR015241.

[a] Russell H. Morgan Department of Radiology and Radiological Science, Johns Hopkins University School of Medicine, 600 North Wolfe Street, Baltimore, MD 21287, USA

[b] Kennedy Krieger Institute, 707 North Broadway, Baltimore, MD 21205, USA

* Corresponding author. Russell H. Morgan Department of Radiology and Radiological Science, Johns Hopkins University School of Medicine, 600 North Wolfe Street, Baltimore, MD 21287.

E-mail address: pbarker2@jhmi.edu

that the elevated Cho signal in brain tumors is due to increased levels of phosphocholine. Cho has also been found to correlate well with the cellular density of the tumor[13] and the degree of tumor infiltration into brain tissue.[14] The use of MRSI to map Cho levels has therefore been suggested as a method for defining tumor boundaries in treatment planning (see later discussion).

Other relatively common metabolic changes in human brain tumors are elevated signals in the lactate and lipid region of the spectrum,[15] and sometimes increased levels of myo-inositol (ml) in short echo time (TE) spectra.[16,17] The increase in lactate is most likely the result of anaerobic glycolysis[5,15,18]; although it could be due to insufficient blood flow leading to ischemia or, possibly, to necrosis. The observation of elevated lipid levels is believed to be associated with necrosis and membrane breakdown.[19–21] Increased levels of ml are believed to reflect increased numbers of glial cells, which have been reported to contain high levels of ml and, in particular, have been reported to be high in grade II gliomas.[16] It has also been reported that patients with gliomatosis cerebri may exhibit elevated inositol levels, even in the absence of increased Cho.[22] Examples of brain tumor spectra are given in Figs. 1 and 2.

TUMOR CLASSIFICATION

Early in the development of MRS of brain tumors, a commonly asked question was whether or not MRS could help to noninvasively diagnose tumor type and grade because this would have an influence on management decisions and prognosis. While MR imaging is without doubt the most sensitive modality available for the detection of brain tumors, its specificity is low, and several different tumor types (as well as lesions with other causes) may share a similar MR imaging appearance. Two particularly important imaging diagnoses are the differentiation between high-grade and low-grade tumors, or between neoplastic and nonneoplastic lesions (see later discussion), respectively. High-grade brain tumors are usually treated more aggressively than low-grade tumors, and so preoperative diagnosis of tumor grade is important for this reason.

In astrocytomas, several studies, but not all, have suggested an association between tumor grade and Cho levels, with the higher grade tumors having greater Cho concentrations.[10,23,24] This would appear consistent with the more aggressive tumors having higher membrane turnover and cellular density. However, some studies

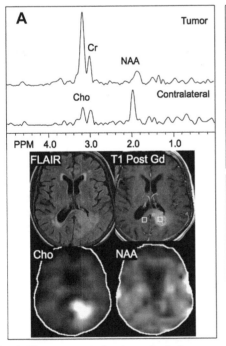
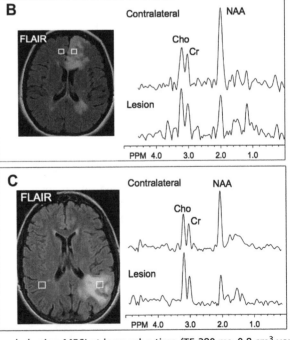

Fig. 1. Three untreated, primary brain tumors recorded using MRSI at long echo time (TE 280 ms, 0.8 cm³ voxel size, 1.5T). (A) GBM involving the left side of the corpus callosum has a large increase in Cho and decrease in NAA compared with the contralateral side. (B) Left frontal WHO grade II oligodendroglioma shows reduced NAA compared with the contralateral side and minimal increase in Cho. (C) Left parietal primary central nervous system lymphoma shows increased Cho and decreased NAA compared with the contralateral hemisphere.

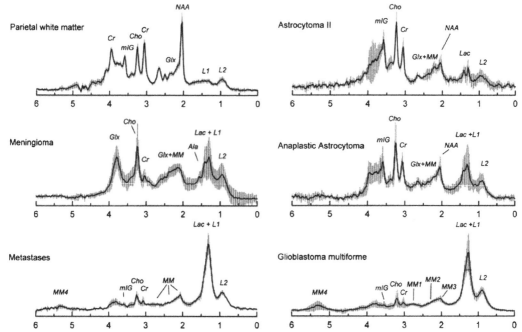

Fig. 2. Group average spectra from normal parietal white matter (n = 6), astrocytoma grade II (n = 5), meningioma (n = 8), anaplastic astrocytoma (grade III) (n = 7), metastases (n = 6), and GBM (grade IV, n = 13) recorded at 1.5T using SV spectroscopy (STEAM, TE = 30 ms, 4–8 cm³ voxel size). All lesions have reduced NAA and also lower creatine (Cr) than normal white matter. Spectra from the necrotic core of metastases and GBM show reduced levels of all metabolites and elevated lipids (in contrast to the GBM spectrum in **Fig. 1** which was non-necrotic). Grade II and III astrocytomas show elevated Cho and lactate signals; grade II astrocytomas also have a prominent mI signal. A signal from alanine (Ala) is assigned in the meningioma spectra. Glx, glutamine plus glutamate; L, lipid; Lac, lactate; mIG, myo-inositol plus; MM, macromolecules. (*Reproduced from* Howe FA, Barton SJ, Cudlip SA, et al. Metabolic profiles of human brain tumors using quantitative in vivo 1H magnetic resonance spectroscopy. Magn Reson Med 2003;49(2):223–32; with permission.)

have found high-grade tumors (eg, grade IV glioblastoma multiforme [GBM]) to have lower levels of Cho than grade II or grade III astrocytoma.[19] This may be due to the presence of necrosis in high-grade tumors, particularly those with necrotic cores, because necrosis is associated with low levels of all metabolites.[25] Since tumors are commonly heterogenous, with necrotic cores, proliferative rims, and invasion of surrounding brain tissue, the spectrum may vary greatly depending on the region that is sampled by MRS (**Fig. 3**).[26] Hence, the region-of-interest chosen for analysis has a large influence on the results and MRSI is generally considered preferable because it allows metabolic heterogeneity to be evaluated and the voxel with the maximum Cho signal to be chosen for analysis.[27] One recent MRSI study used MR perfusion imaging (arterial spin labeling) to guide the spectral measurement location. In regions with elevated flow, Cho (as well as glutamate plus glutamine [Glx] and lactate plus lipid) was found to be higher in high-grade

compared with low-grade gliomas.[28] No metabolic differences between high-grade and low-grade gliomas were found in normal or hypoperfused tumor regions.

Using sophisticated analysis schemes or pattern-recognition techniques, several groups have been able to use proton MRS or MRSI to accurately diagnose different types of neoplasia.[29–32] However, because of lesion variability, heterogeneity, overlap between different tumor types, and dependence on data collection and analysis techniques, these results have proven difficult to replicate in general clinical practice. In most cases, therefore, it is very difficult for a clinician to use MRS alone to diagnose a brain lesion with high confidence. Rather, MRS should perhaps be seen as an adjunct technique that may contribute to differential diagnoses that are being considered on the basis of MR imaging, clinical and other information. For instance, as depicted in **Figs. 1** and **2**, high Cho levels are typically seen in nonnecrotic high-grade brain

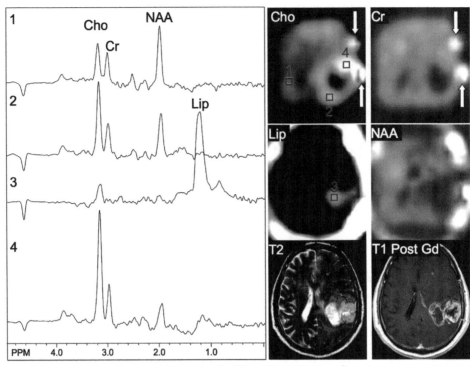

Fig. 3. MRSI (PRESS: TR/TE=1200/135 ms; 24×24 matrix; FOV=200×200x15 mm³) and conventional MR imaging in a 56-year-old man who had chemotherapy after partial surgical resection of a GBM in the left temporal and inferior parietal lobe. The enhancing rim of the lesion is characterized by a high Cho signal (regions 2 and 4), while the central necrotic core (region 3) has elevated lipids and reduced levels of other metabolites. NAA is reduced in all T2-hyperintense regions, including the core and enhancing rim. The bright rim outside the brain in the Lip and NAA images arises from lipid signals in the scalp. Arrows in the Cr and Cho images point to field-inhomogeneity artifact due to surgical staples. Region 1 shows the normal spectrum from the right hemisphere. Lip, Lipid; Post Gd, post-gadolinium contrast agent; PPM, parts per million. (*Data provided courtesy of* Dr Alberto Bizzi, Istituto Neurologica Carlo Besta, Milan, Italy.)

tumors (eg, anaplastic astrocytoma, GBM, primary CNS lymphoma, whereas necrotic GBM and metastases are characterized by low levels of all metabolites and increased lipids). Meningiomas are usually readily diagnosed based on conventional imaging features, but the diagnosis may be additionally confirmed by the presence of a signal from alanine (a doublet centered on ~ 1.47 ppm), which has been reported to be elevated in many meningiomas.[33]

For discriminating solitary metastases from primary brain tumors, it has been suggested that investigation of perienhancing tumor regions may be useful. Whereas gliomas are often invasive lesions that show elevated Cho in surrounding tissue, metastatic lesions tend to be more encapsulated and do not typically show high Cho signals or other abnormalities outside the region of enhancement.[34,35] Metastatic lesions and glioblastomas nearly always show elevated lipid peaks; thus, if the lesion does not exhibit mobile lipid signals, anaplastic glioma is more likely.[36]

TUMORS VERSUS NONNEOPLASTIC LESIONS

If a lesion can be confidently diagnosed as nonneoplastic, an invasive brain biopsy procedure may be avoided and a different treatment course, depending on the cause of the lesion, may be considered. Examples of nonneoplastic lesions that may mimic brain tumors on conventional imaging are infectious (including abscess) or ischemic lesions, or demyelinating lesions (eg, tumefactive demyelination). Differentiation between tumors and nonneoplastic lesions using conventional MR imaging may be challenging. Whereas MR imaging is a sensitive technique for detection of brain lesions, the specificity and capability of conventional MR imaging for distinguishing between benign and malignant lesions is limited.

Low-grade gliomas and many nonneoplastic lesions, such as early stage lesions or diffusely infiltrating lesions, may not exhibit a mass effect. Low-grade gliomas may present as small T_2 hyperintense lesions that may be difficult to differentiate from focal cortical dysplasias or other pathologies.[37] The use of a contrast agent may also not increase diagnostic specificity because various nonneoplastic processes are often associated with disruption of the blood-brain barrier and not all tumors enhance.[38]

Since tumors typically exhibit elevated Cho and decreased NAA, the greatest benefit of adding MRS to a clinical examination may be in including (or excluding) diagnoses with markedly different spectroscopic patterns (eg, strokes or focal cortical dysplasias, neither of which are expected to have increased Cho). Conversely, differentiation between tumors and acute demyelinating lesions based on MRS alone may be difficult as both entities typically present with elevated Cho and decreased NAA, as well as often increased lactate.[39] A combination of conventional MR imaging with modern techniques of physiologic imaging—in particular, perfusion MR imaging—can therefore improve the classification.

Several studies have evaluated the utility of ^{1}H MRS to differentiate between tumors and non-neoplastic lesions[40–44] or have compared spectroscopic characteristics of specific groups of neoplastic and nonneoplastic lesions.[45–47] Two recent retrospective studies evaluated the value of MRSI[38] and SV-MRS[48] to differentiate between brain tumors and nonneoplastic lesions. In the ^{1}H MRSI study performed at a TE of 280ms, 84% of 69 brain lesions (36 tumors) were correctly classified using the ratios NAA/Cho, NAA/creatine (Cr), and Cho and NAA signal areas normalized to signal areas in a control region.[38] There were five cases of tumors misclassified as nonneoplastic lesions: (1) anaplastic astrocytoma, World Health Organization (WHO) grade II; (2) infiltrating astrocytoma, WHO grade III; (3) gliomatosis cerebri, WHO grade II; (4) oligodendroglioma, WHO grade II; and (5) ganglioglioma, WHO grade II. Six nonneoplastic lesions were classified as tumors. The diagnoses included demyelination, radiation necrosis, postsurgical gliosis, and stable lesions not confirmed on pathologic examination. In a subgroup of 32 lesions, perfusion MR imaging also showed significant differences between high-grade and low-grade tumors, and between high-grade tumors and nonneoplastic lesions. By combining both MRSI and perfusion MR imaging, a sensitivity

of 72.2% and specificity of 91.7% in differentiating tumors from nonneoplastic lesions was achieved with cutoff points of NAA/Cho less than or equal to 0.61 and relative cerebral blood volume (rCBV) greater than or equal to 1.50 corresponding to tumor diagnosis.[38] Examples of benign and malignant lesions from this study are shown in **Figs. 4** and **5**. In an SV-MRS study of 84 solid brain masses performed at a short TE (30 ms) and long TE (136 ms), presence of tumor was indicated when mI/NAA ratio (obtained at short TE) was greater than 0.9 and when Cho/NAA ratio (obtained at the long TE) was greater than 1.9.[48] In this study, the group of tumors was represented by gliomas of WHO grade II and III.[48] In a retrospective study of 32 children with primary brain lesions (19 tumors, 13 benign lesions), 78% of originally grouped cases could be correctly classified based on the Cho/Cr ratio.[10]

Typical imaging features of the most common intracranial masses in adults—including primary neoplasms (high-grade and low-grade), secondary (metastatic) neoplasms, lymphoma, tumefactive demyelinating lesions, abscesses, and encephalitis— on perfusion MR imaging, diffusion MR imaging, and proton MR spectroscopy (and examples of individual cases) were summarized in a recent review.[49] The role of commonly used advanced imaging techniques in differentiation among intracranial masses in adults was retrospectively evaluated[49,50] and the accuracy of MR imaging-based strategy to differentiate among histologically confirmed lesions was assessed.[50] A practical MRI-based algorithm, including results from postcontrast MR imaging, diffusion-weighted MR imaging, perfusion MR imaging, and ^{1}H MRSI was proposed to improve the diagnosis and classification of these lesions (**Fig. 6**).[50] The diagnostic strategy was evaluated based on 40 patients who had complete data from all included imaging modalities; to differentiate between tumors and nonneoplastic lesions, the accuracy, sensitivity, and specificity of the classification strategy was 90%, 97%, and 67%.[49,50] These results suggest that integration of advanced imaging techniques with conventional MR imaging may help to improve the reliability of the diagnosis and classification of brain lesions.[51]

Generally, spectra from brain abscesses are quite different from those of high-grade neoplasia—they usually have low Cho signals, as well as decreased NAA and Cr, and often also exhibit increased signals from compounds that are not typically seen in neoplasia (eg, alanine, acetate, acetoacetate, succinate) in variable amounts depending on the source of the primary

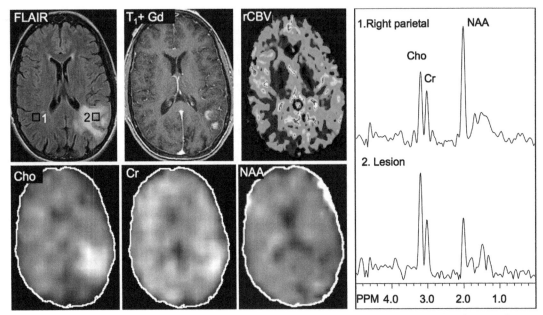

Fig. 4. Example of MR imaging (fluid-attenuated inversion recovery [FLAIR], and T1-weighted post-Gd), MRSI (Cho, Cr and NAA, 1.5T, TE 280 msec) and MR perfusion imaging (rCBV) in a 38-year-old female with left parietal primary CNS lymphoma. This malignant, contrast-enhancing lesion shows both elevated rCBV and Cho, as well as reduced NAA. (*Adapted from* Hourani R, Brant LJ, Rizk T, et al. Can proton MR spectroscopic and perfusion imaging differentiate between neoplastic and nonneoplastic brain lesions in adults? AJNR Am J Neuroradiol 2008;29(2):366–72; with permission.)

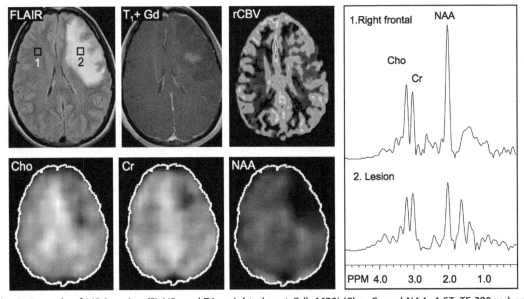

Fig. 5. Example of MR imaging (FLAIR, and T1-weighted post-Gd), MRSI (Cho, Cr and NAA, 1.5T, TE 280 ms) and MR perfusion imaging (rCBV) in a 27-year-old female with left frontal meningoencephalitis. This nonneoplastic, contrast-enhancing lesion shows decreased levels of all metabolites (Cho, Cr, and NAA) suggestive of loss of cellularity and edema. Lesion rCBV is decreased cortically but appears mildly increased in the subcortical white matter. (*Adapted from* Hourani R, Brant LJ, Rizk T, et al. Can proton MR spectroscopic and perfusion imaging differentiate between neoplastic and nonneoplastic brain lesions in adults? AJNR Am J Neuroradiol 2008;29(2):366–72; with permission.)

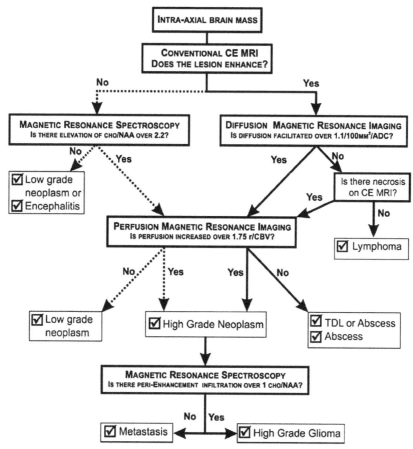

Fig. 6. A flow-chart for determining brain lesion type based on conventional contrast-enhanced MR imaging, diffusion-weighted MR imaging, MR spectroscopy, and MR perfusion imaging; $1.1/100MM^2/ADC = 1.1 \times 10^{-3}$ mm²/sec. ADC, apparent diffusion coefficient; CE, contrast material enhanced; TDL, tumefactive demyelinating lesion. (*Adapted from* Al-Okaili RN, Krejza J, Woo JH, et al. Intraaxial brain masses: MR imaging-based diagnostic strategy—initial experience. Radiology 2007;243(2):539–50; with permission.)

infectious process.[52,53] Therefore, the distinction between abscess and neoplasm should be straightforward using MRS, which may add confidence to the diagnosis made by other techniques (eg, diffusion-weighted imaging[54]).

PREDICTION OF SURVIVAL

Long-term prognosis for patients with high-grade gliomas is poor despite aggressive treatment strategies. Nevertheless, survival time can be quite variable, and is important information for patients and their families. The ability of MRS to predict survival has been evaluated in both adult and pediatric brain tumor populations. A series of papers have evaluated the role of ¹H MRSI in prediction of survival of GBM patients.[55–58] In a recent study, conventional MR imaging, and ¹H MRSI, diffusion, and perfusion MR imaging were used in a group of

grade IV glioma patients (examined before surgery and treatment). Kaplan-Meier survival curves were generated and Cox proportional hazards model was applied to evaluate the utility of selected parameters on patients' survival.[56] Survival was relatively poor in patients with lesions exhibiting large areas of contrast enhancement, abnormal metabolism, or restricted diffusion. Specifically, of the parameters involving tissue volumes, high relative volumes (in the T_2 hyperintense lesion) of (1) combined contrast enhancement and necrosis areas, (2) the region with abnormal (elevated) Cho/NAA index, and (3) the region with apparent diffusion coefficient (ADC) less than 1.5 times of the ADC in normal-appearing white matter were negatively associated with survival. Survival time was also negatively associated with high lactate and lipid levels, and the ADC within the enhancing volume. None of the evaluated perfusion parameters was predictive of survival.[56] In another study, ^{1}H MRSI was applied with MRSI, as well as conventional, diffusion, and perfusion MR imaging in 68 GBM patients with a median age of 58 years, examined after surgery, but before administration of adjuvant radiation treatment and chemotherapy.[55] In this case, all evaluated MR imaging measures, including volume of increased CBV on perfusion MR imaging, were related to survival. As in the previous study, high Cho/NAA ratios and the combined lactate and lipid signal were associated with a higher risk of poor outcome.[55]

In other studies, an inverse relationship between Cho/Cr ratio and survival time was detected in seven patients with gliomatosis cerebri, examined before treatment.[59] A prospective longitudinal study examined 14 patients with high-grade gliomas before radiation treatment, at week 4 of radiation treatment, and 2 months posttreatment.[60] Several spectroscopic indices were associated with unfavorable survival (including lactate [Lac]/NAA at week 4 and the change in normalized Cho/Cr between baseline and the first follow-up). The most significant was a more than 40% decrease in normalized Cho between the first and second follow-up visits in the contrast-enhancing region.[60] However, no spectra were presented in this paper, making it difficult to judge the quality of the primary data that these conclusions were based on. In a retrospective ^{1}H MRSI study (performed at long TE; data collected before treatment) of 51 histopathologically verified cases of supratentorial gliomas, four MRSI indices (maximum value of Cho/Cr, maximum value of Lac/Cr, total number of voxels with NAA/Cr values less than two-thirds of the mean value from the normal appearing contralateral region, and the number of voxels with Lac/Cr ratios ≥ 1) measured in the area of abnormal MR imaging signal were significant predictors of survival.[61] Multivariate analysis of spectra of 21 patients with brain metastases differentiated between patients surviving 5 months and patients with a shorter survival.[62]

However, not all studies have found associations between metabolic indices and prognosis; for instance, in 16 patients with a B-cell lymphoma, presence of Lac and lipids in the spectra collected before treatment was not associated with overall survival.[63] In another prospective ^{1}H MRS study, 50 patients with newly diagnosed low-grade gliomas (WHO grade II) evaluated before surgery showed no relationship between Cho and Cr levels in the tumor and survival.[64]

Several studies have also examined the prognostic value of spectroscopy in pediatric brain tumors. In a ^{1}H MRSI study of 76 children with brain tumors, a low value (<1.8) of an index including Cho and lactate and lipid levels, normalized to contralateral Cr, was found to be a strong predictor of survival.[65] In another study of children with recurrent gliomas, a high Cho/NAA ratio was associated with decreased survival.[66]

TREATMENT PLANNING

Accurate, noninvasive diagnosis in glioma patients is important, as the prognosis and therapeutic plan (including surgery, if any) is often based on the histopathological grade of the tumor.[67,68] Proton MRSI and other physiologic imaging techniques may assist the surgeon in obtaining representative samples of the tumor tissue for histology and surgical resection, by identifying regions of active tumor. As described above, MRSI provides information on tumor heterogeneity, including distinguishing normal tissue, infiltrating tumor, and vasogenic edema.[68] This information is also of great potential value in planning targeted radiotherapy, as well as to help differentiate residual or recurrent tumor from radiation necrosis on follow-up (see discussion below). Multimodality MR imaging, including MRSI, may potentially provide information that may aid in stratifying patients into high- or low-risk groups for clinical trials, and in selecting optimal treatment for individual patients.[56]

MRSI Integration in Multimodality Imaging

Proton MRSI may be readily integrated into a multimodality MR imaging examination for presurgical evaluation of patients with gliomas.[68,69] In one study of 143 newly diagnosed glioma patients, MRSI, and conventional, perfusion, and diffusion MR imaging were performed before any treatment had begun.[69] Analysis of the results suggested that this multimodality approach, with appropriate analysis techniques, could accurately identify tumors of different grade, and hence be used to guide treatment choices.[69]

In another study, multimodality 3T MR imaging (including long TE MRSI) was performed in 31 patients with either high- or low-grade glioma.[68] Using linear discriminant analysis, patterns associated with tumor tissue, edema, and tumor-infiltrated edema in perienhancing regions with abnormal signal on conventional MR imaging, and a pattern of infiltration in perienhancing tissue with normal MR imaging appearance were presented. To differentiate among the patterns in perienhancing regions of high-grade gliomas, the best discrimination was achieved when all MR imaging parameters were used (ie, normalized Cho and NAA, ADC, and rCBV). The regions presumed to be a tumor, had normalized Cho less than 1.3 and Cho/NAA ratio less than 1, and lower ADC and higher rCBV than vasogenic edema. Presumed vasogenic edema had normal Cho/NAA ratio (<1). Presumed tumor-infiltrated edema had Cho levels similar to or lower than normal values, with abnormal Cho/NAA ratio, higher ADC, and lower rCBV than regions defined as tumors, and lower ADC and higher rCBV than vasogenic edema regions. Perienhancing regions with normal appearance were classified as presumed tumor-infiltrated regions (with normalized Cho >1.3 or Cho/NAA ratio >1) or presumably normal regions (with close to normal metabolite levels). Low- and high-grade tumors could be separated based on all examined MR parameters, except ADC. In low-grade tumors, normalized Cho was significantly lower in the tumor margins, normalized NAA higher in the tumor mass and the margins, normalized Cr higher in the tumor mass, and rCBV lower both in the mass and tumor margins. In contrast to high-grade gliomas, spectra of low-grade gliomas did not show an elevated lactate-lipid signal. High- and low-grade tumors and their margins could be differentiated based on the lactate-lipid signal and rCBV. The classification was based only on MR imaging-related parameters as no histologic correlations were performed in the study.[68]

Identification of Active Tumor and Tumor Invasion

The primary therapeutic goal in neuro-oncology is complete removal of the tumor; therefore, it is essential to know the exact tumor borders.[70] However, in high-grade gliomas, the tumor boundaries and the degree of infiltration are difficult to define due to their diffuse growth pattern. By evaluating metabolic abnormalities, proton MRS can also enhance the diagnostic yield of stereotactic brain biopsy, which is usually performed based on anatomic appearance of the lesion or enhancement characteristics.[71] Brain biopsy carries multiple risks, such as bleeding or infection. In high-grade heterogeneous tumors, there is a possibility that an unspecific or lower-grade tumor tissue is sampled or that important functional tracts are damaged. Ideally, regions of increased angiogenesis, vascular permeability and high metabolic activity should be sampled.[72] The role of proton MRS in biopsy guidance is to recognize regions of high metabolic activity: regions of elevated Cho levels (and low NAA levels) indicative of tumor tissue, represent a good target for biopsy.[12,67,71,73–75] Regions with low Cho and

NAA levels may indicate radiation necrosis, astrogliosis, macrophage infiltration, or mixed tissue.[73]

In one study, biopsy samples were obtained in 26 patients from the target tissue identified on MRSI and the utility of MRSI in guiding biopsy was evaluated.[71] In 17 out of 21 patients, who had confirmed neoplasm, Cho was elevated; however, low Cho levels (similar to those observed in necrotic regions) were observed in four patients with tumors. In all patients with necrosis, Cho levels were low.[71] In nine patients with T_2-hyperintense lesions without contrast enhancement suggestive of low-grade glioma on conventional MR imaging, ^1H MRSI was performed presurgically and the area of the highest Cho intensity (or, if not apparent, area from the center of the lesion) was chosen as a biopsy target using a frameless stereotactic system.[67] MRSI correctly classified all four histologically confirmed gliomas WHO grade III and four out of five WHO grade II gliomas.

To assess the degree of tumor infiltration, MRSI data obtained in seven patients with untreated supratentorial gliomas (WHO grades II and III) were fused with 3D-MR imaging data sets and integrated into a frameless stereotactic system for image-guided surgery, in an interactive manner.[76] Tissue samples were obtained from three regions, defined individually in each patient based on the Cho/NAA ratio: (1) spectroscopically normal region, (2) transitional region, and (3) region with maximum spectroscopical abnormality. The biopsy coordinates were labeled in the 3D-MR imaging dataset and metabolic maps for later correlations to histopathology. In all cases, the highest Cho/NAA ratios were obtained in the tumor center, and intermediate values in the regions of low tumor invasion. However, in four subjects, biopsies sampled in regions with normal Cho/NAA ratio showed tumor infiltration. One of the reasons may be low resolution of MRSI with respect to glioma borders.[76] A retrospective study performed in 10 glioma patients, examined the relationship between metabolite levels and histopathologic parameters in the border zone of gliomas.[77] A strong negative correlation was detected between NAA concentration and both absolute and relative measures of tumor infiltration; no correlation for Cho was detected. The study concluded that NAA concentration is the most significant parameter for the detection of low levels of tumor cell infiltration.[77]

Improvement in tissue classification and visualization of tumor spread may be achieved by using methods of pattern recognition.[78–80] A recent MRSI study in patients with gliomas applied independent component analyses to segment the tumor core (cystic and necrotic tissue), infiltrative growth, and normal brain tissue.[80] Diffusion indices (fractional anisotropy and mean diffusivity) were also computed and compared for MRSI voxels in the three evaluated tissue groups. It was concluded that MRSI and diffusion tensor imaging can provide markers of infiltrative tumor growth and that the combination of these two techniques may improve delineation of tumor invasion.

Delineation of the Target Volume for Radiation Therapy

Radiation therapy was the first adjuvant treatment for brain tumors.[81] The aim of localized radiation therapy is to maximize the therapeutic dose to the tumor while delivering minimal doses to surrounding normal tissue.[81] Radiation therapy planning for management of gliomas requires optimization of the radiation doses, time of radiation, and choice of treatment technique, depending on the characteristics of different glioma subtypes.[82] Patients with high-grade gliomas receive high dose to the areas of active tumor (gross total volume, defined based on MR imaging- or CT-contrast enhancement) while the regions suspicious for tumor infiltration (clinical target volumes) are treated with lower doses.[83,84] However, MR imaging metrics such as contrast enhancement or T2-hyperintensity may not reliably identify regions of active tumor or the extent of the tumor.[85] In fact, in many cases they may be associated with necrosis or edema, not active tumor. Therefore, there is a strong rationale for incorporating other modalities, such as ^{1}H MRSI, into the planning process, which may provide more specific information about the location of active tumor growth.[84]

The potential of ^{1}H MRSI to improve the accuracy of target volumes definition based on metabolic information was evaluated in 34 patients with WHO grades II to IV gliomas.[83] Comparison of the extent (and location) of active tumor as defined by MR imaging and MRSI demonstrated differences between the two techniques.[83] This report and later studies documented that the area of metabolic abnormality as defined by MRSI may exceed the area of abnormal T2-weighted signal.[76,83,86] Furthermore, a study in 26 patients with WHO grade IV gliomas treated with gamma knife surgery showed that patients in who the volume of metabolically active lesion defined by ^{1}H MRSI was mostly within the radiosurgically treated volume had a longer survival time than patients with a lesser overlap.[58]

MONITORING OF THERAPY AND POSTTHERAPY EVALUATION
Radiation Therapy

In 3% to 24% of glioma patients receiving adjuvant radiotherapy, radiation necrosis—a focal reaction to radiation—is identified. Typical MR imaging appearance of radiation necrosis is a T_2-hyperintense signal and T_1-enhancement after contrast administration, which is difficult to distinguish from tumor progression or pseudoprogression (a transient increase in edema, mass effect, and contrast enhancement that resolves over time).[87] In glioma patients, clinical MR imaging is typically performed at predetermined intervals, for instance every 3 months after completion of chemotherapy, or 6 weeks, 3 months, 6 months, and 12 months after radio- or chemotherapy in high-grade gliomas. However, early evaluation and prediction of tumor response based on physiologic and functional tumor parameters may be a more beneficial strategy. Availability of surrogate markers that could differentiate between therapy-related necrosis and tumor recurrence would help to decide early in the course of therapy whether the treatment scheme should be continued, adapted, or changed completely.[70] The role of MRSI in assessment of the effect of radiation on the tumor and normal-appearing brain tissue was reviewed recently.[88]

Proton MRS has been applied to differentiate between radiation-induced tissue injury and tumor recurrence in adult and pediatric brain tumor patients postradiation, after gamma knife radiosurgery, and brachytherapy. Increased Cho signal (evaluated as Cho levels relative to Cho signal in normal-appearing tissue, Cho/Cr or Cho/NAA ratios) are suggestive of recurrence, while significantly reduced Cho (and Cr) levels are suggestive of radiation necrosis.[25,89–91] Fig. 7 shows an example of MRSI in a patient with a large right hemisphere astrocytoma treated with radiation. For the most part, the spectra exhibit low metabolite signals consistent with necrosis; however, spread of the tumor (high Cho) is also apparent through the splenium of the corpus callosum into the contralateral hemisphere. Necrotic regions may also show elevated lipid and lactate signals.[92–94] A recent retrospective MRSI study in 31 patients with a previous diagnosis of an intracranial tumor reported a sensitivity of 85%, a specificity of 69% to differentiate between recurrent tumor and radiation necrosis using the Cho/NAA ratio.[95] Comparison with biopsy specimens revealed that MRSI cannot reliably differentiate between tissue containing mixed tumor-radiation necrosis

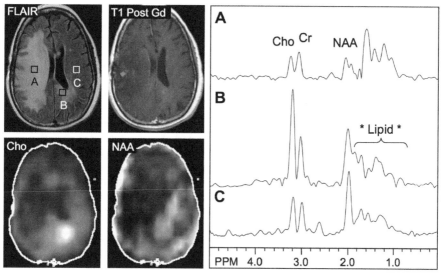

Fig. 7. MR imaging (FLAIR, T1, post-Gd) and MRSI (Cho, NAA) in a 53-year-old female with a right frontal anaplastic astrocytoma previously treated with surgery and radiation. The T2 hyperintense large right hemisphere lesion is characterized by reduced levels of all metabolites (A), consistent with radiation necrosis, while high Cho is observed in the splenium of the corpus callosum crossing into the left hemisphere, consistent with tumor growth (B). A spectrum from a normal-appearing region in the left hemisphere is shown in (C) for comparison. Note that the lipids seen in (A–C) most likely artifacts resulting from head motion during the scan, and also affect the reconstructed NAA image. Small nodules of contrast enhancement are seen in the right hemisphere and the left side of the corpus callosum. The MRSI results were in good accordance with an fluorodeoxyglucose (FDG)-positron emission tomography scan performed contemporaneously.

and either tumor or radiation necrosis, although it did achieve good separation between pure necrosis and pure tumor.[92]

Adding ADC values to MRSI parameters did not improve differentiation between mixed tissue and pure tumor or pure necrosis[96] but did improve differentiation between pure tumor and radiation necrosis (which exhibits higher ADC values than tumors).[96,97] The diagnostic accuracy of MRS in differentiating between radiation necrosis may be improved if spectra of both the abnormal and normal tissue are available pre- and posttreatment.[93] If the spectrum is indeterminate (ie, indicating presence of both residual tumor and radiation change), repeated examination is suggested after an interval of 6 to 8 weeks.[93]

On conventional MR imaging, the evaluation of treatment response and the categorization as stable disease, responder (partial remission) and nonresponder (progression) are usually based predominantly on changes in tumor volumes.[70] Potentially, MRSI may be able to distinguish metabolic changes in the tumor before any change in volume. Following radiotherapy or gamma knife radiosurgery, reduction in Cho may indicate partial remission, while no change or increase in Cho is suggestive of progression.[84,98,99] In a longitudinal study evaluating glioma patients before radiation treatment and up to 2 to 3 months postradiation,

shrinkage of tumor in 6 out of 11 patients was accompanied by a decrease in Cho signal in four patients and increase in Cho in two patients.[100] Disappearance of lactate in three patients was associated with decrease in Cho and in tumor diameter; no changes in NAA were observed.[100] MRSI was able to differentiate patients with stable disease and patients with disease progression (malignant degeneration of a low-grade tumor or tumor recurrence) in a group of 27 patients with grade I to IV gliomas treated with combinations of surgery, chemotherapy, and radiation therapy.[101] The patients were examined at least twice, with a between-studies interval of 8.3 plus or minus 5.1 months, at 49 plus or minus 41 months after time of disease onset. In patients with stable disease (assessed as unchanged clinical status since previous examination), the changes in normalized Cho intensity were smaller than a critical value of 35% (range 33% to 28%). In patients with progressive disease, the between-studies changes in normalized Cho were larger than 45% (range 46%–104%). MRSI categorization also demonstrated an excellent agreement with survival data.[101]

MRSI has also been applied to predict onset of new contrast enhancement on MR imaging after therapy. A prospective clinical trial including patients with GBM sought to compare locations of

MRSI abnormality (Cho/NAA ≥ 2, at TR/TE = 1000/ 135 ms) at baseline with location of new contrast enhancement and abnormal MRSI after treatment with radiation and chemotherapy.[102] At relapse, 82% of the 17 voxels with Cho/NAA greater than or equal to 2 at baseline exhibited either continuing or new contrast enhancement (as compared with 15% of 323 voxels with normal Cho/NAA ratio). The study also showed that combining MRSI and postcontrast T_1 and T_2-weighted MR imaging may better predict regions of relapse after treatment than MR imaging alone.[102]

Finally, radiotherapy planning involves a careful balance between maximizing dose to the tumor while limiting radiotoxicity to surrounding normal brain tissue. Radiation injury may be acute, short term, or long term. Long-term injury is particularly an issue in radiotherapy of children, where radiation may have long-term deleterious effects on the developing brain.[88] MRS has been shown the ability to detect effects of radiation on normal brain, and may have some role in monitoring injury to normal brain tissue. The most commonly reported changes following radiation are decreases in NAA,[103] which can be detected 1 to 4 months after radiation in nontumoral regions receiving between 20 to 50 Gy[104] and decreases in Cho levels.[88]

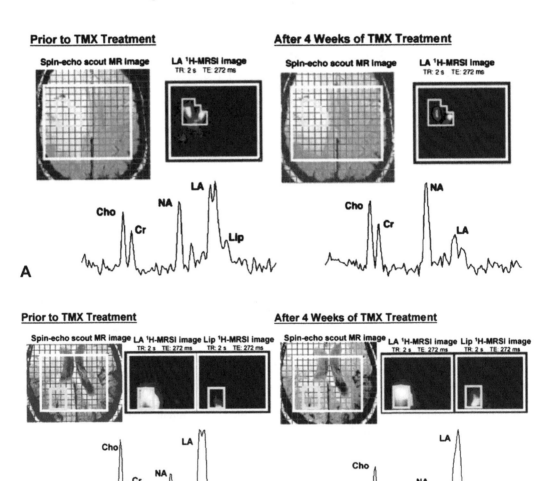

Fig. 8. T2-weighted MR imaging and MRSI in two cases with recurrent glioma before and after response to tamoxifen (TMX) therapy. (*A*) Case A, a recurrent astrocytoma, shows a large decrease in lactate in the lesion at 1 month, which corresponded to a clinical improvement in the patient, while other metabolites (Cho, Cr, NAA) are largely unchanged. (*B*) Case B, a recurrent GBM, did not respond the therapy and had symptom progression. The spectrum after 4 weeks of TMX is similar (in particular unchanged lactate levels) to that pretreatment. LA, lactate; Lip, lipid; NA, N-acetyl compound; TR, repetition time. (*Adapted from* Preul MC, Caramanos Z, Villemure JG, et al. Using proton magnetic resonance spectroscopic imaging to predict in vivo the response of recurrent malignant gliomas to tamoxifen chemotherapy. Neurosurgery 2000;46(2):306–18; with permission.)

Chemotherapy

In patients with gliomas, chemotherapy is often used as the initial treatment after histologic diagnosis in combination with radiation therapy, or at recurrence after surgery and radiation therapy.[105] In patients treated with chemotherapy, proton MRS may provide data on functional response on tumor chemosensitivity to potentially allow for early treatment modification and to avoid unnecessary toxicity.[106] In malignant glioma patients, survival time is short in the absence of effective treatment; therefore, the ability to evaluate chemosensitivity early in the course of treatment would represent a significant advancement in chemotherapy planning.[107]

In an early study of MRSI monitoring of chemotherapy, 16 patients treated with high-dose tamoxifen for recurrent malignant glioma were evaluated with proton MRSI before and during treatment. Starting at week 4 into the tamoxifen therapy, responders had a significantly lower tumor volume and higher Karnofsky score. Using linear discriminant analyses, responders (seven patients) and nonresponders could be differentiated based on five metabolite ratios (Cho, Cr, NAA, lactate, lipids in the tumor—relative to contralateral Cr) obtained before treatment, and at 2 and 4 weeks into treatment. No time-related differences in Cho, Cr, and NAA ratios were detected between responders and nonresponders; however, lactate and lipid ratios decreased over time in responders (**Fig. 8**).[107] In another study, patients with oligodendroglial tumors and anaplastic astrocytomas, increases in the lactate/Cr ratio (in the contrast-enhancing region) and in the Cho/Cr ratio (in regions adjacent to nonenhancing tumor) during treatment, and low baseline NAA/Cr ratio in regions adjacent to nonenhancing tumor, correlated with decreases in progression-free survival time.[108] Fourteen patients included in this retrospective pilot MRSI study were treated with procarbazine, CCNU, and vincristine (the follow-up intervals were 42–146 days); 10 patients also had a previous radiotherapy.[108]

SV spectroscopy has also been applied to assess response to temozolomide treatment in 12 patients with low-grade gliomas.[109] The patients were examined before treatment, and at 3, 6, 9, and 12 months follow-up intervals. Over the course of the treatment, the decrease in Cho signal (normalized to water) paralleled the decrease in tumor volume (ie, metabolite changes did not precede volumetric changes).[109] Reduction in tumor volume and in Cho/Cr ratio (and normalized Cho intensity) was also reported in a WHO grade II astrocytoma patient with tumor recurrence, 3 months after chemotherapy.[110] A preliminary longitudinal study in three patients with GBM also suggested that MRSI is a feasible technique to detect metabolic response in individual patients to treatment with BCNU chemotherapy wafers.[111] Collectively these papers indicate the potential for MRSI to monitor the effects of chemotherapy on brain tumors, although individually they are all small studies. They also highlight the importance (as with MR imaging) of performing serial MRSI scans to monitor changes in metabolite levels over time, rather than looking at a single time point to judge treatment response.

SUMMARY

In using MRS for application to brain tumors, the limited spatial resolution (usually 1 cm^3 or less for MRSI and $\sim$ 4 to 8 cm^3 for SV MRS) and partial volume effects should be kept in mind. For example, in treatment planning, MRSI pixel whose "point-spread function" overlaps both tumor and normal tissue has the potential to be misclassified as tumor invasion into surrounding brain if this issue is neglected. For this reason, use of high as possible spatial resolution is recommended.[76] High-resolution MRSI with good signal-to-noise ratios is best performed using high magnetic field strengths and multichannel phased-array coils, and efficient pulse sequences. Multislice or 3D MRSI techniques that provide full lesion coverage, as well as include surrounding and contralateral brain regions, are also very important.[112] Unfortunately, many previous human brain tumor MRSI studies have used PRESS-based techniques that do not always fulfill these criteria.

Whereas the utility of MRS in diagnosis and evaluation of treatment response to brain tumors has been widely documented, MRS has not been widely accepted as a routine clinical tool. Robust and automated procedures are needed to collect the data, analyze the spectra and display the results in a timely fashion. Standardization across sites and different vendors of acquisition and analysis techniques is also important. Finally, carefully designed, multicenter trials complying with criteria of evidence-based medicine have not yet been completed, and as a result MRS is only relatively occasionally used for tumor evaluation outside of major academic medical centers.[113]

REFERENCES

1. Bottomley PA, Edelstein WA, Foster TH, et al. In vivo solvent-suppressed localized hydrogen

nuclear magnetic resonance spectroscopy: a window to metabolism? Proc Natl Acad Sci U S A 1985;82(7):2148–52.

2. Hanstock CC, Rothman DL, Prichard JW, et al. Spatially localized 1H NMR spectra of metabolites in the human brain. Proc Natl Acad Sci U S A 1988;85(6):1821–5.

3. Frahm J, Bruhn H, Gyngell ML, et al. Localized high-resolution proton NMR spectroscopy using stimulated echoes: initial applications to human brain in vivo. Magn Reson Med 1989;9(1):79–93.

4. Bruhn H, Frahm J, Gyngell ML, et al. Noninvasive differentiation of tumors with use of localized H-1 MR spectroscopy in vivo: initial experience in patients with cerebral tumors. Radiology 1989; 172(2):541–8.

5. Barker PB, Glickson JD, Bryan RN. In vivo magnetic resonance spectroscopy of human brain tumors. Top Magn Reson Imaging 1993;5(1):32–45.

6. Ouwerkerk R, Bleich KB, Gillen JS, et al. Tissue sodium concentration in human brain tumors as measured with 23Na MR imaging. Radiology 2003;227(2):529–37.

7. Bottomley PA. Spatial localization in NMR spectroscopy in vivo. Ann N Y Acad Sci 1987;508: 333–48.

8. Frahm J. Localized proton spectroscopy using stimulated echoes. J Magn Reson 1987;72(3):502–8.

9. Brown TR, Kincaid BM, Ugurbil K. NMR chemical shift imaging in three dimensions. Proc Natl Acad Sci U S A 1982;79(11):3523–6.

10. Hourani R, Horska A, Albayram S, et al. Proton magnetic resonance spectroscopic imaging to differentiate between nonneoplastic lesions and brain tumors in children. J Magn Reson Imaging 2006;23(2):99–107.

11. Langkowski JH, Wieland J, Bomsdorf H, et al. Preoperative localized in vivo proton spectroscopy in cerebral tumors at 4.0 Tesla—first results. Magn Reson Imaging 1989;7(5):547–55.

12. Barker PB. N-acetyl aspartate—a neuronal marker? Ann Neurol 2001;49(4):423–4.

13. Gupta RK, Cloughesy TF, Sinha U, et al. Relationships between choline magnetic resonance spectroscopy, apparent diffusion coefficient and quantitative histopathology in human glioma. J Neurooncol 2000;50(3):215–26.

14. Croteau D, Scarpace L, Hearshen D, et al. Correlation between magnetic resonance spectroscopy imaging and image-guided biopsies: semiquantitative and qualitative histopathological analyses of patients with untreated glioma. Neurosurgery 2001;49(4):823–9.

15. Herholz K, Heindel W, Luyten PR, et al. In vivo imaging of glucose consumption and lactate concentration in human gliomas. Ann Neurol 1992;31(3):319–27.

16. Castillo M, Smith JK, Kwock L. Correlation of myo-inositol levels and grading of cerebral astrocytomas. AJNR Am J Neuroradiol 2000;21(9): 1645–9.

17. Hattingen E, Raab P, Franz K, et al. Myo-inositol: a marker of reactive astrogliosis in glial tumors? NMR Biomed 2008;21(3):233–41.

18. Alger JR, Frank JA, Bizzi A, et al. Metabolism of human gliomas: assessment with H-1 MR spectroscopy and F-18 fluorodeoxyglucose PET. Radiology 1990;177(3):633–41.

19. Howe FA, Barton SJ, Cudlip SA, et al. Metabolic profiles of human brain tumors using quantitative in vivo 1H magnetic resonance spectroscopy. Magn Reson Med 2003;49(2):223–32.

20. Kuesel AC, Sutherland GR, Halliday W, et al. 1H MRS of high grade astrocytomas: mobile lipid accumulation in necrotic tissue. NMR Biomed 1994;7(3):149–55.

21. Di Costanzo A, Scarabino T, Trojsi F, et al. Proton MR spectroscopy of cerebral gliomas at 3 T: spatial heterogeneity, and tumour grade and extent. Eur Radiol 2008;18(8):1727–35.

22. Saraf-Lavi E, Bowen BC, Pattany PM, et al. Proton MR spectroscopy of gliomatosis cerebri: case report of elevated myoinositol with normal choline levels. AJNR Am J Neuroradiol 2003;24(5):946–51.

23. Arnold DL, Shoubridge EA, Villemure JG, et al. Proton and phosphorus magnetic resonance spectroscopy of human astrocytomas in vivo. Preliminary observations on tumor grading. NMR Biomed 1990;3(4):184–9.

24. Gill SS, Thomas DG, Van Bruggen N, et al. Proton MR spectroscopy of intracranial tumours: in vivo and in vitro studies. J Comput Assist Tomogr 1990;14(4):497–504.

25. Preul MC, Leblanc R, Caramanos Z, et al. Magnetic resonance spectroscopy guided brain tumor resection: differentiation between recurrent glioma and radiation change in two diagnostically difficult cases. Can J Neurol Sci 1998;25(1):13–22.

26. Ricci PE, Pitt A, Keller PJ, et al. Effect of voxel position on single-voxel MR spectroscopy findings. AJNR Am J Neuroradiol 2000;21(2):367–74.

27. Senft C, Hattingen E, Pilatus U, et al. Diagnostic value of proton magnetic resonance spectroscopy in the noninvasive grading of solid gliomas: comparison of maximum and mean choline values. Neurosurgery 2009;65(5):908–13 [discussion: 913].

28. Chawla S, Wang S, Wolf RL, et al. Arterial spin-labeling and MR spectroscopy in the differentiation of gliomas. AJNR Am J Neuroradiol 2007;28(9):1683–9.

29. Preul MC, Caramanos Z, Collins DL, et al. Accurate, noninvasive diagnosis of human brain tumors by using proton magnetic resonance spectroscopy. Nat Med 1996;2(3):323–5.

30. Tate AR, Griffiths JR, Martinez-Perez I, et al. Towards a method for automated classification of 1H MRS spectra from brain tumours. NMR Biomed 1998;11(4-5):177–91.

31. De Edelenyi FS, Rubin C, Esteve F, et al. A new approach for analyzing proton magnetic resonance spectroscopic images of brain tumors: nosologic images. Nat Med 2000;6(11):1287–9.

32. Tate AR, Majos C, Moreno A, et al. Automated classification of short echo time in in vivo 1H brain tumor spectra: a multicenter study. Magn Reson Med 2003;49(1):29–36.

33. Demir MK, Iplikcioglu AC, Dincer A, et al. Single voxel proton MR spectroscopy findings of typical and atypical intracranial meningiomas. Eur J Radiol 2006;60(1):48–55.

34. Fan G, Sun B, Wu Z, et al. In vivo single-voxel proton MR spectroscopy in the differentiation of high-grade gliomas and solitary metastases. Clin Radiol 2004;59(1):77–85.

35. Chiang IC, Kuo YT, Lu CY, et al. Distinction between high-grade gliomas and solitary metastases using peritumoral 3-T magnetic resonance spectroscopy, diffusion, and perfusion imagings. Neuroradiology 2004;46(8):619–27.

36. Ishimaru H, Morikawa M, Iwanaga S, et al. Differentiation between high-grade glioma and metastatic brain tumor using single-voxel proton MR spectroscopy. Eur Radiol 2001;11(9):1784–91.

37. Omuro AM, Leite CC, Mokhtari K, et al. Pitfalls in the diagnosis of brain tumours. Lancet Neurol 2006;5(11):937–48.

38. Hourani R, Brant LJ, Rizk T, et al. Can proton MR spectroscopic and perfusion imaging differentiate between neoplastic and nonneoplastic brain lesions in adults? AJNR Am J Neuroradiol 2008; 29(2):366–72.

39. Saindane AM, Cha S, Law M, et al. Proton MR spectroscopy of tumefactive demyelinating lesions. AJNR Am J Neuroradiol 2002;23(8):1378–86.

40. Butzen J, Prost R, Chetty V, et al. Discrimination between neoplastic and nonneoplastic brain lesions by use of proton MR spectroscopy: the limits of accuracy with a logistic regression model. AJNR Am J Neuroradiol 2000;21(7):1213–9.

41. Moller-Hartmann W, Herminghaus S, Krings T, et al. Clinical application of proton magnetic resonance spectroscopy in the diagnosis of intracranial mass lesions. Neuroradiology 2002;44(5): 371–81.

42. Poptani H, Gupta RK, Roy R, et al. Characterization of intracranial mass lesions with in vivo proton MR spectroscopy. AJNR Am J Neuroradiol 1995; 16(8):1593–603.

43. Poptani H, Kaartinen J, Gupta RK, et al. Diagnostic assessment of brain tumours and non-neoplastic brain disorders in vivo using proton nuclear magnetic resonance spectroscopy and artificial neural networks. J Cancer Res Clin Oncol 1999; 125(6):343–9.

44. Rand SD, Prost R, Haughton V, et al. Accuracy of single-voxel proton MR spectroscopy in distinguishing neoplastic from nonneoplastic brain lesions. AJNR Am J Neuroradiol 1997;18(9): 1695–704.

45. De Stefano N, Caramanos Z, Preul MC, et al. In vivo differentiation of astrocytic brain tumors and isolated demyelinating lesions of the type seen in multiple sclerosis using 1H magnetic resonance spectroscopic imaging. Ann Neurol 1998;44(2): 273–8.

46. Venkatesh SK, Gupta RK, Pal L, et al. Spectroscopic increase in choline signal is a nonspecific marker for differentiation of infective/inflammatory from neoplastic lesions of the brain. J Magn Reson Imaging 2001;14(1):8–15.

47. Vuori K, Kankaanranta L, Hakkinen AM, et al. Low-grade gliomas and focal cortical developmental malformations: differentiation with proton MR spectroscopy. Radiology 2004;230(3):703–8.

48. Majos C, Aguilera C, Alonso J, et al. Proton MR spectroscopy improves discrimination between tumor and pseudotumoral lesion in solid brain masses. AJNR Am J Neuroradiol 2009;30(3):544–51.

49. Al-Okaili RN, Krejza J, Wang S, et al. Advanced MR imaging techniques in the diagnosis of intraaxial brain tumors in adults. Radiographics 2006; 26(Suppl 1):S173–89.

50. Al-Okaili RN, Krejza J, Woo JH, et al. Intraaxial brain masses: MR imaging-based diagnostic strategy—initial experience. Radiology 2007; 243(2):539–50.

51. Law M, Hamburger M, Johnson G, et al. Differentiating surgical from non-surgical lesions using perfusion MR imaging and proton MR spectroscopic imaging. Technol Cancer Res Treat 2004; 3(6):557–65.

52. Remy C, Grand S, Lai ES, et al. 1H MRS of human brain abscesses in vivo and in vitro. Magn Reson Med 1995;34(4):508–14.

53. Garg M, Gupta RK. MR Spectroscopy in intracranial infection. In: Gillard JH, Waldman AD, Barker PB, editors. Clinical MR neuroimaging: diffusion, perfusion and spectroscopy. Cambridge (UK): Cambridge University Press; 2004. p. 380–406.

54. Desprechins B, Stadnik T, Koerts G, et al. Use of diffusion-weighted MR imaging in differential diagnosis between intracerebral necrotic tumors and cerebral abscesses. AJNR Am J Neuroradiol 1999;20(7):1252–7.

55. Saraswathy S, Crawford FW, Lamborn KR, et al. Evaluation of MR markers that predict survival in patients with newly diagnosed GBM prior to adjuvant therapy. J Neurooncol 2009;91(1):69–81.

56. Crawford FW, Khayal IS, McGue C, et al. Relationship of pre-surgery metabolic and physiological MR imaging parameters to survival for patients with untreated GBM. J Neurooncol 2009;91(3):337–51.

57. Arslanoglu A, Bonekamp D, Barker PB, et al. Quantitative proton MR spectroscopic imaging of the mesial temporal lobe. J Magn Reson Imaging 2004;20(5):772–8.

58. Chan AA, Lau A, Pirzkall A, et al. Proton magnetic resonance spectroscopy imaging in the evaluation of patients undergoing gamma knife surgery for Grade IV glioma. J Neurosurg 2004;101(3):467–75.

59. Guzman-de-Villoria JA, Sanchez-Gonzalez J, Munoz L, et al. 1H MR spectroscopy in the assessment of gliomatosis cerebri. AJR Am J Roentgenol 2007;188(3):710–4.

60. Alexander A, Murtha A, Abdulkarim B, et al. Prognostic significance of serial magnetic resonance spectroscopies over the course of radiation therapy for patients with malignant glioma. Clin Invest Med 2006;29(5):301–11.

61. Kuznetsov YE, Caramanos Z, Antel SB, et al. Proton magnetic resonance spectroscopic imaging can predict length of survival in patients with supratentorial gliomas. Neurosurgery 2003;53(3):565–74 [discussion: 574–6].

62. Sjobakk TE, Johansen R, Bathen TF, et al. Metabolic profiling of human brain metastases using in vivo proton MR spectroscopy at 3T. BMC Cancer 2007;7:141.

63. Raizer JJ, Koutcher JA, Abrey LE, et al. Proton magnetic resonance spectroscopy in immunocompetent patients with primary central nervous system lymphoma. J Neurooncol 2005;71(2):173–80.

64. Hattingen E, Raab P, Franz K, et al. Prognostic value of choline and creatine in WHO grade II gliomas. Neuroradiology 2008;50(9):759–67.

65. Marcus KJ, Astrakas LG, Zurakowski D, et al. Predicting survival of children with CNS tumors using proton magnetic resonance spectroscopic imaging biomarkers. Int J Oncol 2007;30(3):651–7.

66. Warren KE, Frank JA, Black JL, et al. Proton magnetic resonance spectroscopic imaging in children with recurrent primary brain tumors. J Clin Oncol 2000;18(5):1020–6.

67. Hermann EJ, Hattingen E, Krauss JK, et al. Stereotactic biopsy in gliomas guided by 3-tesla 1H-chemical-shift imaging of choline. Stereotact Funct Neurosurg 2008;86(5):300–7.

68. Di Costanzo A, Scarabino T, Trojsi F, et al. Multiparametric 3T MR approach to the assessment of cerebral gliomas: tumor extent and malignancy. Neuroradiology 2006;48(9):622–31.

69. Chang SM, Nelson S, Vandenberg S, et al. Integration of preoperative anatomic and metabolic physiologic imaging of newly diagnosed glioma. J Neurooncol 2009;92(3):401–15.

70. Weber MA, Giesel FL, Stieltjes B. MRI for identification of progression in brain tumors: from morphology to function. Expert Rev Neurother 2008;8(10):1507–25.

71. Martin AJ, Liu H, Hall WA, et al. Preliminary assessment of turbo spectroscopic imaging for targeting in brain biopsy. AJNR Am J Neuroradiol 2001;22(5):959–68.

72. Klingebiel R, Bohner G. Neuroimaging. Recent Results Cancer Res 2009;171:175–90.

73. Dowling C, Bollen AW, Noworolski SM, et al. Preoperative proton MR spectroscopic imaging of brain tumors: correlation with histopathologic analysis of resection specimens. AJNR Am J Neuroradiol 2001;22(4):604–12.

74. Hall WA, Martin A, Liu H, et al. Improving diagnostic yield in brain biopsy: coupling spectroscopic targeting with real-time needle placement. J Magn Reson Imaging 2001;13(1):12–5.

75. Hall WA, Galicich W, Bergman T, et al. 3-Tesla intraoperative MR imaging for neurosurgery. J Neurooncol 2006;77(3):297–303.

76. Ganslandt O, Stadlbauer A, Fahlbusch R, et al. Proton magnetic resonance spectroscopic imaging integrated into image-guided surgery: correlation to standard magnetic resonance imaging and tumor cell density. Neurosurgery 2005;56(Suppl 2):291–8 [discussion: 291–8].

77. Stadlbauer A, Nimsky C, Buslei R, et al. Proton magnetic resonance spectroscopic imaging in the border zone of gliomas: correlation of metabolic and histological changes at low tumor infiltration—initial results. Invest Radiol 2007;42(4):218–23.

78. Lee MC, Nelson SJ. Supervised pattern recognition for the prediction of contrast-enhancement appearance in brain tumors from multivariate magnetic resonance imaging and spectroscopy. Artif Intell Med 2008;43(1):61–74.

79. Menze BH, Kelm BM, Weber MA, et al. Mimicking the human expert: pattern recognition for an automated assessment of data quality in MR spectroscopic images. Magn Reson Med 2008;59(6):1457–66.

80. Wright AJ, Fellows G, Byrnes TJ, et al. Pattern recognition of MRSI data shows regions of glioma growth that agree with DTI markers of brain tumor infiltration. Magn Reson Med 2009;62(6):1646–51.

81. Robertson PL. Advances in treatment of pediatric brain tumors. NeuroRx 2006;3(2):276–91.

82. Combs SE. Radiation therapy. Recent Results Cancer Res 2009;171:125–40.

83. Pirzkall A, McKnight TR, Graves EE, et al. MR-spectroscopy guided target delineation for high-grade gliomas. Int J Radiat Oncol Biol Phys 2001;50(4):915–28.

84. Nelson SJ, Graves E, Pirzkall A, et al. In vivo molecular imaging for planning radiation therapy of gliomas: an application of 1H MRSI. J Magn Reson Imaging 2002;16(4):464–76.

85. Payne GS, Leach MO. Applications of magnetic resonance spectroscopy in radiotherapy treatment planning. Br J Radiol 2006;79(Spec No 1): S16–26.

86. McKnight TR, von dem Bussche MH, Vigneron DB, et al. Histopathological validation of a three-dimensional magnetic resonance spectroscopy index as a predictor of tumor presence. J Neurosurg 2002; 97(4):794–802.

87. Yang I, Aghi MK. New advances that enable identification of glioblastoma recurrence. Nat Rev Clin Oncol 2009;6(11):648–57.

88. Sundgren PC. MR spectroscopy in radiation injury. AJNR Am J Neuroradiol 2009;30(8):1469–76.

89. Taylor JS, Langston JW, Reddick WE, et al. Clinical value of proton magnetic resonance spectroscopy for differentiating recurrent or residual brain tumor from delayed cerebral necrosis. Int J Radiat Oncol Biol Phys 1996;36(5):1251–61.

90. Wald LL, Nelson SJ, Day MR, et al. Serial proton magnetic resonance spectroscopy imaging of glioblastoma multiforme after brachytherapy. J Neurosurg 1997;87(4):525–34.

91. Chernov MF, Hayashi M, Izawa M, et al. Multivoxel proton MRS for differentiation of radiation-induced necrosis and tumor recurrence after gamma knife radiosurgery for brain metastases. Brain Tumor Pathol 2006;23(1):19–27.

92. Rock JP, Hearshen D, Scarpace L, et al. Correlations between magnetic resonance spectroscopy and image-guided histopathology, with special attention to radiation necrosis. Neurosurgery 2002;51(4):912–9 [discussion: 919–20].

93. Law M. MR spectroscopy of brain tumors. Top Magn Reson Imaging 2004;15(5):291–313.

94. Li X, Vigneron DB, Cha S, et al. Relationship of MR-derived lactate, mobile lipids, and relative blood volume for gliomas in vivo. AJNR Am J Neuroradiol 2005;26(4):760–9.

95. Smith EA, Carlos RC, Junck LR, et al. Developing a clinical decision model: MR spectroscopy to differentiate between recurrent tumor and radiation change in patients with new contrast-enhancing lesions. AJR Am J Roentgenol 2009; 192(2):W45–52.

96. Rock JP, Scarpace L, Hearshen D, et al. Associations among magnetic resonance spectroscopy, apparent diffusion coefficients, and image-guided histopathology with special attention to radiation necrosis. Neurosurgery 2004;54(5):1111–7 [discussion: 1117–9].

97. Zeng QS, Li CF, Liu H, et al. Distinction between recurrent glioma and radiation injury using magnetic resonance spectroscopy in combination with diffusion-weighted imaging. Int J Radiat Oncol Biol Phys 2007;68(1):151–8.

98. Graves EE, Nelson SJ, Vigneron DB, et al. Serial proton MR spectroscopic imaging of recurrent malignant gliomas after gamma knife radiosurgery. AJNR Am J Neuroradiol 2001; 22(4):613–24.

99. Lichy MP, Plathow C, Schulz-Ertner D, et al. Follow-up gliomas after radiotherapy: 1H MR spectroscopic imaging for increasing diagnostic accuracy. Neuroradiology 2005;47(11):826–34.

100. Heesters MA, Kamman RL, Mooyaart EL, et al. Localized proton spectroscopy of inoperable brain gliomas. Response to radiation therapy. J Neurooncol 1993;17(1):27–35.

101. Tedeschi G, Lundbom N, Raman R, et al. Increased choline signal coinciding with malignant degeneration of cerebral gliomas: a serial proton magnetic resonance spectroscopy imaging study. J Neurosurg 1997;87(4):516–24.

102. Laprie A, Catalaa I, Cassol E, et al. Proton magnetic resonance spectroscopic imaging in newly diagnosed glioblastoma: predictive value for the site of postradiotherapy relapse in a prospective longitudinal study. Int J Radiat Oncol Biol Phys 2008;70(3):773–81.

103. Sundgren PC, Nagesh V, Elias A, et al. Metabolic alterations: a biomarker for radiation-induced normal brain injury—an MR spectroscopy study. J Magn Reson Imaging 2009;29(2): 291–7.

104. Esteve F, Rubin C, Grand S, et al. Transient metabolic changes observed with proton MR spectroscopy in normal human brain after radiation therapy. Int J Radiat Oncol Biol Phys 1998;40(2):279–86.

105. Wick W, Weller M. Adjuvant therapy. In: Deimling AV, editor. Gliomas, recent results in cancer research. Heidelberg (Germany): Springer-Verlag; 2009. p. 141–53.

106. Schwarz AJ, Maisey NR, Collins DJ, et al. Early in vivo detection of metabolic response: a pilot study of 1H MR spectroscopy in extracranial lymphoma and germ cell tumours. Br J Radiol 2002;75(900):959–66.

107. Preul MC, Caramanos Z, Villemure JG, et al. Using proton magnetic resonance spectroscopic imaging to predict in vivo the response of recurrent malignant gliomas to tamoxifen chemotherapy. Neurosurgery 2000;46(2):306–18.

108. Balmaceda C, Critchell D, Mao X, et al. Multisection 1H magnetic resonance spectroscopic imaging assessment of glioma response to chemotherapy. J Neurooncol 2006;76(2):185–91.

109. Murphy PS, Viviers L, Abson C, et al. Monitoring temozolomide treatment of low-grade glioma with proton magnetic resonance spectroscopy. Br J Cancer 2004;90(4):781–6.

110. Lichy MP, Bachert P, Henze M, et al. Monitoring individual response to brain-tumour chemotherapy: proton MR spectroscopy in a patient with recurrent glioma after stereotactic radiotherapy. Neuroradiology 2004;46(2):126–9.

111. Dyke JP, Sanelli PC, Voss HU, et al. Monitoring the effects of BCNU chemotherapy Wafers (Gliadel) in glioblastoma multiforme with proton magnetic resonance spectroscopic imaging at 3.0 Tesla. J Neurooncol 2007;82(1):103–10.

112. Golay X, Gillen J, van Zijl PC, et al. Scan time reduction in proton magnetic resonance spectroscopic imaging of the human brain. Magn Reson Med 2002;47(2):384–7.

113. Heerschap A. In vivo magnetic resonance spectroscopy in clinical oncology. In: Shields A, Price P, editors. Cancer drug discovery and development: in vivo imaging of cancer therapy. Totowa (NJ): Humana Press Inc; 2007. p. 241–58.

Advanced Imaging in Brain Tumor Surgery

Robert J. Young, MD[a,b], Nicole Brennan, BA[a],
Justin F. Fraser, MD[c], Cameron Brennan, MD[b,c,d,e],*

KEYWORDS

- Awake mapping • Brain tumor surgery
- Electrocortical stimulation • Functional MR imaging
- Diffusion tensor imaging

The development and validation of advanced anatomic and functional imaging is expanding the toolbox available for neurosurgical planning. Access to functional magnetic resonance (fMR) imaging, diffusion tractography, and intraoperative MR (iMR) imaging can influence neurosurgical decisions before, during, and after surgery. However, the widespread adoption of these techniques in neurosurgical practice remains limited by the lack of standardized methods, the need for validation across institutions, and the unclear cost-effectiveness, particularly for iMR imaging.

Before advanced imaging results can be used therapeutically, it is incumbent on the neurosurgeon and neuroradiologist to develop a working understanding of each technique's strengths and weaknesses, positive and negative predictive values, and modes of failure. For example, language localization maps by fMR imaging can have a complex relationship to positive stimulation points using direct cortical stimulation in the operating room. The performance of fMR imaging is influenced regionally by the effects of tumor and other pathology on vasculature and the coupling of vascular responses to neural activity. Similarly, the fractional anisotropy measured by diffusion tensor imaging is regionally influenced by edema, whereas the 3-dimensional (3D) tractography map is dependent on the computational model used. This article reviews several imaging modalities that are increasingly used in neurosurgical planning. As these techniques are progressively applied to surgery, radiologists, medical physicists, neuroscientists, and engineers will be necessary partners with the treating neurosurgeon to bridge the gap between the experimental and the therapeutic.

INTRAOPERATIVE MAPPING AND MONITORING

Surgical applications of advanced imaging are best considered in the context of standard practice and the neurosurgical "gold standards" for functional localization, which are based on intraoperative neurologic assessment and electrophysiology. These traditional forms of mapping are performed in patients awake under local anesthesia or, in certain circumstances, under light general anesthesia. During awake procedures patients may be monitored continuously as resection approaches functionally eloquent territory—that is, territory in which a focal injury leads to an conspicuous loss of function.

Function can be assessed intraoperatively by direct electrical stimulation of exposed cortical and white matter regions (electrocortical stimulation, ECS). ECS is generally performed with a dual electrode (bipolar) stimulator that limits current spread to less than 1 cm (see Matz

[a] Department of Radiology, Memorial Sloan-Kettering Cancer Center, New York, NY, USA
[b] Brain Tumor Center, Memorial Sloan-Kettering Cancer Center, New York, NY, USA
[c] Department of Neurosurgery, Weill Medical College of Cornell University, New York, NY, USA
[d] Department of Neurosurgery, Memorial Sloan-Kettering Cancer Center, New York, NY, USA
[e] Human Oncology and Pathogenesis Program, Memorial Sloan-Kettering Cancer Center, New York, NY, USA
* Corresponding author. Memorial Sloan-Kettering Cancer Center, 1275 York Avenue Box 71, New York, NY 10065.
E-mail address: cbrennan@mskcc.org

Neuroimag Clin N Am 20 (2010) 311–335
doi:10.1016/j.nic.2010.04.011

and colleagues[1] for a good review of the direct cortical stimulation protocol). ECS may elicit a positive motor sign that is observed directly (eg, hand clench or vocalization) or detected by electromyography (EMG).[2,3] ECS stimulation may also elicit a negative functional sign or loss of function. Examples are speech arrest, word finding, paraphasias, or perseveration detected while the patient is engaged in an active task. Of course, stimulation at a particular site may elicit neither positive nor negative responses even after escalating to the maximal safe current. In that case, the surgeon must consider anatomy and the effects of the underlying pathology to decide whether this "negative result" signifies a safe region to operate through.

Electrocorticography (ECoG) is a related technique that can be used for sensorimotor mapping in sedated or noncooperating patients. Somatosensory evoked potentials (SSEP) are used to attempt localization of the central sulcus. In this technique, a stimulating electrode is placed on the wrist overlying the median nerve and an evoked potential is recorded from the strip electrode oriented perpendicular to the presumed rolandic gyri. The phase of the evoked waveform is "flipped" between electrodes in the frontal and parietal lobes, localizing central sulcus at the reversal point. SSEPs may be distorted or absent in the presence of underlying tumor, limiting the reliability of the technique.

Fig. 1 shows an example of awake language and motor mapping guided by preoperative fMR imaging. Integration of functional and anatomic features in a neuronavigational system allows a reassuring registration of the expected picture with surface anatomy on craniotomy. During intraoperative mapping, sterile paper markers are placed on the cortex at positive stimulation points where behavior was evoked or interrupted by the bipolar stimulation. Note that after the strip electrode is used to establish somatosensory evoked potentials, it remains positioned on the cortex for seizure monitoring (electrocorticography) during bipolar stimulation and throughout the resection. In usual practice, a distance of 1 to 3 cm between the positive stimulation point and the surgical resection margin is respected to avoid deficit.[4,5]

There are several technical limitations of functional mapping by bipolar stimulation. Cortical mapping is restricted to the gyral surface; sulcal function cannot be assessed. Some cortical regions are inconvenient for mapping. For example, lesions that impinge on the precentral motor area for the foot, located in the interhemispheric fissure, can be difficult to access with a cortical stimulator. Cortical sensitivity to stimulation (ie, the threshold current required to elicit responses) varies regionally and may be affected by the level of anesthesia and the effects of tumor and related edema. Stimulation may elicit pathologic afterdischarges or frank seizures that can limit or prevent further mapping. Even when cortical structures are successfully spared, white matter injuries can be devastating. In fact, it has been suggested that white matter injuries may result in more profound and permanent functional deficits than gray matter injuries.[6] Although subcortical bipolar stimulation is becoming more common, it is technically more difficult and is not routinely performed.

Intraoperative mapping has practical limitations as well. Most awake mapping relies on the concerted participation of the patient; an exception is motor mapping by passive observation of movement and/or EMG. Patients can have difficulty awakening from anesthesia, and can be uncooperative or perform so variably that mapping is no longer reliable. In the authors' experience, preoperative deficits often are exacerbated by anesthesia and patients with preoperative deficits can require a longer "wake-up" period to return to baseline performance before mapping. Furthermore, time for functional mapping in the operating room is limited and a balance must be achieved between a complete mapping, with a varied battery of tasks and the time necessary to perform them.

In light of these limitations of intraoperative mapping, preoperative functional imaging offers potentially more complete functional mapping, acquired under controlled conditions. It is important that these results are available before surgery to assess risk, inform discussion with the patient, and aid in surgical planning. In this article the authors consider the use of advanced imaging in brain tumor surgery. Specifically, the discussion focuses on fMR imaging, diffusion tensor imaging (DTI), and iMR imaging, and to what extent they affect treatment planning.

FUNCTIONAL MR IMAGING

The most common application of fMR imaging is to assess risk in patients with lesions in or near language and motor areas. Functional mapping by MR imaging can be done by several techniques. Blood oxygen dependent

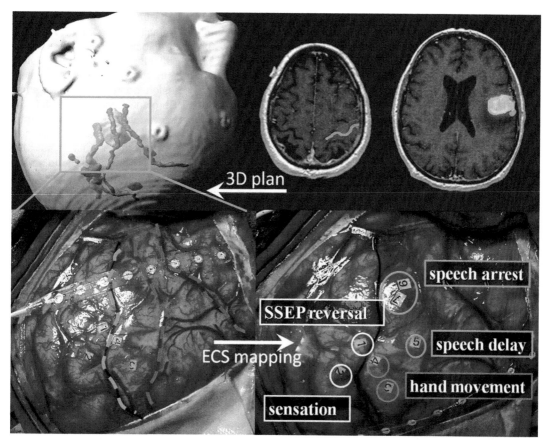

Fig. 1. Integration of functional MR (fMR) imaging with operative plan and electrocortical stimulation (ECS). (*Top*) Frameless neuronavigation software is used to display fMR imaging activation during finger-thumb tapping (*red*), the inferred location of central sulcus (*green*), and cortical veins (*purple*) in relation to the target lesion (*yellow*). These elements are viewed in a 3D volume in the planned operating position. (*Bottom left*) Exposed cortex during craniotomy. Central sulcus (*green dashes*) is determined by somatosensory evoked potential using the 8-channel recording strip is visible superior to the sylvian fissure. Cortical veins are marked for anatomic registration with the preoperative plan (*purple dashes*). (*Bottom right*) Result of electrocortical stimulation during awake craniotomy. Sterile paper tags mark sites of functional response during bipolar cortical stimulation.

functional magnetic resonance imaging (BOLD fMR imaging) is most commonly used and is described more completely by Gupta and colleagues in the article on fMR imaging and DTI elsewhere in this issue. The BOLD signal itself measures differences in magnetic susceptibility between oxy- and deoxyhemoglobin, the ratio of which varies in relation to cortical blood flow and tissue oxygen use. During task performance, cortical regions that experience increased neuronal activity see increased oxyhemoglobin concentrations relative to the resting baseline. This phenomenon is due to (and dependent on) increased perfusion with oxygenated blood resulting from active arteriolar dilation. The observation of

increased regional perfusion with neural activity was first made in humans by the neurosurgeon Wilder Penfield, who noted a red shift in the color of temporal cortical veins during an intraoperative seizure.[7] The shift in oxygenation is detectable by a T2∗ pulse sequence from which quantitative comparisons for task related neural activity can be made.

Cortical activation leads to relatively small BOLD changes of 1% to 2% for most regions and tasks, though sensorimotor tasks can elicit stronger signals from rolandic cortex. As previously described, neurovascular uncoupling is a concern for brain regions affected by tumor burden, prior surgery, or radiation: the arterioles may be maximally dilated at baseline as a result of pathology. Weaker BOLD signals are susceptible to scanner artifacts and head motion, and this can lead to false-negative predictions. Arguably the single greatest concern when applying fMR imaging results in surgery is managing the risk of acting on a false-negative result. Therefore, significant attention has been directed at validating fMR imaging and understanding the modes of failure.

Functional MR Imaging Concordance with Direct Electrocortical Stimulation

One-way fMR imaging is evaluated for neurosurgical planning is by testing concordance with intraoperative direct cortical stimulation. To date, fMR imaging has shown varied degrees of agreement with direct cortical stimulation depending on the modality being tested. fMR imaging localization of the motor gyrus has achieved very good concordance in correlative studies.[8,9] In fact, in the authors' experience fMR imaging of the primary motor gyrus has been more reliable than intraoperative SSEP measurements in patients with peri-rolandic tumors.[10] Krings and colleagues,[11] in an investigation of 103 patients (194 functional scans), found that fMR imaging was able to correctly identify the motor gyrus in 85% of cases. fMR imaging failed to localize any functional motor information in 30 fMR imaging scans. In 11 patients no functional activation was seen in any motor scan performed. The investigators concluded that fMR imaging failure in these cases was predominantly a result of head motion. Roux and colleagues[12] found that although fMR imaging overestimated the spatial extent of a cortical area required to elicit a positive motor response, it was highly concordant with ECS in brain tumor patients with various pathologies.

The experience of the authors in brain tumor patients supports that despite tumor-induced sensitivity loss of the BOLD fMR imaging signal, the motor gyrus can be identified correctly if the fMR imaging study is technically successful (ie, rolandic activation is seen).[10,13] In practice, fMR imaging prediction of central sulcus is considered together with anatomic predictions. Interrater agreement on the location of central sulcus based on anatomic MR imaging alone in healthy volunteers has been reported to be low (76%) and would be expected to diminish in cases with rolandic tumor distorting anatomy.[14] **Fig. 2** shows a typical case of central sulcus localization by BOLD fMR imaging. The lesion (glioblastoma

multiforme, GBM) is imposing significant mass effect and is effacing the central sulcus, making functional localization by anatomic markers alone difficult. fMR imaging localizes the motor gyrus in this case and places the majority of the lesion posterior to the primary motor gyrus. Surgical resection within or through the sensory cortex of the postcentral gyrus is far less likely to cause weakness than within the precentral gyrus. It is often useful to perform multiple motor paradigms to activate different portions of the motor homunculus using a tongue motor (inferolateral aspect of the motor gyrus), hand motor (lateral aspect), and foot motor (medial aspect) task. A typical finger-tapping paradigm can activate premotor, primary motor, and postcentral (sensory) cortices simultaneously, making motor localization sometimes difficult using a single fMR imaging task.

Concordance with Language Function

Compared with the sensorimotor system, language function is more broadly distributed and language tasks elicit smaller BOLD signals overall than do motor tasks. Intraoperative mapping by ECS is limited by the time and patient cooperation required to accurately detect subtle language errors across a panel of tests. Not surprisingly, fMR image mapping appears overall to be less concordant with ECS for language function.[15,16] Some forms of discordance are systematic, and for these it is useful to investigate why the functional study failed to predict intraoperative findings.

Sometimes the failure of concordance between fMR imaging and direct cortical stimulation is traceable to a mismatch between MR imaging and intraoperative testing paradigms. One of the main behavioral signs used during intraoperative ECS to localize essential expressive language territory is speech arrest. fMR imaging activation during covert (nonverbal) expressive language tasks might extend over broad territory, but would be expected to include these sites of intraoperative speech arrest. In a study of patients undergoing awake language mapping, it was found that silent speech fMR imaging correctly predicted sites of language disturbance with ECS in the inferior and middle frontal gyri but failed to predict observed sites of speech arrest in the precentral motor gyrus.[10] In normal controls, vocalized speech not only enlisted the classical Broca's area (in the inferior frontal gyrus) but also the inferior aspect of the motor

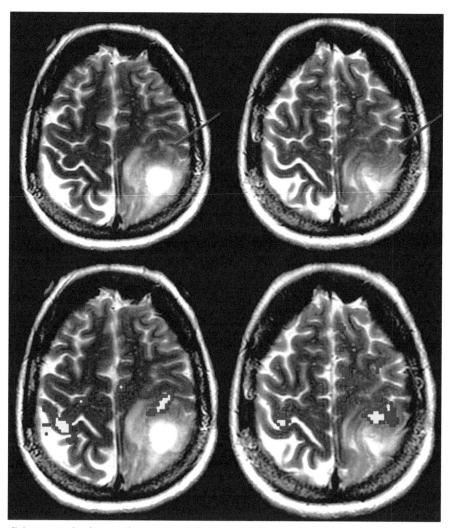

Fig. 2. Localizing central sulcus in the presence of tumor. A 62-year-old with a glioblastoma multiforme. (*Top panels*) Significant mass effect is effacing sulci making discrimination of central sulcus difficult. (*Bottom panels*) fMR imaging places the majority of the lesion within the sensory gyrus . The red line indicates the position of the central sulcus.

gyrus. Because interruption of vocalized speech (speech arrest) is a principal finding during ECS mapping, it follows that having the patient perform at least one fMR imaging speech task aloud should support better concordance between the testing protocols. However, vocalized speech paradigms are challenging to employ for fMR imaging, as they require the subject to keep his or her head still while speaking. This rigidity requires a level of concentration that may be unsustainable for sick patients. Head motion can degrade the study and can lead to false positives if motion is correlated with the stimulus.

Functional MR Imaging Determination of Hemispheric Dominance for Language

The left hemisphere is the dominant seat of language in nearly all right-handed patients as well as the majority of left-handed patients. It is important in neurosurgical practice to be able to identify the exceptions: patients with language dominance in the right hemisphere or shared between hemispheres ("codominant"). The intracarotid amobarbital test (or Wada test) has historically been the gold standard test to determine which hemisphere predominantly controls language (language laterality). This test employs transient anesthesia of each hemisphere separately to determine language laterality.[17,18] Language lateralization using fMR imaging has achieved good but imperfect concordance with the Wada procedure.[19–22] Reasons for the discordance are multifaceted depending on whether Wada or fMR imaging predicted language dominance correctly. For example, in epilepsy patients concordance between fMR imaging and the Wada test has been shown to reach 91%.[20,22] Because fMR imaging laterality measures are based on quantitative comparisons, they may be particularly sensitive to subtle effects of neurovascular uncoupling on the pathology-bearing side.[23–25] Ulmer and colleagues[26] found that of 85 functional areas tested (in 50 patients with brain lesions), 23 (27%) areas showed perilesional (within 5 mm) decreases in fMR imaging signal. This finding led to incorrect measurements of dominance. Patients with previous surgery are another cohort at risk of false-negative fMR imaging signals as a result of signal dropout imposed by blood products and surgical staples. This risk may be reduced by using a hemispheric region of interest to calculate language laterality in order to minimize regional susceptibility artifacts.[27] Increasing refinement of laterality measure by fMR imaging will hopefully lead to standards by which studies can be made comparable and quality measures can reduce the risk of false prediction.[9,28–30]

In clinical practice, all patients with left-sided lesions in potential language areas are considered for awake mapping because the majority will be left-dominant. fMR imaging measures of hemispheric dominance are most valuable when they indicate unexpected or atypical results that are clinically actionable. For example, when fMR imaging indicates right hemispheric dominance or split dominance, either a Wada test can be ordered or the potentially translocated/reorganized area in question can be mapped intraoperatively. These cases are uncommon. More typically, in the authors' experience brain tumor patients exhibit either the expected left hemisphere laterality on fMR imaging or varying degrees of bilateral activation, depending in part on how the study is processed.[31]

The functional significance of bilateral fMR imaging activation is not yet clear and as a result, it is not prudent to infer functional codominance without confirmatory testing. A study by Knecht and colleagues[32] investigated transcranial magnetic stimulation (TMS) to validate the fMR imaging measurement of hemispheric dominance. TMS uses extracranial magnetic pulses during speech production tasks to map function much the same way direct electrocortical stimulation is employed in the operating room. This study tested control subjects with varying degrees of putative hemispheric dominance predicted by fMR imaging laterality (completely left dominant, codominant, and completely right dominant). In individuals with bilateral fMR imaging activation, TMS identified speech interruption sites in both hemispheres more often than for well-lateralized counterparts. However, whether this pattern of speech distribution provides any protection against surgical injury is unknown.

Unlike invasive mapping techniques, fMR imaging is well suited to fine-mapping language codominance or split dominance and to follow changes in the dominance pattern over time. In rare cases, split dominance appears to be consistent with cortical compensation and/or translocation of function in the context of progressive injury from tumor growth and treatment.[33–35]

Issues with Functional MR Imaging Interpretation for Surgical Use

In addition to the problem of neurovascular uncoupling, the interpretation of BOLD fMR imaging in brain tumor patients suffers from 2 other central issues: thresholding and essential versus nonessential function. These issues, in turn, affect the way the fMR imaging map is trusted in the operating room.

Thresholding refers to the choice of statistical cutoff applied during the analysis, which affects the apparent pattern of a functional activation. If the statistical significance is lenient, the functional activation is more extensive and includes a higher chance of false positives; stringent thresholds risk false-negative calls. There is no single optimum statistical threshold that can be applied patient to patient. BOLD signal, task performance, artifacts, and noise vary individually, regionally, and from study to study.[31,36]

There have been many attempts to address the thresholding problem. Voyvodic and colleagues[37] proposed a method to localize the motor strip using the most statistically active voxels, achieved by normalizing statistical t-test maps to peak amplitudes of voxels within functional regions. Another study has similarly suggested using the first appearance of a fixed number of active voxels as a more stable measure of language laterality than the traditional statistical thresholding.[38] All things considered, thresholding is a weakness in laterality measurements and localization of weak BOLD signals, and the clinician should be mindful when interpreting fMR imaging data.

It is surprising that although the BOLD phenomenon is well established, the relationship between BOLD signal and the underlying cortical circuit—that is, what *kind* of activity BOLD signal is measuring—is not at all clear (see review by Logothetis[39] for sobering detail). Among the complications to consider are that inhibitory neurons outnumber excitatory neurons in the central nervous system and their function adds to metabolic demand; and that synaptic potentials (representing, in part, cortical input) lead to far larger ion fluxes and metabolic demand than action potentials (representing output). Even when a stimulus is known to generate cortical activation and excitatory output from a particular region, there is no general rule regarding the neurologic effects of injury to that region. For instance, fMR imaging activation of the motor strip in a finger-thumb tapping task is associated with cortical output and predicts weakness if the area is injured. However, activation of Heschl's gyrus in an auditory-driven task is also associated with cortical output and yet injuries to this site may have no discernible effects. Therefore, even with "true positive" fMR imaging activation, it is impossible to know which areas are essential versus supportive for the function tested. This issue is particularly relevant in neurosurgical planning because only a subset of the fMR imaging localizations, when stimulated with a bipolar stimulator, will actually show interruption of function. Accordingly, fMR imaging (particularly for language studies) is most commonly used as a moderate preoperative estimator of risk and a guide to intraoperative cortical stimulation. In practical terms this use of FMR imaging has been shown to reduce mapping time in the operating room.[40]

Functional MR Imaging and Clinical Outcomes

The historical view of neurosurgical outcomes suggests that new technologies lead to incremental improvements rather than dramatic advances. In light of the cost of preoperative fMR imaging, there is great interest in measuring the effect on clinical outcomes. At present there are only data on intermediate or technical outcomes, such as influence on surgical technique or correlations with neurologic morbidity. Petrella and colleagues,[40] in a case series of 39 patients, found that treatment plans for 19 patients were changed in light of the preoperative functional imaging; they also found that fMR imaging resulted in reduced surgical mapping in 22 patients, a more aggressive resection in 6 patients, and a smaller exposure in 2 patients. A study of patients with seizure disorders concluded that fMR imaging helped avoid further clinical testing (including the Wada test) in 63% of patients.[41] In the same study fMR imaging

altered intraoperative mapping procedures in 52% and altered surgical plans in 42%.

The predictive value of fMR imaging for recovery from stroke and other neurologic injuries is also being investigated.[42-44] A recent study of stroke recovery found that fMR imaging was a significant predictor, along with age and neuropsychological performance, of whether a patient would significantly regain language performance 6 months after the event, together achieving 86% accuracy.[45] Another study found that temporal lobe epilepsy patients with ipsilateral temporal lobe fMR imaging activation versus contralateral activation had greater memory decline following mesial temporal lobe resection.[46] Thus, the value of clinical fMR imaging has the potential to be significant as its use is refined.

Future Directions for Functional Imaging for Presurgical Planning

Arterial spin labeling (ASL) is an alternative approach to fMR imaging, which measures activity-dependent blood flow changes directly by tracking the passage of arterial blood that has been spin-labeled in the carotid artery. The advantages of ASL include higher specificity than BOLD, less vulnerability to head motion, less variability in spatial localizations in test/retest studies, and fewer artifacts from magnetic susceptibility.[47,48] The major drawback is limited sensitivity (signal magnitudes are between half and a quarter that of BOLD fMR imaging).

Resting state fMR imaging, where very slow fluctuations of the BOLD signal are measured during prolonged resting state, has recently reemerged as an alternative approach to task-driven imaging in clinical applications.[49,50] The practical advantage is that the behavioral constraints in these studies are lifted because intrinsic network connectivity/integrity is measured while patients are at rest in the scanner. This technique is still in its early stages and will need significant validation before it can be used for neurosurgical planning.

Multimodality mapping is also gaining traction in neurosurgical planning. Complementary techniques like magnetoencephalography add temporal resolution to the BOLD signal. TMS has the potential to validate fMR imaging maps, characterize clinically ambiguous fMR imaging studies, and clarify the functional significance of bilateral language activation by allowing relatively unrestricted stimulation compared with what is available intraoperatively. TMS can achieve spatial precision when used with a stereotactic navigational system, lending information about the essential versus supportive nature of fMR imaging activations preoperatively.[51]

DIFFUSION TENSOR IMAGING

fMR imaging and DTI play complementary roles in operative planning. As discussed in this issue by Gupta and colleagues in the article on fMR imaging and DTI elsewhere in this issue, DTI infers the pathway of major white matter tracts by their impact on the directionality and magnitude of water diffusion. Water diffusion in the brain tends to track along bundles of white matter fibers, and the portion of overall diffusion that is directional (as opposed to random) is referred to as fractional anisotropy (FA). The most commonly used representation of DTI is the directionally encoded color FA map. The FA map encodes the magnitude of anisotropy in signal brightness and fiber orientation in 3 standard colors: transverse in red, anteroposterior in green, and craniocaudal in blue. **Fig. 3** shows a typical FA map for neurosurgical planning. The FA map can be coregistered with conventional anatomic imaging to provide a preoperative map of functional anatomy and identify major fiber tracts at risk during surgery. In the case shown, preoperative DTI was useful to direct white matter stimulation to the anteromedial margin.

As a general statement, fMR imaging has been described as being more useful in the planning phase and DTI in the resection phase.[52] In practice, fMR imaging mapping of cortical function informs about resectability, risk, and cortical window of approach, whereas DTI mapping of white matter often becomes most relevant later in the resection. Gulati and colleagues[53] described fMR imaging and DTI as facilitating identification of functional areas in 91% and 94% of cases, respectively.

Diffusion Tensor Tractography

The FA map serves as an atlas of the major fiber bundles and allows for comparison between tumor-bearing and healthy hemispheres. Because it shows the magnitude and direction of anisotropy voxel by voxel, it is the most reliable representation of DTI for general interpretation. However, tracts that run a long distance, run obliquely, or change orientation along their course can be difficult to follow on the FA map. Diffusion tensor tractography (DTT; also known as fiber tracking) is an additional analysis step that reconstructs the probable course of fiber tracts using a computer model based on the FA map. Tractography is typically generated by drawing seed regions of interest (ROIs) along the white matter tract of interest. Tracts are estimated by moving voxel to voxel along the major axis of anisotropy in both directions. In this way, DTT can also be used to localize eloquent gray matter centers. By placing a seed ROI in the cerebral peduncle to reconstruct the corticospinal tract, the primary motor area (Brodmann's area 4) was identified in 9 patients with brain lesions in the precentral gyrus in whom fMR imaging and/or somatosensory evoked magnetic field localization had failed.[54] Another

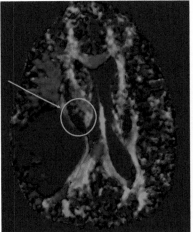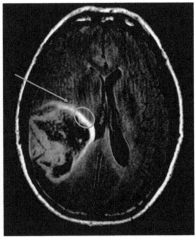

Fig. 3. Diffusion tensor imaging in a patient with right frontoparietal tumor predicts corticospinal tract displacement. (*Left*) The directionally encoded or color fractional anisotropy (FA) map encodes orientation of diffusion of water, corresponding to major white matter tracts: transverse left-right (*red*), anteroposterior (*green*), and craniocaudal (*blue*). Major medial craniocaudal pathway suggests displacement of corticospinal tract. (*Right*) Preoperative fluid-attenuated inversion recovery MR imaging from navigational system showing approximate location of positive white matter stimulation: 12-mA bipolar current elicited leg paresthesias.

study noted that similar results could be achieved for localization of the precentral gyrus.[55]

Because tractography is influenced by operator-defined parameters and reconstruction algorithms, it may be considered less reliable than the color-encoded FA maps. Bürgel and colleagues[56] compared 4 popular fiber tractography programs using data from a normal subject, and found disparate tracking results for the corticospinal tract. Further divergence and inaccuracies are expected in the presence of tumor and edema that distort normal anatomy and can reduce FA. These effects may be ameliorated as more sophisticated algorithms are developed. While still potentially useful, tractography is in need of further validation testing. In the authors' practice, the FA map is used for presurgical planning in the tumor vicinity and tractography is primarily used to illustrate major pathways that are not distorted by tumor. **Fig. 4** shows several common representations of a typical DTI study as it might be incorporated into a neuronavigational system for use in the operating room. In this example, the DTI signal (anisotropy) appears to be attenuated in the tumor hemisphere on the FA map. Comparison with the contralateral side suggests that the corticospinal tracts may be pushed medially and anteriorly. Tractography preferentially marks a more posterior descending tract. If tractography were viewed in isolation, it would be easy to misinterpret the study as showing posterior displacement of the corticospinal tract.

Intraoperative Incorporation of Diffusion Tensor Imaging

Both fMR imaging and DTI datasets are easily integrated in commercially available neuronavigation software suites, with the caveat that gradient images register imperfectly with spin-echo–based anatomic navigational datasets. The overall error of DTI coregistration into the 3D navigational dataset has been estimated to be less than 2 mm, which is only slightly more than the error of the navigational system itself at 1.2 mm.[55] Concordance between subcortical electrical stimulation and corticospinal tractography, including errors in the tracking algorithm, errors in the neuronavigational system, and dissipation of the electrical current has been estimated at 8.7 ± 3.1 mm (mean distance).[57] A recent study compared results from subcortical stimulation and DTI in 10 patients with low-grade gliomas,[58] in which 17 of 21 positive subcortical stimulation points were concordant with DTI language tract localizations (concordance defined as 6 mm or less from the DTI prediction). Four positive white matter stimulation sites were not located in the vicinity of a DTI fiber tract.

Accurate fiber tracking of the corticospinal tract has been confirmed by subcortical electrical stimulation and motor evoked potentials (MEPs), with MEPs usually elicited within 1 cm of the reconstructed tracts.[59,60] Preliminary validation of tractography of the visual pathway has been suggested by Kamada and colleagues,[60] who confirmed functional connections of reconstructed

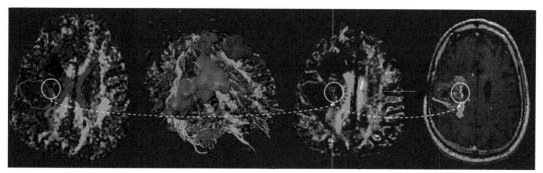

Fig. 4. Tractography derived from FA map may be misleading if considered in isolation. (*Left to right*) (1) A typical DTI FA map in a patient with frontoparietal glioblastoma. Tumor contour is outlined (*pink*) and a region of craniocaudal fibers (*blue FA color*) is visible on the anteromedial border (*white circle*). Comparison with the left hemisphere suggests attenuation of the FA signal near the tumor mass. (2) 3D volumetric view of integrated data including DTI tractography, tumor mass (*pink*), central sulcus (*green*), and fMR imaging activation (*purple*). (3) Axial slice of tractography showing tracts seeded from a region of interest in the cerebral peduncle. The dominant descending tracts appear to be posterior to the tumor. (4) Segmentation of craniocaudal tracts for import into neuronavigation display in the operating room. At this stage, the information needed to interpret the quality of tractography has been stripped from the study, and there is a risk of misinterpreting the large posterior bundle as posterior displacement of the corticospinal tract when in fact there is anterior displacement.

optic radiations using intraoperative visual evoked potentials (VEP). The DTI and DTT data may be used to avoid essential white matter tracts, which may be displaced, infiltrated, or destroyed by tumor. In a study of 12 patients with primary brain tumors, Talos and colleagues[61] described infiltration by tumor into adjacent white matter tracts by a median 21%, even when the anatomic images suggested simple mass effect and displacement rather than infiltration. This information, obtained preoperatively, can be valuable to plan a safe resection volume, to discuss risk and surgical goals with the patient, and to direct subcortical stimulation during surgery if needed.

Diffusion Tensor Imaging for Motor Tracts

The corticospinal tract is a common target for DTI mapping, and has been compared with cortical and subcortical bipolar stimulation testing during awake craniotomy. Whereas cortical stimulation allows the surgeon to localize the motor gyrus prior to resection, subcortical stimulation is used to assess the proximity of the corticospinal tract by monitoring the patient's motor response to stimulation of exposed white matter during the operation. This procedure is occasionally done with the additional use of MEPs.[60] However, unlike the cortical folds, deep white matter tracts are not discernible visually and may fail to stimulate reliably with reasonable currents. Postoperative motor deficits have been described as more common after successful subcortical stimulation.[62] This apparent paradox likely reflects a bias caused by closer proximity of the surgery to the motor tract and the sensitivity of the tract to manipulation, local cautery, and other sources of injury.

Subcortical Stimulation of Language Tracts

Subcortical stimulation for the localization of language-related white matter tracts is becoming an increasingly important adjunct to cortical stimulation mapping during resection, and DTI can guide the surgeon regarding where to stimulate and when to commence during resection. Subcortical stimulation is being used to avoid iatrogenic deficit and to characterize language pathways with increasing behavioral specificity. For example, Duffau and colleagues,[63] in developing the subcortical language stimulation technique, were able to broadly attribute the subcallosal fasciculus to initiation disorders, the periventricular white matter to dysarthric disturbances, and the arcuate fasciculus and insular connections to anomia in a series of 20 patients. Like its direct cortical stimulation counterpart, data on the

reliability of subcortical stimulation testing in speech mapping is accruing as technical aspects are worked out.[64–66]

The authors' experience with subcortical stimulation testing has been varied, with results depending on many factors including the extent of pathology (and edema), the tract in question, and the depth of tract localization. Subcortical stimulation is less reliable overall at eliciting responses than cortical stimulation, and no study has systematically addressed the false-negative rate. Negative responses may indicate that the tract of interest is not near the stimulation point, that the tract is not functional, or that current must be escalated to establish a true negative result. As a result of these and other difficulties with the technique, there is a need for additional measures of anatomic/functional localization and risk. Because DTI can be performed both presurgically and intraoperatively, it may be an attractive noninvasive way to delineate specific white matter tracts to help the neurosurgeon maintain a safe margin from these eloquent structures. Further, in cases where the patient cannot tolerate the awake procedure, it is especially useful to have a surrogate marker of white matter tract localization like DTI.

Diffusion Tensor Imaging and Clinical Outcomes

The predictive value of DTI is currently being characterized and validated against subcortical language[64,66] and motor testing[67] intraoperatively. Several studies report success using DTI to drive surgical planning and/or subcortical stimulation testing (similar to fMR imaging data for eloquent cortex).[57,62,66] Romano and colleagues[68] reported that preoperative plans for 80% of their 25 patients were modified after review of the DTI data by the neurosurgeon, 16% of which were due to changes in surgical approach.

The best data available on the impact of DTI on clinical outcomes come from a prospective, randomized study of neuronavigation incorporating DTI data in 238 patients with cerebral gliomas involving the corticospinal tracts.[69] Patients were randomized to have surgery guided either by conventional neuronavigation (control) or DTI integrated with 3D anatomic imaging. Patients in the DTI group were more likely to receive gross total resection of high-grade (but not low-grade) gliomas (74% vs 33%), have preservation of postoperative motor function (85% vs 67%), and maintain 6-month Karnofsky scores (86 vs 74). For high-grade gliomas there was an impact on median survival of 7 months (hazard ratio 0.57).

There are several questions raised by these results: the combination of higher extent of resection and lower motor morbidity has not been seen in other studies, and the effect on survival appears higher than what is typically seen for gross total resection by other means. The reason for lack of benefit in extent of resection for lower grade tumors is unclear. The study is uniquely valuable as the sole prospective randomized study, and as a guide to these unresolved questions.

TUMOR RESECTION: SCENARIOS BY PATHOLOGY

In this section the utility of presurgical functional imaging and DTI is framed from the perspective of common surgical scenarios in neuro-oncology. The type of pathology often determines if and how preoperative functional imaging will be used. **Fig. 5** shows examples of common tumor types and how functional imaging might be used if the tumors were located in or around regions of eloquent function. There are 3 common scenarios.

Superficial circumscribed or extra-axial lesion. Examples include meningioma, hemangiopericytoma, and dural-based metastases. These lesions are immediately visible on craniotomy and generally there are no ambiguities with regard to surgical entry point, trajectory, or resection margin. However, preoperative functional imaging is useful to inform discussion with the patient about the potential for neurologic deficits from surgery or complications (stroke, hemorrhage, seizure, and so forth). During resection, the functional areas (cortical and white matter) will be approached with greater caution. If the tumor is focally adherent or invasive, the surgeon may use the functional map to gauge the risk of attempting total versus subtotal resection.

Deep circumscribed lesion. This presentation is a common one for brain metastases. Functional imaging can be used in the same way as described above. In addition, in this scenario the tumor is below the cortical surface and choice of surgical trajectory includes balancing the shortest distance with the lowest risk of neurologic injury. If the preoperative studies suggest that the best trajectory will pass through or near a functional region, the surgeon may decide to perform the procedure awake to validate the map intraoperatively and to choose the safest entry point with high confidence.

Infiltrative lesion. This pattern is typical of glioma or radiation necrosis. The key distinction is that the margin is ill-defined and invasive into normal parenchyma. In addition to the aforementioned uses, functional imaging can be helpful for deciding preoperatively on how much may be safely resected (or whether only biopsy is safe), whether to plan intralesional mapping and/or awake assessment during resection, and whether to use intraoperative MR imaging.

INTRAOPERATIVE MR IMAGING

iMR imaging is increasingly used to obtain images during the course of surgery. The main utility of iMR imaging in neurosurgical oncology is to identify residual tumor during resection, to localize this in relation to surrounding anatomy that may shift during the course of surgery, and to update neurosurgical navigation systems to help achieve safe and complete resection. iMR imaging systems differ primarily in their field strength and physical configuration: whether the surgeon is operating within the magnet, swinging the operating table into the bore, or bringing the machine to the patient. iMR imaging is most commonly used for anatomic imaging, although advanced modalities such as DTI, spectroscopy, perfusion, or fMR imaging can be obtained with high field strength systems of 1.5 to 3 Tesla, clinical use of which, however, is rare.

The capital expense for purchasing and installing high field magnets in an operating room environment is significantly higher than for outpatient scanners, and annual maintenance costs for dedicated intraoperative systems are not offset by the throughput of an outpatient scanner. These economics, coupled with the complexity of operating iMR imaging systems, have limited the deployment of high-field iMR imaging technology and have driven a lively debate about the true value of the technology. During its decade of development, iMR imaging has been subjected to greater scrutiny than other technologies broadly adopted in neurosurgical practice, such as the operating microscope, ultrasound, and neuronavigational systems.

Intraoperative MR Imaging for Neuronavigation

Bringing MR imaging to the operating room was an inevitable step in the continuous advancement of neurosurgical navigation. Navigation techniques have evolved from the use of anatomic references such as the Schaltenbrand-Bailey stereotactic atlas to modern systems that integrate multimodal imaging results for preoperative planning and navigation in real time during surgery.[70] Computer-based navigation systems allow the surgeon to directly reference and correlate the preoperative MR imaging images to the operative field with millimeter accuracy. Intraoperative neuronavigation

	Common Examples	Decision support by functional imaging (fMRI, DTI)						
		Perioperative Risk Assessment	Tumor margins requiring extra caution	Surgical approach, trajectory	Plan awake craniotomy, mapping	Plan resection volume or biopsy	Plan intralesional mapping	Plan intra-op MRI
Superficial circumscribed or extra-axial lesion	meningioma, dural metastases (Figure 5a)	✓	✓					
Deep circumscribed lesion	metastases (Figure 5b)	✓	✓	✓	✓			
Infiltrative lesion	glioma, radiation necrosis (figure 5c)	✓	✓	✓	✓	✓	✓	✓

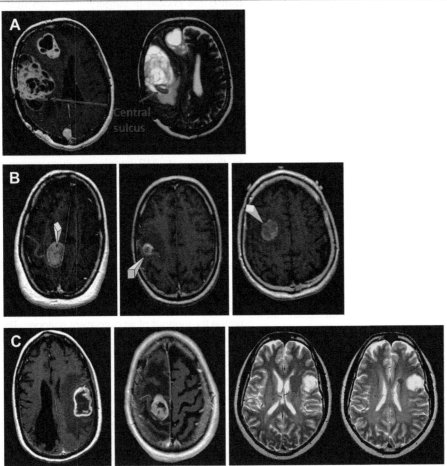

Fig. 5. Common scenarios for the use of functional imaging (fMR imaging and DTI) in surgical planning. For lesions in or near functional regions, the type of pathology often dictates how preoperative imaging is used to support surgical decisions. (A–C) Examples corresponding to superficial circumscribed, deep circumscribed, and infiltrative lesions, respectively. (A) A superficial extra-axial hemangiopericytoma surrounds and displaces the central sulcus as determined by preoperative fMR imaging. This information was useful to estimate the risk of surgery preoperatively and to mark the posterior medial margin for particular attention during resection. (B) Functional imaging can inform the decision on optimal trajectory for deep tumors. Shown are 3 cases of metastatic tumor near the central sulcus. In each case, central sulcus was identified by fMR imaging preoperatively (*red curves*) and this information was used to design an approach and decide on awake motor mapping. (C) Three examples of infiltrative/invasive pathology for which preoperative functional imaging helped to define neurologic risk, surgical trajectory, operative goals, and use of awake mapping and/or intraoperative MR imaging. Left: this lesion was safely approached from a posterior parietal entry and resected to the central sulcus (*red curve*) without additional deficit. Middle: Radiation necrosis, planned subtotal resection based on proximity to precentral lower extremity motor representation, and descending corticospinal tract. Procedure was planned awake. Right: Low-grade glioma surrounded by fMR imaging activation in Boston Naming task. Speech arrest was elicited by cortical stimulation anterior and posterior to the lesion. Subtotal resection was performed.

based solely on preoperative imaging has become routine in modern neuro-oncologic surgery and has been associated with more complete resection, although case comparative studies are confounded by selection bias.[71–73]

The principal limitation of stereotactic neuronavigation comes from referencing a static set of preoperative images to a constantly changing operative field. As the anatomy changes from cerebrospinal fluid (CSF) loss, manipulation, retraction, and resection, preoperative images gradually lose their relevance. **Fig. 6** demonstrates the brain shift associated with tumor resection and loss of buoyancy when the skull is opened. Brain shift is highly variable and may easily overwhelm the automated adjustments that are possible using commercially available neuronavigational software, rendering navigation useless or misleading when the surgeon is most in need of an accurate map to target the last remnants of tumor.[74] In this setting, iMR imaging is indisputably valuable for updating the neuronavigational system and reevaluating the operative field for residual tumor. The next sections review low-field and high-field iMR imaging systems separately.

Low-Field Intraoperative MR Imaging: Lessons Learned

Initial attempts to incorporate MR imaging involved low-field magnets (0.2 to 0.5 Tesla) that were added into existing operative suites. Wirtz and colleagues[75] published the first series of patients in which the iMR imaging data were used intraoperatively to update neuronavigation planning software. Early reports noted that the image quality was limited but sufficient to identify residual tumor in many cases, and that iMR imaging was particularly useful for resections where pathology involved lesions that were

cystic and/or nearby ventricles.[76,77] In such tumors, the resection cavity and brain surface would collapse early and significantly during the course of the operation.[76] The same group published their first 200 patients in whom 0.5-Tesla iMR imaging was used (111 craniotomies): iMR imaging detected 2 significant perioperative hemorrhages in the region of the pathology that underwent evacuation before the end of the operative procedure.[78] McClain and colleagues[79] discovered unexpected intracranial hemorrhages via iMR imaging in 2 pediatric patients undergoing craniotomy for tumor; an epidural hematoma from Mayfield pin placement occurred in one, while a subdural hematoma contralateral to the craniotomy was detected in another.

These results provided some foundation for using iMR imaging to improve tumor resection and survival. In a study of 38 patients with high-grade glioma undergoing resection, Knauth and colleagues[80] demonstrated that 0.2-Tesla iMR imaging significantly improved extent of tumor resection; use of iMR imaging improved their rate of gross total resection (GTR) from 36.6% to 75.6%. Schneider and colleagues[81] produced similar findings, demonstrating an improvement in GTR. Furthermore, there was a significant difference in survival between patients who had GTR (537 days) versus subtotal resection (STR; 237 days, $P = .0037$), which is consistent with other published studies.[81–83]

Limitations of low-field iMR imaging became apparent in published results of their use. Zimmermann and colleagues,[84] in describing the use of 0.5-Tesla iMR imaging in 34 craniotomies of patients with tumors near eloquent brain regions, noted that GTR was achieved in 28 cases. In 3 of 6 subtotal resections, residual tumor was not visible on intraoperative images (but was identified

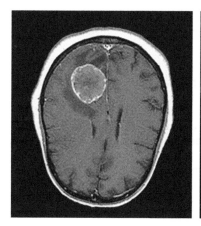
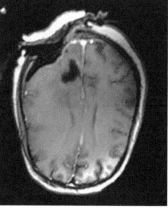

Fig. 6. Example of brain shift during tumor resection tracked by intraoperative MR (iMR) imaging. Brain shift occurs to varying degree as soon as the calvarium is opened and natural buoyancy from cerebrospinal fluid is lost. Shift continues during tumor resection as the cavity collapses. iMR imaging allows the neuronavigational system to be updated with an accurate map during surgery.

on early diagnostic follow-up MR imaging).[84] Nimsky and colleagues[85] also noted some difficulty in visualizing completeness of resection with a 0.2-Tesla system, especially in cases of low-grade gliomas. In comparing this with another imaging modality (3D ultrasonography), Tronnier and colleagues[86] noted that low-field MR was more easily interpreted, but better visibility of 1 case (in 35) of low-grade glioma was noted using ultrasonography over low-field MR. Thus, although low-field iMR imaging provides real-time imaging in the perioperative period, can identify hematoma, and allows for neuronavigational recalibration, it is limited in the ability to detect residual tumor (especially in cases of low-grade glioma) and to incorporate more complex neuroimaging modalities.

High-Field Intraoperative MR Imaging: Mechanics and Safety

High-field iMR imaging is gaining in popularity despite cost and complexity. High-field magnets require significant engineering to build into an operating room: magnetic and radiofrequency shielding, ventilation, safety monitoring systems, and some amount of MR-compatible equipment depending on configuration.[87–89] In most installations either the operating table or the MR scanner moves into and out of the scanning position when needed. The advantage of such systems is that operations can be performed using conventional, non-MR imaging compatible instruments and equipment. The main disadvantage is that more time is required to obtain a scan and real-time imaging is unavailable. Fig. 7 shows the intraoperative MR imaging suite at Memorial Sloan Kettering Cancer Center. During the operative portion of the case the surgeons, staff, patient, and equipment remain outside the 5-gauss line. When an MR imaging scan is desired, instruments are removed from the patient and counted, electrocautery grounding pads are removed, and the patient is draped and moved into the scanner. With an adjacent control room and integrated neuronavigational software, the images can be immediately used to update the navigation software without significantly delaying the ongoing procedure. While the workflow has a definite learning curve, the establishment of a regulated protocol with a knowledgable team engenders efficiency and safety.

Intraoperative Functional Imaging

Intraoperative BOLD fMR imaging may be performed on high-field iMR imaging systems with online statistical analysis tools to update the neuronavigational system and compensate for brain shift.[90] Despite being technically feasible, intraoperative fMR imaging is rarely necessary in clinical practice and may not be advantageous to intraoperative mapping by ECS. However, intraoperative DTI has a potentially valuable role: brain shift during surgery is a critical issue for deep white matter structures, as these are often approached late in resection, may be infiltrated with tumor, and are vulnerable to injury. In a series of patients with intraoperative DTI, white matter tracts were found to show a relatively modest mean outward shift of 2.7 mm, but maximal outward shifts of up to 15 mm (62.2%) and inward shifts up to 8 mm (29.7%).[91] In these situations, DTI may provide invaluable information to update the neuronavigational system. Fig. 8 shows the use of intraoperative anatomic and DTI imaging to aid in the complete resection of a deeply located pilocytic astrocytoma.

A current limitation of intraoperative DTI relates to the tilt and rotation of the patient's head necessary for brain surgery. The directionally encoded color FA maps are based on rigid x, y, and z axes aligned to the MR imaging scanner, and remain constant after aligning the images to standard orthogonal planes—the white matter fibers and reconstructed tracts are correct but displayed in the wrong color scheme (Fig. 9). The directionally encoded color FA maps may be recalculated after manually recalculating the angles of rotation, but this process requires an offline workstation and time that is not conducive to the operating suite. Intraoperative MR imaging perfusion may also be performed, to maximize resection of perfusion determined high-grade tumor while not limited by brain shift.[92]

Additional Applications for Intraoperative MR imaging

While one major focus of iMR imaging applications has been craniotomy resection of intraparenchymal tumors, there are several other operative procedures into which iMR imaging has been integrated.

Stereotactic biopsy

Stereotactic biopsy and catheter placement may benefit from accuracy with the use of iMR imaging, particularly if the position of the burr hole or a transventricular trajectory allow for CSF release and brain shift. If the surgery is performed within the magnet, the trajectory can be dynamically tracked. For systems designed for out-of-field surgery, iMR imaging can be used to update the navigation system after a burr hole is made. In the authors'

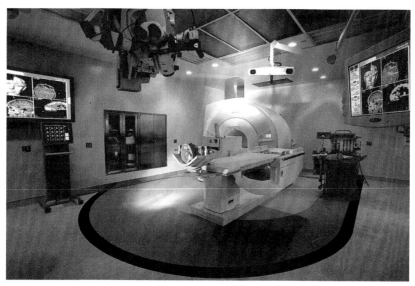

Fig. 7. The iMR imaging at Memorial Sloan Kettering Cancer Center uses a 1.5-Tesla wide-bore magnet and a robotic operating table. In this configuration, cranial operations are performed outside the 5-gauss safety line, permitting the use of conventional instruments (including ferromagnetic construction) and routine equipment such as operating microscope and ultrasound. To obtain an intraoperative scan, the table is rotated into the bore.

practice using such a system, iMR imaging is obtained after burr hole placement if the target is small and deep. A second scan is obtained while the initial biopsy core is reviewed in pathology; this permits confirmation of the needle tract in most cases and assessment for potential complications such as hematoma.

Transphenoidal resection

Transphenoidal surgery is especially well suited to iMR imaging. The surgical exposure is limited and it is difficult to assess residual tumor in many cases; downward shift of the brain and chiasm present a risk of injury. The first patient series was reported in 2001 by Bohinski and

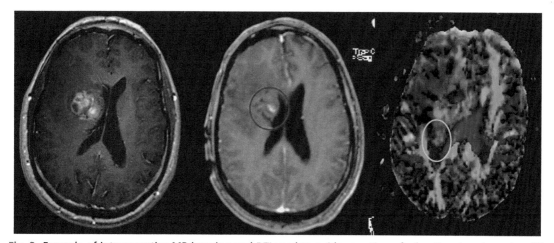

Fig. 8. Example of intraoperative MR imaging and DTI used to guide resection of pilocytic astrocytoma in a 39-year-old man. (Left) preoperative scan shows a heterogeneously enhancing mass in the deep frontal white matter. Resection was performed from a frontal approach using deep retractors. (Middle) Intraoperative MR imaging reveals residual enhancing and nonenhancing tumor requiring continued resection. (Right) Intraoperative DTI suggests posterior displacement of corticospinal tracts. The navigation system was updated and the remaining tumor was resected.

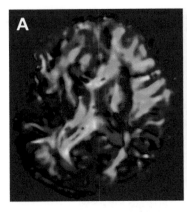 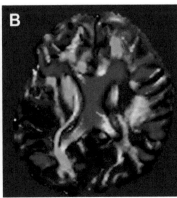

Fig. 9. Intraoperative directionally encoded color FA map. (A) Due to nonstandard head positioning, the color axes are off-axis (note green color of transversely oriented fibers of the genu of the corpus callosum, which is usually red). (B) Corrected image after manual calculations of head angle and rotation.

colleagues,[93] who described results of 30 patients who had iMR imaging-guided transphenoidal surgery using a low-field system. Residual tumor identified in 66% of cases led to further resection. Several other groups have subsequently published their experience with low-field and high-field iMR imaging systems. Most transphenoidal surgery is performed for pituitary adenoma. The requirements for iMR imaging guidance are different than for glioma resection in that, for the purpose of safe and thorough debulking, large adenomas can be tracked by low-field systems reasonably well.[87,93–98] However, where complete resection is medically required, as for growth-hormone–secreting adenomas, or where the tumors are small, high-field systems appear to be advantageous.[99,100] Fig. 10 illustrates the use of iMR imaging in resection of a pituitary macroadenoma through a microscopic

transphenoidal approach. The superior and lateral margins pose the greatest risk of injury to the optic apparatus and carotid arteries, yet are not well visualized from this approach. iMR imaging is particularly useful to facilitate complete resection safely.

Laser thermal ablation

Laser interstitial thermal therapy (LITT) is a technique by which high-energy laser illumination is delivered directly to brain tumors using a stereotactically placed optical conduit. If sufficient energy can be delivered, tissue temperatures can be raised above a threshold of viability, defined by a function of temperature and time. If this threshold is reached the tissue will undergo necrosis. Although the technique is not new, only recently has it been possible to track temperatures spatially and temporally

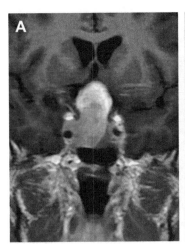 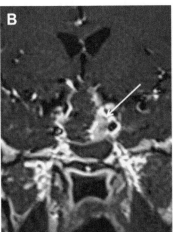 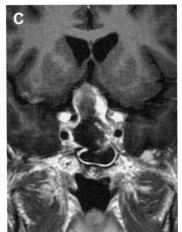

Fig. 10. Coronal contrast T1-weighted images in a patient with a pituitary macroadenoma. (A) Preoperative image shows invasion of bilateral cavernous sinuses and the suprasellar cistern. (B) Intraoperative image reveals resection of most of the tumor, including the right cavernous sinus component, with a small component remaining along the left sellar margin (arrow). (C) Postoperative image confirms successful resection of the left sellar residual component, although resection remains subtotal with residual tumor in the left cavernous sinus.

during the procedure using MR imaging. Two devices are currently approved by the Food and Drug Administration and are in their first large-scale clinical studies.[101–103] Both rely on dynamic MR imaging thermometry to determine the treatment margin within which tissue is predicted to necrose. Results to date are preliminary, but the technique has promise as an option for lesions that are deep and/or surgically unapproachable.

Intraoperative MR imaging: completion scans

In addition to confirming maximal resections, completion iMR imaging scans performed at the end of the surgery may be useful in revealing neurosurgical complications that otherwise would not be discovered until the routine postoperative MR imaging obtained around 24 hours. For example, expansile hematomas that compress the adjacent brain may be drained at the same operating room and anesthesia setting, and potentially reduce any negative effects on morbidity or mortality (**Fig. 11**). The postoperative MR imaging is usually obtained within 24 hours because enhancing granulation tissue develops after 24 hours; any enhancement before that time likely represents enhancing tumor. An example of this is seen in **Fig. 12**.

Intraoperative MR Imaging and Outcomes

Despite case series to date, little can be ascertained at this point regarding clinical outcomes of iMR imaging–guided surgery. One might anticipate that iMR imaging would be most advantageous for low-grade tumors that are infiltrative or otherwise difficult to resect completely, such as certain astrocytomas, oligodendrogliomas, and ependymomas. In a study of 156 patients with supratentorial low-grade gliomas resected using intraoperative MR imaging from 1997 to 2003, Claus and colleagues[104] reported high rates of GTR compared with historical controls, and measured a significant impact of GTR on survival. Low-grade gliomas are rare compared with glioblastoma, however, and for GBM the survival advantage of gross total resection is modest.[105–107] Low-grade gliomas are also relatively rare compared with meningiomas and metastases, most of which are encapsulated and for which iMR imaging offers little aid to GTR anyway. Therefore, it may be necessary in the short term to study the impact of iMR imaging on the extent of resection as a surrogate end point. It is then reasonable to anticipate a survival benefit (or absence of benefit) comparable to that determined by larger dedicated series of conventional surgery.

The authors retrospectively reviewed the literature to identify the subset of studies that measured residual tumor before and after intraoperative scan was obtained. **Tables 1** and **2** summarize these studies, citing degree-of-resection outcomes from 1999 to 2006, excluding studies with overlapping patient cohorts. Because well-circumscribed tumors are less likely to benefit from iMR imaging, the subset of gliomas is considered. While there were heterogeneous tumor histologies among the published studies, high-grade gliomas were

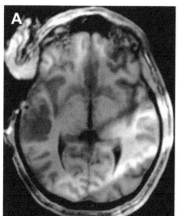 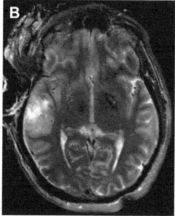 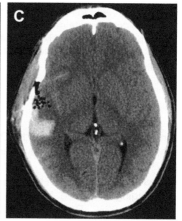

Fig. 11. Low-grade oligodendroglioma in the frontal operculum (not shown). Intraoperative (*A*) T1-weighted and (*B*) T2-weighted images reveal an acute hematoma below the operative site in the right temporal lobe. The hematoma was partially evacuated before the patient left the operating suite. (*C*) CT scan performed 8 hours later demonstrates a smaller temporal lobe hematoma, as well as subarachnoid hemorrhage in a few hemispheric sulci.

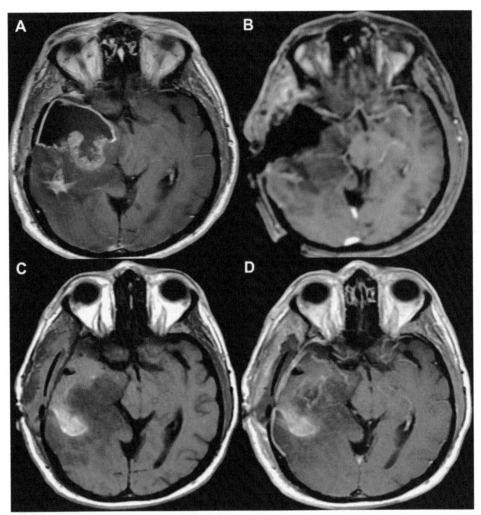

Fig. 12. Recurrent glioblastoma in the right temporal lobe. (*A*) Contrast T1-weighted image shows previous craniotomy with a large heterogeneously enhancing mass expanding most of the temporal lobe. (*B*) Intraoperative contrast T1-weighted image shows near total resection of the enhancing components, aside from small residual enhancing tumor in the posterior temporal lobe. (*C*) Noncontrast and (*D*) contrast T1-weighted images obtained at 48 hours demonstrate new curvilinear enhancement at the margins of the surgical cavity consistent with granulation tissue. Without the iMR imaging showing absent enhancement at the margins, this could be mistaken for residual enhancing tumor. Note that the posterior temporal enhancement is now obscured by hyperintense blood products.

represented in all but one study. Overall, the use of iMR imaging improved the extent of resection in 17% to 92% of cases. When the data for gliomas are analyzed separately, the use of iMR imaging improved the extent of resection in 24% to 92%. Perhaps unsurprisingly, GTR rates overall and for glioma-only were increased by iMR imaging in all studies that reported the data.[108] Bohinski and colleagues[109] reported the greatest success with iMR imaging, increasing their glioma GTR rate from 47.5%

to 97.5%. There were no complications related to the use of iMR imaging in any series. These results suggest that in some cases glioma resection is technically limited with neuronavigation alone, and iMR imaging is safe and generally sensitive for localizing residual tumor that might otherwise have been found only on postoperative scan. However, these results are potentially misleading. Selection bias is an issue in nonrandomized studies. Also, despite best intentions surgeons might stop resection earlier

Table 1
Demographics of select studies reporting extent of residual tumor at the time of iMR imaging and after further MR imaging–guided resection

Study	Field Strength (Tesla)	N (Tumors)	Age (yr) Mean	Age (yr) (Range)	Gender: N (%) Female	Glioma: N (%) High Grade	Glioma: N (%) Low Grade
Knauth et al, 1999[80]	0.2	41	N/A	N/A	N/A	38 (100)	0 (0)
Bohinski et al, 2001[109]	0.3	40	44	(18–75)	15 (37.5)	30 (75.0)	10 (25.0)
Schneider et al, 2001[108]	0.5	12	37	(20–63)	N/A	0 (0)	12 (100)
Nimsky et al, 2002[85]	0.2	230	40.9	(2–85)	122 (39.4)	48 (20.9)	47 (20.4)
Schulder and Carmel, 2003[110]	0.12	112	47	(3–81)	N/A	25 (22.3)	12 (10.7)
Hirschberg et al, 2005[111]	0.5	32	60.5	(38–77)	10 (31.3)	32 (100)	0 (0)
Schneider et al, 2005[81]	0.5	31	58.8	(39–75)	12 (38.7)	31 (100)	0 (0)
Muragaki et al, 2006[112]	0.3	96	39	(6–78)	46 (47.9)	63 (65.6)	30 (31.3)
Martin et al, 2000[113]	1.5	30	35	(14–70)	12 (40.0)	12 (40.0)	7 (23.3)
Nimsky et al, 2006[114]	1.5	137	47.1	(6–77)	55 (40.1)	98 (71.5)	39 (28.5)

Abbreviation: N/A, data not available.

Table 2
Extent of MR imaging–guided resection

Study	Improvement in Resection Completion: N (%)		Gross Total Resection Overall: N (%)		Gross Total Resection Glioma Only: N (%)		Complications Due to iMR Imaging
	Overall	Glioma Only	Pre-iMR Imaging	Post-iMR Imaging	Pre-iMR Imaging	Post-iMR Imaging	
Knauth et al, 1999[80]	17 (41.5)	17 (41.5)	15 (36.6)	31 (75.6)	15 (36.6)	31 (75.6)	0
Bohinski et al, 2001[109]	21 (52.5)	21 (52.5)	19 (47.5)	39 (97.5)	19 (47.5)	39 (97.5)	0
Schneider et al, 2001[108]	11 (91.7)	11 (91.7)	1 (8.3)	6 (50.0)	0 (0.0)	6 (50.0)	0
Nimsky et al, 2002[85]	40 (17.4)	23 (24.2)	56 (24.3)	82 (35.7)	35 (36.8)	49 (51.6)	0
Schulder and Carmel, 2003[110]	40 (35.7)	N/A	N/A	N/A	N/A	N/A	0
Hirschberg et al, 2005[111]	14 (43.8)	14 (43.75)	5 (15.6)	19 (59.4)	5 (15.6)	19 (59.4)	0
Schneider et al, 2005[81]	25 (80.6)	25 (80.6)	2 (6.5)	11 (35.5)	2 (6.5)	11 (35.5)	0
Muragaki et al, 2006[112]	N/A	N/A	N/A	44 (45.8)	N/A	N/A	0
Martin et al, 2000[113]	17 (56.7)	N/A	N/A	24 (80.0)	N/A	16 (84.2)	0
Nimsky et al, 2006[114]	56 (40.9)	56 (40.9)	37 (27.0)	55 (40.1)	37 (27.0)	55 (40.1)	0

when an iMR image is anticipated, with the expectation that residual tumor will be identified and localized to complete the resection.

SUMMARY

Whereas the advent of anatomic imaging truly revolutionized the practice of neurosurgery, the advanced imaging techniques outlined in this content are only slowly establishing their place in surgical practice. Surgical decision-making is necessarily conservative, and in this context even a low risk of false information is unacceptable. Still, as more validation studies and greater experience accrue, surgeons are becoming more comfortable weighing the quality of information from functional imaging studies. Results can vary by patient, paradigm, analysis approach and institution. It is imperative that surgeons, neuroradiologists, physicists and technicians work together to define their own standards of quality, interpretation and reporting and most of all to know when a study has failed. Advanced imaging information is highly complementary to established surgical "good practice" such as anatomic planning, awake craniotomy and ECS. However, the greatest impact of advanced imaging is perhaps on how neurosurgery is planned and discussed before the patient is ever brought to the operating room.

REFERENCES

1. Matz PG, Cobbs C, Berger MS. Intraoperative cortical mapping as a guide to the surgical resection of gliomas. J Neurooncol 1999;42(3):233–45.

2. Berger MS, Ojemann GA. Intraoperative brain mapping techniques in neuro-oncology. Stereotact Funct Neurosurg 1992;58(1–4):153–61.

3. Kombos T, Suss O. Neurophysiological basis of direct cortical stimulation and applied neuroanatomy of the motor cortex: a review. Neurosurg Focus 2009;27(4):E3.

4. Roux FE, Boulanouar K, Ranjeva JP, et al. Usefulness of motor functional MRI correlated to cortical mapping in Rolandic low-grade astrocytomas. Acta Neurochir (Wien) 1999;141(1):71–9.

5. Sunaert S. Presurgical planning for tumor resectioning. J Magn Reson Imaging 2006;23(6):887–905.

6. Martin PI, Naeser MA, Ho M, et al. Overt naming fMRI pre- and post-TMS: two nonfluent aphasia patients, with and without improved naming post-TMS. Brain Lang 2009;111(1):20–35.

7. Penfield W. The evidence for a cerebral vascular mechanism in epilepsy. Ann Intern Med 1933;7:303–10.

8. Hirsch J, Ruge MI, Kim KH, et al. An integrated functional magnetic resonance imaging procedure for preoperative mapping of cortical areas associated with tactile, motor, language, and visual functions. Neurosurgery 2000;47(3):711–21 [discussion: 721–2].

9. Tomczak RJ, Wunderlich AP, Wang Y, et al. fMRI for preoperative neurosurgical mapping of motor cortex and language in a clinical setting. J Comput Assist Tomogr 2000;24(6):927–34.

10. Petrovich N, Holodny AI, Tabar V, et al. Discordance between functional magnetic resonance imaging during silent speech tasks and intraoperative speech arrest. J Neurosurg 2005;103(2):267–74.

11. Krings T, Reinges MH, Erberich S, et al. Functional MRI for presurgical planning: problems, artefacts, and solution strategies. J Neurol Neurosurg Psychiatry 2001;70(6):749–60.

12. Roux FE, Boulanouar K, Ranjeva JP, et al. Cortical intraoperative stimulation in brain tumors as a tool to evaluate spatial data from motor functional MRI. Invest Radiol 1999;34(3):225–9.

13. Kim MJ, Holodny AI, Hou BL, et al. The effect of prior surgery on blood oxygen level-dependent functional MR imaging in the preoperative assessment of brain tumors. AJNR Am J Neuroradiol 2005;26(8):1980–5.

14. Sobel DF, Gallen CC, Schwartz BJ, et al. Locating the central sulcus: comparison of MR anatomic and magnetoencephalographic functional methods. AJNR Am J Neuroradiol 1993;14(4):915–25.

15. Ojemann G, Ojemann J, Lettich E, et al. Cortical language localization in left, dominant hemisphere. An electrical stimulation mapping investigation in 117 patients. J Neurosurg 1989;71(3):316–26.

16. Herholz K, Reulen HJ, von Stockhausen HM, et al. Preoperative activation and intraoperative stimulation of language-related areas in patients with glioma. Neurosurgery 1997;41(6):1253–60 [discussion: 1260–2].

17. Wada J, Rasmussen T. Intracarotid injection of sodium amytal for the lateralization of cerebral speech dominance. 1960. J Neurosurg 1960;17:266–82.

18. Branch C, Milner B, Rasmussen T. Intracarotid sodium amytal for the lateralization of cerebral speech dominance; observations in 123 patients. J Neurosurg 1964;21:399–405.

19. Kho KH, Leijten FS, Rutten GJ, et al. Discrepant findings for Wada test and functional magnetic resonance imaging with regard to language function: use of electrocortical stimulation mapping to confirm results. Case report. J Neurosurg 2005;102(1):169–73.

20. Fernandez G, Specht K, Weis S, et al. Intrasubject reproducibility of presurgical language lateralization and mapping using fMRI. Neurology 2003; 60(6):969–75.

21. Woermann FG, Jokeit H, Luerding R, et al. Language lateralization by Wada test and fMRI in 100 patients with epilepsy. Neurology 2003;61(5): 699–701.

22. Arora J, Pugh K, Westerveld M, et al. Language lateralization in epilepsy patients: fMRI validated with the Wada procedure. Epilepsia 2009;50(10): 2225–41.

23. Hou BL, Bradbury M, Peck KK, et al. Effect of brain tumor neovasculature defined by rCBV on BOLD fMRI activation volume in the primary motor cortex. Neuroimage 2006;32(2):489–97.

24. Fujiwara N, Sakatani K, Katayama Y, et al. Evoked-cerebral blood oxygenation changes in false-negative activations in BOLD contrast functional MRI of patients with brain tumors. Neuroimage 2004; 21(4):1464–71.

25. Sakatani K, Murata Y, Fujiwara N, et al. Comparison of blood-oxygen-level-dependent functional magnetic resonance imaging and near-infrared spectroscopy recording during functional brain activation in patients with stroke and brain tumors. J Biomed Opt 2007;12(6):062110.

26. Ulmer JL, Hacein-Bey L, Mathews VP, et al. Lesion-induced pseudo-dominance at functional magnetic resonance imaging: implications for preoperative assessments. Neurosurgery 2004;55(3):569–79 [discussion: 580–1].

27. Peck KK, Bradbury M, Petrovich N, et al. Presurgical evaluation of language using functional magnetic resonance imaging in brain tumor patients with previous surgery. Neurosurgery 2009;64(4):644–52 [discussion: 652–3].

28. Wilke M, Lidzba K, Staudt M, et al. Comprehensive language mapping in children, using functional magnetic resonance imaging: what's missing counts. Neuroreport 2005;16(9):915–9.

29. Rutten GJ, Ramsey NF, van Rijen PC, et al. Development of a functional magnetic resonance imaging protocol for intraoperative localization of critical temporoparietal language areas. Ann Neurol 2002;51(3):350–60.

30. Ruge MI, Victor J, Hosain S, et al. Concordance between functional magnetic resonance imaging and intraoperative language mapping. Stereotact Funct Neurosurg 1999;72(2–4):95–102.

31. Ruff IM, Petrovich Brennan NM, Peck KK, et al. Assessment of the language laterality index in patients with brain tumor using functional MR imaging: effects of thresholding, task selection, and prior surgery. AJNR Am J Neuroradiol 2008; 29(3):528–35.

32. Knecht S, Floel A, Drager B, et al. Degree of language lateralization determines susceptibility to unilateral brain lesions. Nat Neurosci 2002;5(7): 695–9.

33. Petrovich NM, Holodny AI, Brennan CW, et al. Isolated translocation of Wernicke's area to the right hemisphere in a 62-year-man with a temporo-parietal glioma. AJNR Am J Neuroradiol 2004;25(1): 130–3.

34. Holodny AI, Schulder M, Ybasco A, et al. Translocation of Broca's area to the contralateral hemisphere as the result of the growth of a left inferior frontal glioma. J Comput Assist Tomogr 2002; 26(6):941–3.

35. Plaza M, Gatignol P, Leroy M, et al. Speaking without Broca's area after tumor resection. Neurocase 2009;15(4):294–310.

36. Chang CY, Peck KK, Brennan NM, et al. Functional MRI in the presurgical evaluation of patients with brain tumors: characterization of the statistical threshold. Stereotact Funct Neurosurg 2010;88(1): 35–41.

37. Voyvodic JT, Petrella JR, Friedman AH. fMRI activation mapping as a percentage of local excitation: consistent presurgical motor maps without threshold adjustment. J Magn Reson Imaging 2009;29(4):751–9.

38. Abbott DF, Waites AB, Lillywhite LM, et al. fMRI assessment of language lateralization: an objective approach. Neuroimage 2010;50(4):1446–55.

39. Logothetis NK. What we can do and what we cannot do with fMRI. Nature 2008;453(7197):869–78.

40. Petrella JR, Shah LM, Harris KM, et al. Preoperative functional MR imaging localization of language and motor areas: effect on therapeutic decision making in patients with potentially resectable brain tumors. Radiology 2006;240(3):793–802.

41. Medina LS, Bernal B, Dunoyer C, et al. Seizure disorders: functional MR imaging for diagnostic evaluation and surgical treatment—prospective study. Radiology 2005;236(1):247–53.

42. Bassett SS, Yousem DM, Cristinzio C, et al. Familial risk for Alzheimer's disease alters fMRI activation patterns. Brain 2006;129(Pt 5):1229–39.

43. Wang L, Laviolette P, O'Keefe K, et al. Intrinsic connectivity between the hippocampus and posteromedial cortex predicts memory performance in cognitively intact older individuals. Neuroimage 2010;51(2):910–7.

44. Richardson MP, Strange BA, Thompson PJ, et al. Pre-operative verbal memory fMRI predicts postoperative memory decline after left temporal lobe resection. Brain 2004;127(Pt 11):2419–26.

45. Saur D, Ronneberger O, Kummerer D, et al. Early functional magnetic resonance imaging activations

predict language outcome after stroke. Brain 2010; 133(Pt 4):1252–64.

46. Powell HW, Richardson MP, Symms MR, et al. Preoperative fMRI predicts memory decline following anterior temporal lobe resection. J Neurol Neurosurg Psychiatry 2008;79(6):686–93.

47. Liu TT, Brown GG. Measurement of cerebral perfusion with arterial spin labeling: part 1. Methods. J Int Neuropsychol Soc 2007;13(3):517–25.

48. Detre JA, Wang J. Technical aspects and utility of fMRI using BOLD and ASL. Clin Neurophysiol 2002;113(5):621–34.

49. Kim JH, Lee JM, Jo HJ, et al. Defining functional SMA and pre-SMA subregions in human MFC using resting state fMRI: functional connectivity-based parcellation method. Neuroimage 2010; 49(3):2375–86.

50. Kokkonen SM, Nikkinen J, Remes J, et al. Preoperative localization of the sensorimotor area using independent component analysis of resting-state fMRI. Magn Reson Imaging 2009;27(6):733–40.

51. Julkunen P, Saisanen L, Danner N, et al. Comparison of navigated and non-navigated transcranial magnetic stimulation for motor cortex mapping, motor threshold and motor evoked potentials. Neuroimage 2009;44(3):790–5.

52. Rasmussen IA Jr, Lindseth F, Rygh OM, et al. Functional neuronavigation combined with intra-operative 3D ultrasound: initial experiences during surgical resections close to eloquent brain areas and future directions in automatic brain shift compensation of preoperative data. Acta Neurochir (Wien) 2007;149(4):365–78.

53. Gulati S, Berntsen EM, Solheim O, et al. Surgical resection of high-grade gliomas in eloquent regions guided by blood oxygenation level dependent functional magnetic resonance imaging, diffusion tensor tractography, and intraoperative navigated 3D ultrasound. Minim Invasive Neurosurg 2009;52(1):17–24.

54. Kamada K, Sawamura Y, Takeuchi F, et al. Functional identification of the primary motor area by corticospinal tractography. Neurosurgery 2007; 61(Suppl 1):166–76 [discussion: 176–7].

55. Nimsky C, Grummich P, Sorensen AG, et al. Visualization of the pyramidal tract in glioma surgery by integrating diffusion tensor imaging in functional neuronavigation. Zentralbl Neurochir 2005;66(3): 133–41.

56. Bürgel U, Madler B, Honey CR, et al. Fiber tracking with distinct software tools results in a clear diversity in anatomical fiber tract portrayal. Cen Eur Neurosurg 2009;70(1):27–35.

57. Berman JI, Berger MS, Chung SW, et al. Accuracy of diffusion tensor magnetic resonance imaging tractography assessed using intraoperative

subcortical stimulation mapping and magnetic source imaging. J Neurosurg 2007;107(3):488–94.

58. Leclercq D, Duffau H, Delmaire C, et al. Comparison of diffusion tensor imaging tractography of language tracts and intraoperative subcortical stimulations. J Neurosurg 2010;112(3):503–11.

59. Mikuni N, Okada T, Enatsu R, et al. Clinical impact of integrated functional neuronavigation and subcortical electrical stimulation to preserve motor function during resection of brain tumors. J Neurosurg 2007;106(4):593–8.

60. Kamada K, Todo T, Morita A, et al. Functional monitoring for visual pathway using real-time visual evoked potentials and optic-radiation tractography. Neurosurgery 2005;57(Suppl 1):121–7 [discussion: 121–7].

61. Talos IF, Zou KH, Kikinis R, et al. Volumetric assessment of tumor infiltration of adjacent white matter based on anatomic MRI and diffusion tensor tractography. Acad Radiol 2007;14(4):431–6.

62. Keles GE, Lundin DA, Lamborn KR, et al. Intraoperative subcortical stimulation mapping for hemispherical perirolandic gliomas located within or adjacent to the descending motor pathways: evaluation of morbidity and assessment of functional outcome in 294 patients. J Neurosurg 2004; 100(3):369–75.

63. Duffau H, Capelle L, Sichez N, et al. Intraoperative mapping of the subcortical language pathways using direct stimulations. An anatomo-functional study. Brain 2002;125(Pt 1):199–214.

64. Henry RG, Berman JI, Nagarajan SS, et al. Subcortical pathways serving cortical language sites: initial experience with diffusion tensor imaging fiber tracking combined with intraoperative language mapping. Neuroimage 2004;21(2):616–22.

65. Gil Robles S, Gatignol P, Capelle L, et al. The role of dominant striatum in language: a study using intraoperative electrical stimulations. J Neurol Neurosurg Psychiatry 2005;76(7):940–6.

66. Bello L, Gambini A, Castellano A, et al. Motor and language DTI Fiber Tracking combined with intraoperative subcortical mapping for surgical removal of gliomas. Neuroimage 2008;39(1):369–82.

67. Duffau H. Intraoperative direct subcortical stimulation for identification of the internal capsule, combined with an image-guided stereotactic system during surgery for basal ganglia lesions. Surg Neurol 2000;53(3):250–4.

68. Romano A, Ferrante M, Cipriani V, et al. Role of magnetic resonance tractography in the preoperative planning and intraoperative assessment of patients with intra-axial brain tumours. Radiol Med 2007;112(6):906–20.

69. Wu JS, Zhou LF, Tang WJ, et al. Clinical evaluation and follow-up outcome of diffusion tensor imaging-based functional neuronavigation: a prospective,

controlled study in patients with gliomas involving pyramidal tracts. Neurosurgery 2007;61(5):935–48 [discussion: 948–9].

70. Housepian EM. Stereotactic surgery: the early years. Neurosurgery 2004;55(5):1210–4.

71. Kurimoto M, Hayashi N, Kamiyama H, et al. Impact of neuronavigation and image-guided extensive resection for adult patients with supratentorial malignant astrocytomas: a single-institution retrospective study. Minim Invasive Neurosurg 2004; 47(5):278–83.

72. Wirtz CR, Albert FK, Schwaderer M, et al. The benefit of neuronavigation for neurosurgery analyzed by its impact on glioblastoma surgery. Neurol Res 2000;22(4):354–60.

73. Yoshikawa K, Kajiwara K, Morioka J, et al. Improvement of functional outcome after radical surgery in glioblastoma patients: the efficacy of a navigation-guided fence-post procedure and neurophysiological monitoring. J Neurooncol 2006;78(1):91–7.

74. Hall WA, Truwit CL. Intraoperative MR imaging. Magn Reson Imaging Clin N Am 2005;13(3): 533–43.

75. Wirtz CR, Bonsanto MM, Knauth M, et al. Intraoperative magnetic resonance imaging to update interactive navigation in neurosurgery: method and preliminary experience. Comput Aided Surg 1997;2(3–4):172–9.

76. Alexander E 3rd, Moriarty TM, Kikinis R, et al. The present and future role of intraoperative MRI in neurosurgical procedures. Stereotact Funct Neurosurg 1997;68(1–4 Pt 1):10–7.

77. Black PM, Moriarty T, Alexander E 3rd, et al. Development and implementation of intraoperative magnetic resonance imaging and its neurosurgical applications. Neurosurgery 1997;41(4):831–42 [discussion: 842–5].

78. Schwartz RB, Hsu L, Wong TZ, et al. Intraoperative MR imaging guidance for intracranial neurosurgery: experience with the first 200 cases. Radiology 1999;211(2):477–88.

79. McClain CD, Soriano SG, Goumnerova LC, et al. Detection of unanticipated intracranial hemorrhage during intraoperative magnetic resonance image-guided neurosurgery. Report of two cases. J Neurosurg 2007;106(Suppl 5):398–400.

80. Knauth M, Wirtz CR, Tronnier VM, et al. Intraoperative MR imaging increases the extent of tumor resection in patients with high-grade gliomas. AJNR Am J Neuroradiol 1999;20(9):1642–6.

81. Schneider JP, Trantakis C, Rubach M, et al. Intraoperative MRI to guide the resection of primary supratentorial glioblastoma multiforme—a quantitative radiological analysis. Neuroradiology 2005; 47(7):489–500.

82. Keles GE, Anderson B, Berger MS. The effect of extent of resection on time to tumor progression

and survival in patients with glioblastoma multiforme of the cerebral hemisphere. Surg Neurol 1999;52(4):371–9.

83. Lacroix M, Abi-Said D, Fourney DR, et al. A multivariate analysis of 416 patients with glioblastoma multiforme: prognosis, extent of resection, and survival. J Neurosurg 2001;95(2):190–8.

84. Zimmermann M, Seifert V, Trantakis C, et al. Open MRI-guided microsurgery of intracranial tumours in or near eloquent brain areas. Acta Neurochir (Wien) 2001;143(4):327–37.

85. Nimsky C, Ganslandt O, Tomandl B, et al. Low-field magnetic resonance imaging for intraoperative use in neurosurgery: a 5-year experience. Eur Radiol 2002;12(11):2690–703.

86. Tronnier VM, Bonsanto MM, Staubert A, et al. Comparison of intraoperative MR imaging and 3D-navigated ultrasonography in the detection and resection control of lesions. Neurosurg Focus 2001;10(2): E3. PMID:1674975.

87. Jones J, Ruge J. Intraoperative magnetic resonance imaging in pituitary macroadenoma surgery: an assessment of visual outcome. Neurosurg Focus 2007;23(5):E12.

88. Maciunas RJ, Dean D, Lewin J, et al. Integration of neurosurgical image guidance and an intraoperative magnetic resonance scanner. The University Hospitals of Cleveland experience. Stereotact Funct Neurosurg 2003;80(1–4):136–9.

89. Samdani A, Jallo GI. Intraoperative MRI: technology, systems, and application to pediatric brain tumors. Surg Technol Int 2007;16:236–43.

90. Gasser T, Ganslandt O, Sandalcioglu E, et al. Intraoperative functional MRI: implementation and preliminary experience. Neuroimage 2005;26(3): 685–93.

91. Nimsky C, Ganslandt O, Hastreiter P, et al. Preoperative and intraoperative diffusion tensor imaging-based fiber tracking in glioma surgery. Neurosurgery 2005;56(1):130–7 [discussion: 138].

92. Ulmer S, Helle M, Jansen O, et al. Intraoperative dynamic susceptibility contrast weighted magnetic resonance imaging (iDSC-MRI)—technical considerations and feasibility. Neuroimage 2009;45(1): 38–43.

93. Bohinski RJ, Warnick RE, Gaskill-Shipley MF, et al. Intraoperative magnetic resonance imaging to determine the extent of resection of pituitary macroadenomas during transsphenoidal microsurgery. Neurosurgery 2001;49(5):1133–43 [discussion: 1143–4].

94. Ahn JY, Jung JY, Kim J, et al. How to overcome the limitations to determine the resection margin of pituitary tumours with low-field intra-operative MRI during trans-sphenoidal surgery: usefulness of gadolinium-soaked cotton pledgets. Acta Neurochir (Wien) 2008;150(8):763–71 [discussion: 771].

95. Darakchiev BJ, Tew JM Jr, Bohinski RJ, et al. Adaptation of a standard low-field (0.3-T) system to the operating room: focus on pituitary adenomas. Neurosurg Clin N Am 2005;16(1):155–64.

96. Fahlbusch R, Ganslandt O, Buchfelder M, et al. Intraoperative magnetic resonance imaging during transsphenoidal surgery. J Neurosurg 2001;95(3): 381–90.

97. Gerlach R, du Mesnil de Rochemont R, Gasser T, et al. Feasibility of Polestar N20, an ultra-low-field intraoperative magnetic resonance imaging system in resection control of pituitary macroadenomas: lessons learned from the first 40 cases. Neurosurgery 2008;63(2):272–84 [discussion: 284–5].

98. Schwartz TH, Stieg PE, Anand VK. Endoscopic transsphenoidal pituitary surgery with intraoperative magnetic resonance imaging. Neurosurgery 2006;58(Suppl 1):ONS44–51 [discussion: ONS44–51].

99. Nimsky C, Ganslandt O, von Keller B, et al. Intraoperative high-field MRI: anatomical and functional imaging. Acta Neurochir Suppl 2006;98:89–95.

100. Fahlbusch R, Keller B, Ganslandt O, et al. Transsphenoidal surgery in acromegaly investigated by intraoperative high-field magnetic resonance imaging. Eur J Endocrinol 2005;153(2):239–48.

101. Carpentier A, McNichols RJ, Stafford RJ, et al. Real-time magnetic resonance-guided laser thermal therapy for focal metastatic brain tumors. Neurosurgery 2008;63(1 Suppl 1):ONS21–8 [discussion: ONS28–29].

102. Schwarzmaier HJ, Eickmeyer F, von Tempelhoff W, et al. MR-guided laser-induced interstitial thermotherapy of recurrent glioblastoma multiforme: preliminary results in 16 patients. Eur J Radiol 2006;59(2):208–15.

103. Schwarzmaier HJ, Eickmeyer F, von Tempelhoff W, et al. MR-guided laser irradiation of recurrent glioblastomas. J Magn Reson Imaging 2005;22(6): 799–803.

104. Claus EB, Horlacher A, Hsu L, et al. Survival rates in patients with low-grade glioma after intraoperative magnetic resonance image guidance. Cancer 2005;103(6):1227–33.

105. Whittle IR. Surgery for gliomas. Curr Opin Neurol 2002;15(6):663–9.

106. Sanai N, Berger MS. Glioma extent of resection and its impact on patient outcome. Neurosurgery 2008;62(4):753–64 [discussion: 764–6].

107. Stummer W, Reulen HJ, Meinel T, et al. Extent of resection and survival in glioblastoma multiforme: identification of and adjustment for bias. Neurosurgery 2008;62(3):564–76 [discussion: 564–76].

108. Schneider JP, Schulz T, Schmidt F, et al. Gross-total surgery of supratentorial low-grade gliomas under intraoperative MR guidance. AJNR Am J Neuroradiol 2001;22(1):89–98.

109. Bohinski RJ, Kokkino AK, Warnick RE, et al. Glioma resection in a shared-resource magnetic resonance operating room after optimal image-guided frameless stereotactic resection. Neurosurgery 2001;48(4):731–42 [discussion: 742–4].

110. Schulder M, Carmel PW. Intraoperative magnetic resonance imaging: impact on brain tumor surgery. Cancer Control 2003;10(2):115–24.

111. Hirschberg H, Samset E, Hol PK, et al. Impact of intraoperative MRI on the surgical results for high-grade gliomas. Minim Invasive Neurosurg 2005; 48(2):77–84.

112. Muragaki Y, Iseki H, Maruyama T, et al. Usefulness of intraoperative magnetic resonance imaging for glioma surgery. Acta Neurochir Suppl 2006;98: 67–75.

113. Martin AJ, Hall WA, Liu H, et al. Brain tumor resection: intraoperative monitoring with high-field-strength MR imaging-initial results. Radiology 2000;215(1):221–8.

114. Nimsky C, Ganslandt O, Buchfelder M, et al. Intraoperative visualization for resection of gliomas: the role of functional neuronavigation and intraoperative 1.5 T MRI. Neurol Res 2006;28(5):482–7.

Imaging of Brain Tumors: Perfusion/ Permeability

Gerard Thompson, MB ChB, MRCS*,
Samantha Jane Mills, MB ChB, MRCP, FRCR,
Stavros Michael Stivaros, MB ChB, FRCR,
Alan Jackson, PhD, FRCP, FRCR, FBIR

KEYWORDS

- Brain tumor • Glioma • Dynamic imaging
- Perfusion • Permeability

Most current clinical CT and MR imaging systems are capable of acquiring images with high temporal and spatial resolution data. Improvements in entry-level MR imaging technology have allowed for routine clinical use of certain relatively complex imaging sequences previously restricted to research studies.[1] Parallel developments at the vanguard of imaging technology have similarly facilitated the development and refinement of techniques aimed at quantification of dynamic physiological processes. Quantitative images of physiological parameters, such as blood flow, should, theoretically, be independent of the imaging modality or the individual system used.[2,3] Although this is rarely the case in practice (discussed later), the paradigm of clinically acceptable quantitative imaging with sufficient repeatability and reproducibility represents a shift in the approach to radiologic investigations. Such imaging measures are designated as biomarkers: "characteristics that are objectively measured and evaluated as an indicator of a normal biologic processes or pathogenic processes or pharmacologic responses to therapeutic intervention."[4] The minimally invasive description of physiological and pathophysiological processes has clear use in screening, diagnosis, prognostication, and treatment monitoring. Examples of currently accepted biomarkers include circulating tumor markers, such as prostate-specific antigen and CA 125. The performance characteristics of any measurement under consideration as a biomarker are key. Sensitivity, specificity, repeatability, reproducibility, and logistics must be taken into consideration. Unfortunately, the development of imaging biomarkers is more complex than that of circulating biomarkers, and standardization is currently lacking. Analyzing the same data with a variety of the commercially available software can result in significant discrepancies[5] and when considering additional variations in scanner age, make, model, software version, and acquisition parameters, standardization can seem even more challenging. Despite these issues, certain imaging biomarkers are now widely used in clinical trials and increasingly finding routine clinical use. Oncology is an area with intense interest in imaging biomarkers. Although histopathology remains the gold standard diagnostic and prognostic tool, it is, by definition, invasive, precludes true longitudinal follow-up, and is subject to significant sampling bias. Given the importance of angiogenesis in tumor development,[6] imaging biomarkers able to characterize the vascular microenvironment within tissues have been the subject of extensive research, largely driven by the development of antiangiogenic and vascular targeting agents for cancer treatment.[3] This

School of Cancer and Imaging Sciences, Wolfson Molecular Imaging Centre, The University of Manchester, 27 Palatine Road, Manchester, England M20 3LJ, UK
* Corresponding author.
E-mail address: gerard.thompson@manchester.ac.uk

neuroimaging.theclinics.com

article reviews the imaging biomarkers of micro-vascular structure and function in common use and describes their potential clinical use.

POTENTIAL MICROVASCULAR IMAGING BIOMARKERS FOR NEURO-ONCOLOGY

Tumor growth is dependent on angiogenesis with consequent development of tumoral neo-vasculature. The angiogenic neovasculature commonly exhibits increased endothelial perme-ability to medium- and large-sized molecules[7,8] as a direct effect of cytokine stimulation, which can be rapidly reversed by inhibition of the angiogenic pathway.[9] In tumors, neoangiogene-sis commonly leads to the development of distorted vascular beds, characterized by an excessive proportion of blood vessels and abnormal blood vessel morphology and flow characteristics.[10] The development of pertinent imaging biomarkers has consequently focused on the estimation of capillary endothelial perme-ability and methods to characterize vascular density, vascular tortuosity, and other morpho-logic abnormalities, which represent the cumula-tive effects of the unchecked angiogenic process. Blood flow within the tumor vascula-ture, for example, reflects the structure of the vascular bed and also is affected by interstitial pressure, the arterial input vessel hierarchy, and local arteriovenous pressure difference.[11,12] Although the measurement of blood flow char-acteristics is often referred to in the literature as perfusion or perfusion-weighted imaging, a distinction must be made between these two distinct properties. Perfusion is the process by which blood flow through a tissue provides nutrition and removes metabolic by-products. Blood flow through a tissue, or voxel, can occur without contributing to capillary perfusion and high flow is not always metabolically useful.[11] Notwithstanding this distinction, imaging tech-niques used to directly quantify perfusion include $H_2^{15}O$ positron emission tomography (PET)[13] and xenon-enhanced CT.[14] These tech-niques are considered gold standard measure-ments of perfusion because the tracers have a high transfer coefficient and their concentra-tion in brain tissue can be considered entirely dependent on vascular concentration and flow. Their use is logistically limited and alternative methods to estimate perfusion or other compo-nents of regional blood flow are more commonly used. Delivery models of freely diffusible tracers also preclude determination of permeability characteristics, and other approaches, therefore, are required.

IMAGING TECHNIQUES FOR MICROVASCULAR CHARACTERIZATION

A detailed description of the range of imaging and image analysis techniques used to produce biomarkers of microvascular structure and func-tion is beyond the scope of this article; interested readers are directed to recent comprehensive review articles.[2,15-17] In practice, three generic approaches are in common use: (1) dynamic contrast-enhanced (DCE) imaging; (2) arterial spin labeling (ASL); and (3) vascular space occu-pancy (VASO) imaging.

An overview of each of these approaches is presented, highlighting those aspects of the tech-niques that enhance understanding of potential clinical applications.

DCE Imaging

DCE techniques are the most commonly applied imaging techniques for the characterization of microvascular structure and function.[2] Rapid, serial images are acquired during the administra-tion of an intravenous contrast agent (**Fig. 1**). These techniques can be applied to MR imaging (DCE–MRI) and CT (DCE-CT). The design of acqui-sition protocols is dependent on the image anal-ysis approach chosen,[15] which requires minimal standards of signal-to-noise ratio and temporal resolution. To achieve these goals, significant compromises may have to be made in spatial resolution or volume coverage.

The radiation doses of DCE-CT have restricted its application in drug trials, where repeated imaging is required. In clinical practice, however, DCE-CT is rapidly becoming a routine investiga-tion, aided by the availability of modern CT equip-ment, the quantitative characteristics of the Hounsfield unit (or CT number), and the relation-ship between the attenuation and concentration of iodinated contrast media. DCE–MRI is osten-sibly performed through the off-license use of clinically approved gadolinium-based contrast agents, although superparamagnetic and larger molecular weight agents are used in research. Two approaches are common, exploiting the susceptibility or relaxivity effects of the contrast media on the signal echo. It is worth mentioning at this point that the terminology in dynamic MR imaging can cause confusion. While DCE-MRI is a generic term for dynamic contrast-enhanced MR imaging, the terms dynamic relaxivity contrast enhanced (DRCE) and dynamic susceptibility contrast enhanced (DSCE) are not widely used to distinguish the two approaches. Instead, DCE-MRI is used to refer to T_1-weighted relaxivity imaging, while dynamic susceptibility contrast

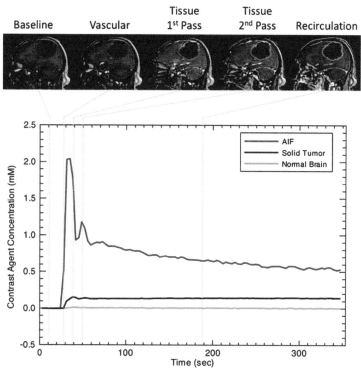

Fig. 1. Time series of DCE images and the resulting concentration-time curve. The dynamic series of images shows the passage of the contrast agent bolus over a given time course. The changes in signal intensity are converted to changes in contrast agent concentration. The graph depicts changes in contrast agent concentration for 3 given regions of interest: artery (*red*), solid enhancing tumor (*blue*), and normal-appearing white matter (*green*).

(DSC)-MRI is used to refer to T2- or T2*-weighted susceptibility imaging. T_1-weighted acquisitions are also frequently referred to as permeability imaging, while T2- or T2*-weighted techniques and CT are referred to as perfusion imaging due to their primary uses. As a result, perfusion weighted imaging (PWI) and perfusion CT (PCT) are sometimes used to refer to DSC-MRI and DCE-CT respectively. Furthermore, a dual echo MR approach which aims to provide susceptibility and relaxivity based measures in a single acquisition has been developed, and is usually prefixed by DE (dual echo).[18] DSC–MR imaging has been widely applied in neuro-oncology, its acceptance promoted over CT by less onerous acquisition and postprocessing requirements. There are, however, several significant issues that should be appreciated: T2*-weighted acquisitions commonly have significant T_1 sensitivity, such that any contrast leakage produces artifactual elevations in the signal time course curve.[10,19] Because the susceptibility effects manifest themselves as reductions in signal-echo intensity, relaxivity effects counter these and produce misleading signal changes. This is particularly problematic in tumors where blood-brain barrier breakdown has occurred. Acquisitions must,

therefore, be designed to minimize the T_1 effect. The most common solution is the use of low flip angle gradient-echo sequences, which have low T_1 sensitivity. This has an adverse effect, however, on the signal-to-noise ratio. A full discussion of these issues is given in the article by Kassner and colleagues.[10] Leakage correction can also be applied to minimise susceptibility effects by pre-dosing with gadolinium prior to acquisition—thereby saturating the extravascular extracellular space—by using software methods such as gamma variate fitting and baseline correction, or by a combination of all of these.[20–22]

DCE-MRI utilises T_1-weighted acquisitions in which relaxivity effects dominate. The major drawback of this approach is the difficulty in resolving the signal change effects resulting from intravascular contrast, contrast leakage, and contrast dispersion within the extravascular extracellular space (EES). Resolution of these and other issues has driven the development of a range of analysis approaches, which are discussed briefly.

Analysis of DCE Data

Early DCE–MRI studies used simple measurements of MR signal change over a specific time course or the change in morphology of the enhancement-time curve.[23,24] Such parameters are unpredictably dependent on the scanning protocol and do not distinguish signal changes due to variations in blood flow (*F*), blood volume (*V*), and contrast leakage.[25] Nonetheless, semi-quantitative techniques provide clear clinical benefit in certain applications. To improve reproducibility and repeatability, the majority of more recent techniques involve the conversion of signal change to contrast agent concentration change over time, which is derived from the primary acquisitions. As alluded to previously, for CT data this is straightforward because the relationship between iodinated contrast agent concentration and the change in attenuation is linear. For DSC–MRI, the relation is nonlinear but easily calculated. The calculation of contrast concentration images from DCE–MRI data requires at least the accurate measurement of local tissue longitudinal relaxivity before contrast administration.[15] As with all facets of MR imaging, the accuracy of T_1 measurement is a function of the imaging parameters used and can involve a trade-off with acquisition time on busy clinical scanners.

Contrast concentration time course data can be analyzed using a range of approaches, including pharmacokinetic models. The simplest of these is the initial area under the contrast concentration curve (IAUC). The IAUC is widely used in DCE analysis despite having little physiological specificity because it is highly reproducible and easy to calculate. The most commonly used approaches beyond this are designed to calculate physiological parameters, such as blood flow. The profusion of analysis approaches can be confusing, because many seem superficially to measure the same parameter (eg, flow) but do so in sometimes subtly distinct ways, such that results are not directly comparable.

As a result of the increasing adoption of disparate pharmacokinetic models, an attempt has been made to standardize the symbolic notation and nomenclature of the pertinent parameters. A selection of these is shown in **Table 1**. The most complete of the extant approaches is the adiabatic tissue homogeneity model (AATH),[26] which produces estimates of blood flow (*F*), capillary endothelial permeability surface area product per unit mass of tissue (*PS*), fractional blood-plasma volume (v_p), and volume of extravascular, extracellular space (EES) per unit volume of tissue (v_e). Although such physiological specificity is appealing, the demands on data quality in terms of signal-to-noise ratio and temporal resolution are highly restrictive. Consequently, simpler pharmacokinetic models, which are less specific but

exhibit other desirable performance characteristics, are more widely used. Many of these combine the effects of *F* and *PS* into a single variable: the volume transfer constant between plasma and the EES (K^{trans}). Although the usefulness of K^{trans} is widely published, comparison of literature values is difficult due to the high dependence on the pharmacokinetic model and image acquisition parameters used. The result is that K^{trans} estimates in different publications may represent different combinations of underlying physiological variables and, in addition, it is impossible to reliably determine which of these physiological characteristics dominate observed variations in K^{trans}.[2]

Using DSC-MRI, calculation of cerebral blood flow (CBF) can be performed by comparison of the contrast concentration time course changes in a feeding artery (the arterial input function) with the changes in individual tissue voxels. The most common approach uses a deconvolution analysis to estimate CBF, cerebral blood volume (CBV), and mean transit time (MTT).[27] Although widely used in ischemic cerebrovascular disease, this approach is less satisfactory in neuro-oncology due to regional variation in arterial flow characteristics within the tumor. Relative measures of CBV, CBF and MTT can be more simply derived from the DSC-MRI intensity-time curves based on the area under the curve—related to volume—and the time taken for the bolus to complete the first pass—related to MTT and therefore to CBF. First pass gamma-variate fitting is often used for this approach. For those individuals wishing further information on novel approaches to absolute flow measurement from DCE-MRI analysis, simple graphic analysis techniques to estimate flow based on the microsphere theorem are also used as described by Vallee and colleagues,[28] although their usefulness in neuro-oncology is not yet clear.

Vascular Space Occupancy Imaging

In light of the technical problems associated with dynamic MR imaging, recent work has addressed the use of other tissue contrast mechanisms for examining tumor vascularity. VASO imaging is a T_1-weighted technique, which differentiates blood from tissue to interrogate blood volume. It was originally used to calculate blood volume changes in experimental cortical functional magnetic resonance imaging (fMRI)[29,30] but has since been applied to tumor imaging.[31] While usually employing an inversion pulse to null intravascular T_1-weighted signal, a simple approach to VASO, whereby T_1-weighted images before and after contrast administration are subtracted and weighted, produces appropriate measures of

Table 1
Commonly used parameters and the agreed international abbreviations and units are listed

Symbol	Short Name	Unit
Measured Quantities		
C_p	Tracer concentration in arterial blood plasma—arterial input function (MR imaging or CT)	mM
C_a	Tracer concentration in arterial blood—arterial input function (PET)	kBq/mL
C_t	Concentration of contrast agent at time, t, in every voxel	mM or kBq/mL
Estimated or predetermined quantities		
MTT	Mean transit time	S
T	Capillary transit time	S
Calculated quantities		
F	Blood flow	mL g^{-1} min^{-1}
CBF	Cerebral blood flow	mL g^{-1} min^{-1}
P	Total capillary-wall permeability	cm min^{-1}
PS	Permeability surface area product per unit mass of tissue	mL g^{-1} min^{-1}
E	Extraction fraction	None
K^{trans}	Volume transfer constant between plasma and EES	Min^{-1}
K_{ep}	Rate constant between EES and plasma	Min^{-1}
K_i	Unidirectional influx constant	Min^{-1}
CBV	Cerebral blood volume	mL
v_p	Fractional blood-plasma volume	None
V_a	Fractional blood volume	None
v_e	Volume of EES per unit volume tissue	None
V_D	Volume of distribution of tracer	None
IAUC	Initial area under gadolinium contrast agent concentration–time curve	mM min

Abbreviation: EES, extravascular, extracellular space.
Reproduced from O'Connor JP, Jackson A, Asselin MC, et al. Quantitative imaging biomarkers in the clinical development of targeted therapeutics: current and future perspectives. Lancet Oncol 2008;9(8):766–76; with permission.

relative (rCBV) or absolute cerebral blood volume in non-leaky tissues.[32] In diseases such as tumors, where BBB breakdown has occurred, the signal increase reflects both blood volume and permeability.[33] The values in normal tissue may be useful, however, for the calibration of CBV in other techniques.

Arterial Spin Labeling

ASL techniques exploit the differences in magnetization between static tissues and labeled blood water molecules produced by having a labeling slab or slice positioned over the feeding arterial supply. This produces pairs of flow-sensitized and control images in which the static tissue signals are identical but where the magnetization of the inflowing blood differs. The subtraction of control from labeled images yields a signal difference, which directly reflects local perfusion. The signal difference depends on many parameters including blood flow, the T_1 of blood and tissue, and the time taken for labelled blood to reach the imaging region (labeling delay). Signal differences can be as low as 1%, however conspicuity can be improved by employing inversion pulses to null the signal from static tissue before and after labelling. Despite the plethora of acronyms found in the ASL literature, there are two main classes of ASL techniques: continuous ASL (CASL) and pulsed ASL (PASL).[34–36] In CASL, the supplying blood is continuously labeled below the imaging slab, until the tissue magnetization reaches a steady state. The PASL approach labels a thick slab of arterial blood at a single instance in time, and the imaging is performed after a sufficient delay to allow distribution in the tissue of interest. As with other dynamic imaging techniques, the final interpretation of ASL flow measurements depends on the labeling process and the subsequent analysis.[17] Each has particular strengths and weaknesses and, therefore, lends itself to different imaging problems, although a compromise approach, known as pseudo- or pulsed CASL, has been developed, which may have benefits for more general use. Despite the challenges associated with ASL, it remains a desirable technique due to the absolute measures of cerebral blood flow it produces, and the fact that endogenous gadolinium contrast agents are not required.

COMMON BIOMARKERS IN NEURO-ONCOLOGY

A few potentially available imaging biomarkers have been identified that enjoy increasingly wide use in neuro-oncologic applications for reasons of practicality and performance. Those of particular importance are discussed.

CBV

CBV can be measured from DCE or VASO imaging data using simple and robust analysis techniques. Values of CBV from different scanners and analysis packages vary less than other imaging biomarkers. Consequently, there has been considerable clinical application of CBV as a microvascular imaging biomarker. Most analysis techniques produce unitless scalar maps of rCBV. Calibration by comparison to normal-appearing white matter in which the CBV is given unit value is common, but the absolute estimation of CBV by calibration to a large venous structure in which CBV is assumed to be 100% is often preferred if practicable. Considerable confusion can be engendered by the use of the term, *regional* cerebral blood volume—also abbreviated to rCBV—and as with all studies of imaging based biomarkers, the reader is strongly encouraged to review the particular acquisition methods and analysis techniques employed when assessing the literature. Current evidence suggests that measurements of CBV DSC-MRI and DSC-MRI are comparable, and therefore provide commensurate clinical information.[37]

K^{trans}

K^{trans} can be derived from any form of DCE data, although it is unusual to estimate this from DSC–MRI due to technical limitations. As discussed previously, the physiological meaning of K^{trans} estimates are entirely dependent on the pharmacokinetic model used to derive them. In general

terms, models can be divided by their complexity into three main groups with decreasing physiological specificity: those that estimate F, PS and v_p separately (eg, AATH)[26]; those that estimate v_p but combine F and PS into K^{trans} (eg, Tofts and colleagues)[38]; and those that combine v_p, F and PS into K^{trans} (eg, Tofts and Kermode).[39] Increasing physiological specificity may be offset by more stringent acquisition requirements, and greater difficulty in accurate model fitting to the experimental data. K^{trans} should, therefore, be measured using an approach which strikes a balance between the need for specificity and the availability of resources given the individual goal that is to be achieved.

Estimates of Flow

Estimate of flow (F) can be derived using DSC-MRI, DCE-MRI, DCE-CT, or ASL. Different techniques analyze slightly different components of the flow process and are, in general terms, not comparable. In neuro-imaging, the flow is often couched in the tissue-specific term, CBF, mirroring nomenclature for blood volume. Again, the lower case 'r' prefix most commonly denotes a relative measure calibrated to normal-appearing white matter. Other terms that may be encountered include blood flow, tumor blood flow, and their relative equivalents. Scrutiny of the acquisition and analysis methods must be made before comparison with published values or deciding on the most suitable technique to implement locally.

Interpreting Parametric Image Data

As with the techniques used to generate them, parametric image data can be analyzed and interpreted in a variety of ways. Some investigators advocate limiting analysis to a defined region of interest containing voxels encompassing a tumor or the enhancing portion of a tumor. This approach—often referred to as hot-spot analysis—produces a single value, such as maximum rCBV (rCBV$_{max}$), to describe a region of interest that may possess high spatial heterogeneity. Advocates cite simplicity and reproducibility of such techniques, although this level of data reduction may be excessive, resulting in loss of usable information. Full voxel-by-voxel analysis—while retaining maximal spatial information—is problematic because it is more prone to noise and model-fitting errors. This has resulted in the increased use of summary measures, which describe the morphology and properties of the parameter distribution histogram,[40–43] or other summary descriptors, such as fractals, which retain greater information regarding spatial distribution.[44] These approaches represent a compromise between data reduction and immunity to noise and have been shown to possess desirable performance characteristics as diagnostic and response biomarkers.

APPLICATIONS OF IMAGING BIOMARKERS IN NEURO-ONCOLOGY

The biomarkers of microvascular structure and function are increasingly demonstrating clinical potential in a variety of roles. Two of the major diagnostic challenges in neuroimaging—the differential diagnosis of the solitary enhancing lesion and the subtyping of gliomas—have been addressed through the use of vascular biomarkers.

Differential Diagnosis of Cerebral Tumors

Differentiating abscess and tumor
Several investigators have demonstrated discrimination between abscess and cerebral tumor based on maps of CBV. CBV values in abscesses are lower than normal white matter (<1% compared with approximately 2%) whereas values in high-grade gliomas and metastases are generally higher (>3%, P<.01).[45,46] As with many imaging biomarkers, performance is improved if used in conjunction with other parameters, and specificity is increased if CBV is combined with calculations from diffusion-weighted imaging of the apparent diffusion coefficient, which is lower in the center of abscesses.[45,47,48] More recent work has suggested that analysis using more complex models, capable of producing estimates of K^{trans}, may also be justified on the basis of increased discriminative power.[49]

Differentiating lymphoma and glioma
The absence of tumor neovascularization in malignant lymphoma leads to low rCBV in comparison with high-grade glioma (HGG) (**Fig. 2**).[50–52] Liao and colleagues[53] found that the rCBV$_{max}$ ratio of primary intracranial lymphomas was 1.72 ± 0.59 whereas that of HGG was 4.86 ± 2.18 ($P = .001$). Early studies with ASL have shown that the significantly higher tumor blood flow in glioblastoma multiforme (GBM) compared with cerebral lymphomas allows effective discrimination with a threshold value of 1.2 for CBF, providing clinically useful performance characteristics (sensitivity of 97%, specificity of 80%, positive predictive value of 94%, and negative predictive value of 89%).[54]

Differentiating primary and secondary brain tumors
Perfusion MR imaging may also be helpful in differentiating primary HGG from solitary cerebral metastases (see **Fig. 2**). Although the tumors themselves exhibit some differences with higher values of mean rCBV in HGG (1.7 ± 0.37) than for metastases (0.54 ± 0.18), considerable improvement in discrimination is provided by examining the peritumoral region where the differences in mechanisms underlying peritumoral edema effect the microvascular environment. Edema surrounding metastatic tumors is predominantly vasogenic edema, that is, increased interstitial water content due to microvascular extra-vasation of plasma fluid and proteins.[55,56] In contrast, the peritumoral region in HGG represents a variable combination of vasogenic edema, cytotoxic edema, and infiltrating tumor cells.[55,57] Cha and colleagues[58,59] demonstrated higher CBV values around HGG than around metastases. They subsequently demonstrated that the first-pass bolus peak height and percentage recovery of signal in the peritumoural region on T2*-weighted DSC images could differentiate between HGG and solitary metastases.[60] This observation is in line with the biologic features of the tumors and is valuable because the measurements can be performed on signal time course curve data. By obviating more complex analysis, certain key performance characteristics, including repeatability and reproducibility, can be improved to a degree that outweighs potential reductions in sensitivity, specificity, precision, and accuracy. Logistic regression analysis showed that a percentage signal recovery less than 66% within the contrast-enhancing region of the tumor had a specificity of 100% and a sensitivity of 69% in correctly identifying that a tumor is not a GBM. Similar findings have also been reported with ASL, where CBF was significantly higher in peritumoral, nonenhancing, T2-hyperintense regions of GBM compared with metastases.[54] A threshold value of 0.5 for CBF provided sensitivity, specificity, positive predictive value, and negative predictive value of 100%, 71%, 94%, and 100%, respectively.

Applications in other intracranial lesions
Comparisons of common intracranial extra-axial with enhancing intra-axial tumors have shown that the extra-axial masses typically have higher values of CBV (see **Fig. 2**).[52] Meningiomas, as expected, exhibit higher values of rCBV than those seen in neurinomas or schwannomas.[7,22,61,62] In addition, measurements of volume of EES per unit v_e from DCE–MRI data were higher in

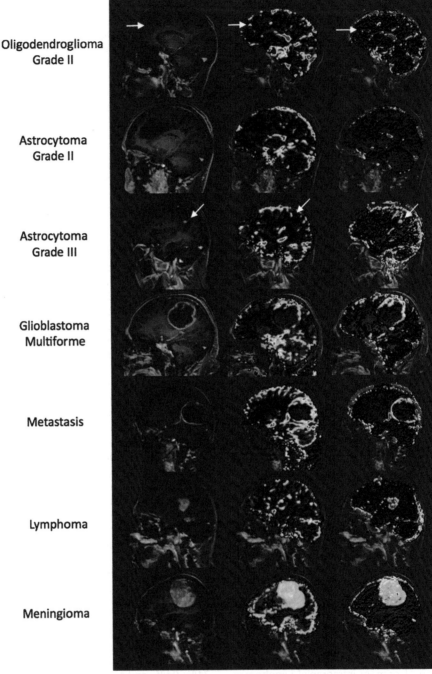

Oligodendroglioma
Grade II

Astrocytoma
Grade II

Astrocytoma
Grade III

Glioblastoma
Multiforme

Metastasis

Lymphoma

Meningioma

Fig. 2. Examples of perfusion and permeability maps for a variety of histologically distinct intracranial tumors. Post-contrast T_1-weighted images (*left column*) with overlaid DSC-MRI rCBV (*centre column*) and DCE-MRI K^{trans} (*right column*) for: oligodendroglioma (grade II)—there are focal increases in rCBV and K^{trans} within the tumor (*white arrows*) when compared with normal-appearing white matter; astrocytoma (grade II)—rCBV and K^{trans} within the tumor are similar normal-appearing white matter; anaplastic astrocytoma (grade III)—marked increase in K^{trans} and small increase in rCBV (*white arrows*) is seen within the tumor when compared with normal-appearing white matter; GBM (grade IV)—the tumor exhibits high rCBV and high K^{trans} within the solid enhancing component, with low/zero rCBV and K^{trans} within the necrotic core; metastasis (primary breast carcinoma)—rCBV and K^{trans} are elevated in comparison with normal-appearing white matter; lymphoma—K^{trans} is elevated within the tumor mass whereas the rCBV remains comparable with normal-appearing white matter; and meningioma (grade I)—the extremely high values of rCBV and K^{trans} within the tumor in comparison with normal-appearing white matter reflect the dural blood supply of the lesion, lying outside the blood-brain barrier.

meningioma than in glioma but were consistently highest in vestibular schwannoma ($P<.001$).[22] These results are in concordance with histologic studies, which have demonstrated large extracellular spaces in schwannomas.[63] It has also been suggested that DCE–MRI may have a role in differentiating meningiomas with atypical conventional MR imaging findings from malignant intra-axial tumors[64] and in the prospective characterization of meningiomas. Yang and colleagues[65] found mean rCBV values lower (8.02 ± 4.74) in typical meningiomas (n = 15) than in atypical meningiomas (10.50 ± 2.1, n = 7). In this same group of patients, K^{trans} was lower in the typical group (0.0016 s^{-1} ± 0.0012) than the atypical group (0.0066 s^{-1} ± 0.0026). Zhang and colleagues[66] found significant differences in $rCBV_{max}$ and relative mean time to enhancement (rMTE—a temporal descriptor of dynamic data) in the edema adjacent to benign and malignant meningiomas. Benign and malignant meningiomas showed maximal values of rCBV of 1.05 ± 0.96 and 3.82 ± 1.39, respectively, and maximal values of rMTE of 0.91 ± 0.25 and 1.24 ± 0.35. Cha and colleagues[58] also identified DSC–MRI as a useful diagnostic tool in differentiating tumefactive demyelinating lesions from intracranial neoplasms. The rCBV values of tumefactive demyelinating lesions ranged from 0.22 to 1.79 (n = 12), with a mean SD of 0.88 ± 0.46, compared with rCBV values of 1.55 to 19.20 (n = 11), with a mean of 6.47 ± 6.52 in intracranial neoplasms (P = .009).

Glial Cell Tumors

Predicting glioma grade

The most commonly published research examining the role of microvascular imaging biomarkers in neuro-oncology addresses the relationship between biomarker values and tumor grade. In practice, all suspicious tumors are biopsied and imaging prediction of histopathological grade has limited apparent clinical benefit. These studies do, however, serve to validate potential biomarkers. In practice, many tumors are undergraded due to inherent sampling error in histopathologic techniques (especially in the setting highly heterogenous GBM) and the dangers of repeat biopsy. Imaging biomarkers are the only tool capable of demonstrating this regional variability, thereby providing biopsy guidance to reduce sampling error, and identifying regional characteristics, which might indicate a need to clinically increase the tumor grade, even in the absence of repeat biopsy. Furthermore, imaging biomarkers studies—in particular those based on MR imaging—possess a substantially better safety profile than repeat biopsy and can be repeated as frequently as is practicable to provide true longitudinal data. Early studies demonstrated that the CBV, as measured by DSC–MRI, is strongly correlated to tumor grade (see Fig. 2).[67–73] Recently, this relationship has been reinforced using CBV measured by VASO imaging[33] and by DCE–CT.[74,75] More importantly, rCBV maps from DSC-MRI can identify areas of malignant transformation or tumor dedifferentiation in at risk primary low grade lesions before they are visible on conventional imaging. This allows for more accurate targeting of stereotactic biopsies, and potentially more accurate estimation of tumor grade.[70,76] An independent relationship between tumor grade and measurements of K^{trans} has also been demonstrated (see Fig. 2),[77,78] although the correlation is less strong than that between grade and CBV. Recent work has suggested that measurement of K^{trans} may allow differentiation between grade III and IV glioma,[79] which previous studies using other vascular parameters have failed to demonstrate, however this requires further validation. In glioma, measurements of blood flow using ASL also correlate with microvascular density (MVD)—a well-established histopathological measure of tumor microvascularity—and can distinguish low- from high-grade tumors.[80–82] The relationship with grade is strengthened if measurements of tumor blood flow are compared with age-dependent mean brain perfusion.[80] Comparisons with histologic studies demonstrate correlations between rCBV and histologic features indicative of tumor aggression, including mitotic activity and vascularity.[69,83–85] MVD has been shown to correlate with the steepest slope of the first pass phase in DCE-MRI (see Fig. 1, for example)[86] and also with CBV when histological measures are corrected for slice thickness effects.[87] Direct comparison of rCBV mapping with other indicators of malignancy, such as fluorodeoxyglucose-PET, shows close agreement between local rCBV values and glucose uptake, and moderately significant correlation between maximal glucose uptake and rCBV (n = 21; r = 0.572; P = .023).[67] Comparison of CBV with ^{11}C-methionine PET also shows a close correlation between the techniques,[88] which is of potential value since methionine PET demonstrates tumor extension beyond that revealed by conventional MR imaging.

Predicting glioma type

There is increasing recognition that several prognostically important genetic and molecular biomarkers allow the identification of subtypes of glioma indistinguishable by simple histologic grading. Oligodendroglial tumors represent more than 30% of glial tumors in adults and are an important subgroup characterized by longer survival, better chemotherapy response, and characteristic genetic alterations.[89] Allelic losses of chromosomes 1p and 19q are a molecular signature of oligodendrogliomas and occur in 50% to 70% of low-grade and anaplastic tumors.[90] Crucially, this genotype is strongly associated with chemosensitivity. Unlike nonoligodendroglial gliomas, tumor contrast enhancement and CBV do not vary significantly between low- and high-grade oligodendrogliomas.[91,92] rCBV values are generally higher, however, in oligodendroglioma than in other benign brain tumors (see **Fig. 2**)[92,93] and, depending on the study, rCBV is elevated in 1p/19q loss of heterogeneity or 1p loss only, although the relationships to chemosensitivity in these cases are unclear.[94–96]

Predicting transformation of LGG

The management of patients with low-grade glioma (LGG) currently requires regular imaging to detect the development of malignant dedifferentiation at the earliest stage possible. It is now established that larger tumors have a greater risk of dedifferentiation and that areas of raised CBV within LGG are more likely to show high-grade histology.[70,97] Recent studies have shown high values of CBV in patients with LGG associated with poor prognosis (**Fig. 3**)[97,98] and that in transforming LGG, susceptibility-weighted MR perfusion imaging can demonstrate significant

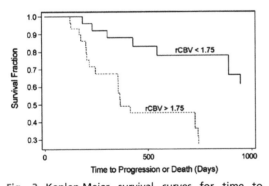

Fig. 3. Kaplan-Meier survival curves for time to progression in patients with LGG. Patients with LGG with low rCBV at baseline have a probable median time to progression of 889 days, whereas the median time to progression among subjects with high rCBV is 365 days. (*From* Caseiras GB, Chheang S, Babb J, et al. Relative cerebral blood volume measurements of low-grade gliomas predict patient outcome in a multi-institution setting. Eur J Radiol 2010;73[2]:215–20; with permission.)

increases in rCBV up to 12 months before contrast enhancement is apparent on T_1-weighted MR imaging, a significant improvement in lead time (**Fig. 4**).[99]

Predicting therapeutic response and prognosis in HGG

Early studies demonstrated an association between delayed contrast uptake in glioma and improved survival.[100] Subsequent pharmacokinetic studies have shown that data from DCE-MRI prior to and during radiotherapy could identify patients who showed subsequent decreases in tumor volume.[101] Several groups have since demonstrated a relationship between CBV in glioma and overall survival.[93,98,102,103] In 2006, Mills and colleagues[104] showed that this relationship mirrors the ability of CBV to predict tumor grade but that measurements of tumor K^{trans} predict survival in HGG independent of CBV. Recent studies using ASL have demonstrated that measurements of tumor blood flow can predict response to surgical treatment, although it is unclear whether or not this is simply a correlation with the relationship between grade and survival.[81] There has been considerable interest in the use of imaging biomarkers to predict radiotherapy response, and MR perfusion techniques seem particularly promising in this regard.[3] Cao and colleagues[102] demonstrated that the percentage of the tumor showing high perfusion before radiotherapy and the fluid-attenuated inversion recovery imaging tumor volume were predictors for survival ($P = .01$). Changes in tumor CBV during the early treatment course also predicted survival, better outcomes being associated with a decrease in fractional low-CBV tumor volume at week one of radiotherapy. Unlike radiotherapy, there is no conclusive value of perfusion imaging for the detection or prediction of response to temozolomide (the current standard chemotherapy in HGG treatment).[105] Treatment-induced changes in microvascular and diffusional characteristics occur regionally within the tumor, and identification of the proportion of tumor showing early response is predictive of overall outcome.[106–108] Recent work has shown that regional changes in CBV and/or CBF that occur early during treatment can be used to construct a parametric response map (PRM), which can predict overall survival in HGG, and may even distinguish pseudoprogression in temozolomide-treated GBM.[106,109]

Novel treatment strategies are increasingly introducing the use of antiangiogenic drugs, which have been shown to have significant survival benefits in patients with glioma.[110–112] Imaging

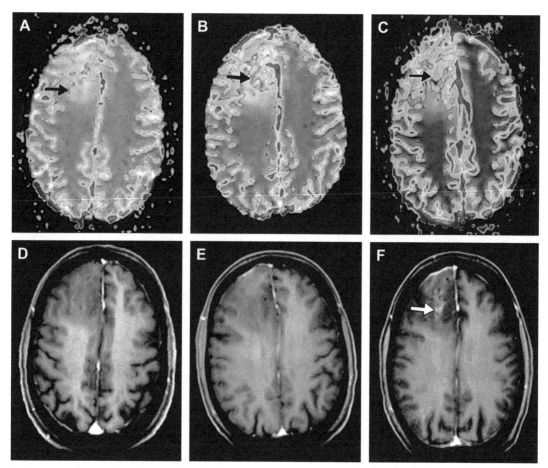

Fig. 4. Images from serial MR perfusion studies in 30-year-old patient with oligodendroglioma showing progression to high-grade tumor 18 months after study entry. (*A–C*) Transverse rCBV overlay images. (*D–F*) Transverse reformatted images obtained with double-dose, contrast-enhanced, volumetric, T_1-weighted sequence (spoiled gradient echo, 14.4/6.4; inversion time, 650 ms). (*A*) rCBV map at baseline shows small area of elevated rCBV (*arrow*) measuring up to 4.52. (*B*) rCBV map 6 months before transformation shows larger area of increased rCBV (*arrow*) measuring up to 8.32. (*C*) rCBV map at transformation shows further increase in area with elevated rCBV (*arrow*), which now reaches a maximum value of 12.04. (*D*) Baseline contrast-enhanced T_1-weighted image shows a hypointense tumor without pathologic enhancement. (*E*) Six months before transformation, there is no evidence of pathologic intratumoral enhancement, despite a markedly increased rCBV. (*F*) At transformation, there is irregular enhancement in center of the tumor (*arrow*); the area of pathologic enhancement is much smaller than the region of increased rCBV. (*From* Danchaivijitr N, Waldman AD, Tozer DJ, et al. Low-grade gliomas: do changes in rCBV measurements at longitudinal perfusion-weighted MR imaging predict malignant transformation? Radiology 2008;247[1]:170–8; with permission.)

biomarkers from DCE techniques have been widely used in clinical trials of antiangiogenic and vascular targeting agents outside the head.[113] These markers show early evidence of biologic activity and commonly show significant relationship with progression-free and overall survival— a prerequisite for clinical surrogacy. As such, microvascular imaging biomarkers have become a standard component of most clinical trials of novel antiangiogenic therapies. Trials of carboplatin and thalidomide, which have an anti-angiogenic activity, have shown significant decreases in rCBV and an association between larger decreases and response.[114] A small-scale study examining the effect of AZD2171 an oral tyrosine kinase inhibitor of vascular endothelial growth factor (VEGF) receptors demonstrated clinical responses and significant prognostic changes in CBV and K^{trans}. This study also demonstrated normalization of mean vessel diameter, which has been previously reported only from histologic studies of antiangiogenic therapy.[111]

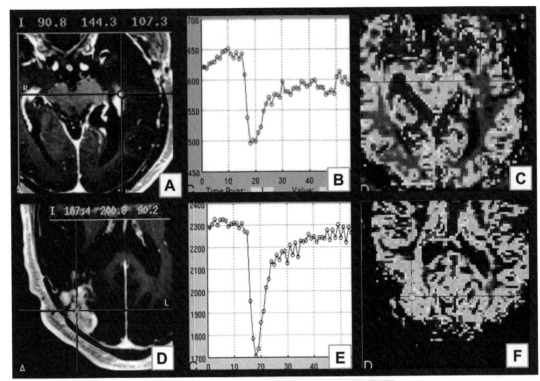

Fig. 5. Representative cases of a histologically diagnosed radiation necrosis (*top panel*) and GBM (*bottom panel*) showing the neuronavigational screen-capture image with documentation of the surgical tissue specimen location (*red target lines*). (*A, D*) Postcontrast images; (*B, E*) signal-intensity time course from the lesion; and (*C, F*) coregistered DSC source image with placement of a region of interest (*blue target lines*) at the specimen location with corresponding (*C*) and color rCBV map (*D*). (*From* Hu LS, Baxter LC, Smith KA, et al. Relative cerebral blood volume values to differentiate high-grade glioma recurrence from posttreatment radiation effect: direct correlation between image-guided tissue histopathology and localized dynamic susceptibility-weighted contrast-enhanced perfusion MR imaging measurements. AJNR Am J Neuroradiol 2009;30[3]:552–8; with permission.)

Further studies of MR microvascular biomarkers in GBM treated with antiangiongenic therapy are underway.[19]

Distinguishing tumor recurrence and radiation necrosis

Conventional treatment of high-grade glioma consists of conformal radiotherapy (60 Gy in 30 fractions) with concurrent and adjuvant temozolomide.[115] As described in brief earlier, the phenomenon of pseudoprogression in this setting has not been fully explored in the setting of perfusion or permeability imaging. One of the major problems in the clinical management of these patients is in the subsequent differentiation between postradiation changes and tumor recurrence/growth. Some workers have suggested that DCE techniques may be helpful in differentiating between tumor recurrence, characterized by high CBV and K^{trans}, and radiation necrosis, characterized by low values of both parameters.[116–119] A recent study[120] demonstrated CBV values in areas of radiation necrosis

ranging from 0.21 to 0.71, with values in recurrent tumor ranging from 0.55 to 4.64. Nonetheless, 8.3% of tumor CBV values fell within the radiation necrosis group range. A threshold value of 0.71 optimized differentiation of the histopathologic groups with a sensitivity of 91.7% and a specificity of 100% (**Fig. 5**). Radiation necrosis represents a heterogeneous process with features resembling inflammation. Immature vessels may grow into previously necrotic areas,[121] and viable tumor cells may still be found in the areas with decreased blood volume so that sites of active recurrence may be overlooked.[52] As with other applications of vascular imaging techniques, diagnostic specificity is considerably increased by the addition of diffusion-weighted imaging, which shows greater specificity for the identification of radiation necrosis than DCE methods.[122]

SUMMARY

The use of biomarkers of microvascular structure and function from perfusion and permeability imaging is now well established in neuro-oncological research. There remain significant challenges to be overcome before these techniques and related biomarkers can find general acceptance. Core to this is the standardization of acquisition and processing protocols for robust use across multiple clinical sites. Certain microvascular imaging biomarkers, such as rCBV, are relatively amenable to widespread implementation and standardization, while others remain the subject of active, ongoing methodological research. Nevertheless, the potential clinical benefits of these approaches to quantify tumor perfusion and permeability are already becoming clear, particularly in the setting of novel antiangiogenic therapies. With an increasing body of evidence in the scientific literature, and with a steadily falling barrier to entry, the coming decade should see rapid developments in imaging biomarkers, and facilitate their transition into routine clinical practice.

REFERENCES

1. Jackson A, Stivaros S, Moore EA. Advances in magnetic resonance imaging. Imaging 2006;18: 97–109.

2. O'Connor JP, Jackson A, Asselin MC, et al. Quantitative imaging biomarkers in the clinical development of targeted therapeutics: current and future perspectives. Lancet Oncol 2008;9(8):766–76.

3. Herholz K, Coope D, Jackson A. Metabolic and molecular imaging in neuro-oncology. Lancet Neurol 2007;6(8):711–24.

4. Biomarkers Definitions Working Group. Biomarkers and surrogate endpoints: preferred definitions and conceptual framework. Clin Pharmacol Ther 2001; 69(3):89–95.

5. Goh V, Halligan S, Bartram CI. Quantitative tumor perfusion assessment with multidetector CT: are measurements from two commercial software packages interchangeable? Radiology 2007; 242(3):777–82.

6. Folkman J. Tumor angiogenesis: therapeutic implications. N Engl J Med 1971;285(21):1182–6.

7. Uematsu H, Maeda M, Sadato N, et al. Vascular permeability: quantitative measurement with double-echo dynamic MR imaging—theory and clinical application. Radiology 2000;214(3):912–7.

8. Knopp MV, Weiss E, Sinn HP, et al. Pathophysiologic basis of contrast enhancement in breast tumors. J Magn Reson Imaging 1999;10(3):260–6.

9. Jayson GC, Zweit J, Jackson A, et al. Molecular imaging and biological evaluation of HuMV833 anti-VEGF antibody: implications for trial design of antiangiogenic antibodies. J Natl Cancer Inst 2002;94(19):1484–93.

10. Kassner A, Annesley DJ, Zhu XP, et al. Abnormalities of the contrast re-circulation phase in cerebral tumors demonstrated using dynamic susceptibility contrast-enhanced imaging: a possible marker of vascular tortuosity. J Magn Reson Imaging 2000; 11(2):103–13.

11. Thacker NA, Scott ML, Jackson A. Can dynamic susceptibility contrast magnetic resonance imaging perfusion data be analyzed using a model based on directional flow? J Magn Reson Imaging 2003;17(2):241–55.

12. Jayson GC, Parker GJ, Mullamitha S, et al. Blockade of platelet-derived growth factor receptor-beta by CDP860, a humanized, PEGylated di-Fab', leads to fluid accumulation and is associated with increased tumor vascularized volume. J Clin Oncol 2005;23(5):973–81.

13. de Langen AJ, Lubberink M, Boellaard R, et al. Reproducibility of tumor perfusion measurements using 15O-labeled water and PET. J Nucl Med 2008;49(11):1763–8.

14. Mullins ME. Stroke imaging with xenon-CT. Semin Ultrasound CT MR 2006;27(3):219–20.

15. Jackson A, Buckley DL, Parker GJM. Dynamic contrast-enhanced magnetic resonance imaging in oncology. Berlin: Springer; 2005.

16. Leach MO, Brindle KM, Evelhoch JL, et al. Assessment of antiangiogenic and antivascular therapeutics using MRI: recommendations for appropriate methodology for clinical trials. Br J Radiol 2003;76(Spec No 1):S87–91.

17. Golay X, Hendrikse J, Lim TC. Perfusion imaging using arterial spin labeling. Top Magn Reson Imaging 2004;15(1):10–27.

18. Uematsu H, Maeda M. Double-echo perfusion-weighted MR imaging: basic concepts and application in brain tumors for the assessment of tumor blood volume and vascular permeability. Eur Radiol 2006;16(1):180–6.

19. Jackson A, Kassner A, Annesley-Williams D, et al. Abnormalities in the recirculation phase of contrast agent bolus passage in cerebral gliomas: comparison with relative blood volume and tumor grade. AJNR Am J Neuroradiol 2002;23(1):7–14.

20. Hu LS, Baxter LC, Pinnaduwage DS, et al. Optimized preload leakage-correction methods to improve the diagnostic accuracy of dynamic susceptibility-weighted contrast-enhanced perfusion MR imaging in posttreatment gliomas. AJNR Am J Neuroradiol 2010;31(1):40–8.

21. Paulson ES, Schmainda KM. Comparison of dynamic susceptibility-weighted contrast-enhanced MR methods: recommendations for measuring relative cerebral blood volume in brain tumors. Radiology 2008;249(2):601–13.

22. Zhu XP, Li KL, Kamaly-Asl ID, et al. Quantification of endothelial permeability, leakage space, and

blood volume in brain tumors using combined T1 and T2* contrast-enhanced dynamic MR imaging. J Magn Reson Imaging 2000;11(6):575–85.

23. Stack J, Redmond O, Codd M, et al. Breast disease: tissue characterization with Gd-DTPA enhancement profiles. Radiology 1990;174:491–4.

24. Flickinger F, Allison J, Sherry R, et al. Differentiation of benign from malignant breast masses by time-intensity evaluation of contrast enhanced MRI. Magn Reson Imaging 1993;11:617–20.

25. Roberts C, Issa B, Stone A, et al. Comparative study into the robustness of compartmental modeling and model-free analysis in DCE-MRI studies. J Magn Reson Imaging 2006;23(4):554–63.

26. St Lawrence K, Lee T. An adiabatic approximation to the tissue homogeneity model for water exchange in the brain: I. Theoretical derivation. J Cereb Blood Flow Metab 1998;18:1365–77.

27. Ostergaard L, Chesler D, Weisskoff R, et al. Modelling cerebral blood flow and flow heterogeneity from magnetic resonance residue data. J Cereb Blood Flow Metab 1999;19:690–9.

28. Vallee JP, Lazeyras F, Khan HG, et al. Absolute renal blood flow quantification by dynamic MRI and Gd-DTPA. Eur Radiol 2000;10(8):1245–52.

29. Lu H, Golay X, Pekar JJ, et al. Functional magnetic resonance imaging based on changes in vascular space occupancy. Magn Reson Med 2003;50(2):263–74.

30. Lu H, van Zijl PC, Hendrikse J, et al. Multiple acquisitions with global inversion cycling (MAGIC): a multislice technique for vascular-space-occupancy dependent fMRI. Magn Reson Med 2004;51(1):9–15.

31. Donahue MJ, Blakeley JO, Zhou J, et al. Evaluation of human brain tumor heterogeneity using multiple T1-based MRI signal weighting approaches. Magn Reson Med 2008;59(2):336–44.

32. Lu H, Law M, Johnson G, et al. Novel approach to the measurement of absolute cerebral blood volume using vascular-space-occupancy magnetic resonance imaging. Magn Reson Med 2005;54(6):1403–11.

33. Lu H, Pollack E, Young R, et al. Predicting grade of cerebral glioma using vascular-space occupancy MR imaging. AJNR Am J Neuroradiol 2008;29(2):373–8.

34. Edelman RR, Siewert B, Adamis M, et al. Signal targeting with alternating radiofrequency (STAR) sequences: application to MR angiography. Magn Reson Med 1994;31(2):233–8.

35. Kwong KK, Chesler DA, Weisskoff RM, et al. MR perfusion studies with T1-weighted echo planar imaging. Magn Reson Med 1995;34(6):878–87.

36. Kim HS, Kim SY. A prospective study on the added value of pulsed arterial spin-labeling and apparent diffusion coefficients in the grading of gliomas. AJNR Am J Neuroradiol 2007;28(9):1693–9.

37. Haroon HA, Patankar TF, Zhu XP, et al. Comparison of cerebral blood volume maps generated from T2* and T1 weighted MRI data in intra-axial cerebral tumours. Br J Radiol 2007;80(951):161–8.

38. Tofts PS, Brix G, Buckley DL, et al. Estimating kinetic parameters from dynamic contrast-enhanced T(1)-weighted MRI of a diffusable tracer: standardized quantities and symbols. J Magn Reson Imaging 1999;10(3):223–32.

39. Tofts PS, Kermode AG. Measurement of the blood-brain barrier permeability and leakage space using dynamic MR imaging. 1. Fundamental concepts. Magn Reson Med 1991;17(2):357–67.

40. Emblem KE, Nedregaard B, Nome T, et al. Glioma grading by using histogram analysis of blood volume heterogeneity from MR-derived cerebral blood volume maps. Radiology 2008;247(3):808–17.

41. Emblem KE, Scheie D, Due-Tonnessen P, et al. Histogram analysis of MR imaging-derived cerebral blood volume maps: combined glioma grading and identification of low-grade oligodendroglial subtypes. AJNR Am J Neuroradiol 2008;29(9):1664–70.

42. Law M, Young R, Babb J, et al. Histogram analysis versus region of interest analysis of dynamic susceptibility contrast perfusion MR imaging data in the grading of cerebral gliomas. AJNR Am J Neuroradiol 2007;28(4):761–6.

43. Young R, Babb J, Law M, et al. Comparison of region-of-interest analysis with three different histogram analysis methods in the determination of perfusion metrics in patients with brain gliomas. J Magn Reson Imaging 2007;26(4):1053–63.

44. Rose CJ, Mills SJ, O'Connor JP, et al. Quantifying spatial heterogeneity in dynamic contrast-enhanced MRI parameter maps. Magn Reson Med 2009;62(2):488–99.

45. Erdogan C, Hakyemez B, Yildirim N, et al. Brain abscess and cystic brain tumor: discrimination with dynamic susceptibility contrast perfusion-weighted MRI. J Comput Assist Tomogr 2005;29(5):663–7.

46. Holmes TM, Petrella JR, Provenzale JM. Distinction between cerebral abscesses and high-grade neoplasms by dynamic susceptibility contrast perfusion MRI. AJR Am J Roentgenol 2004;183(5):1247–52.

47. Bink A, Gaa J, Franz K, et al. Importance of diffusion-weighted imaging in the diagnosis of cystic brain tumors and intracerebral abscesses. Zentralbl Neurochir 2005;66(3):119–25.

48. Mascalchi M, Filippi M, Floris R, et al. Diffusion-weighted MR of the brain: methodology and

clinical application. Radiol Med (Torino) 2005; 109(3):155–97.

49. Haris M, Gupta RK, Singh A, et al. Differentiation of infective from neoplastic brain lesions by dynamic contrast-enhanced MRI. Neuroradiology 2008; 50(6):531–40.

50. Calli C, Kitis O, Yunten N, et al. MR imaging in enhancing malignant cerebral tumors. Eur J Radiol 2006;58(3):394–403.

51. Lee IH, Kim ST, Kim HJ, et al. Analysis of perfusion weighted image of CNS lymphoma. Eur J Radiol 2009 June 3. [Online].

52. Sugahara T, Korogi Y, Shigematsu Y, et al. Value of dynamic susceptibility contrast magnetic resonance imaging in the evaluation of intracranial tumors. Top Magn Reson Imaging 1999;10(2):114–24.

53. Liao W, Liu Y, Wang X, et al. Differentiation of primary central nervous system lymphoma and high-grade glioma with dynamic susceptibility contrast-enhanced perfusion magnetic resonance imaging. Acta Radiol 2009;50(2):217–25.

54. Weber MA, Zoubaa S, Schlieter M, et al. Diagnostic performance of spectroscopic and perfusion MRI for distinction of brain tumors. Neurology 2006; 66(12):1899–906.

55. Strugar JG, Criscuolo GR, Rothbart D, et al. Vascular endothelial growth/permeability factor expression in human glioma specimens: correlation with vasogenic brain edema and tumor-associated cysts. J Neurosurg 1995;83(4):682–9.

56. Strugar J, Rothbart D, Harrington W, et al. Vascular permeability factor in brain metastases: correlation with vasogenic brain edema and tumor angiogenesis. J Neurosurg 1994;81(4):560–6.

57. Rollin N, Guyotat J, Streichenberger N, et al. Clinical relevance of diffusion and perfusion magnetic resonance imaging in assessing intra-axial brain tumors. Neuroradiology 2006;48(3):150–9.

58. Cha S, Knopp EA, Johnson G, et al. Intracranial mass lesions: dynamic contrast-enhanced susceptibility-weighted echo-planar perfusion MR imaging. Radiology 2002;223(1):11–29.

59. Cha S, Law M, Johnson G, et al. Peritumoral region: differentiation between primary high-grade neoplasma and solitary metastasis using dynamic contrast-enhanced T2*-weighted echo-planar perfusion MR imaging. In: Proceeding of the 38th Annual Meeting of the American Society of Neuroradiology. Atlanta (GA): American Society of Neuroradiology; 2000. p. 22.

60. Cha S, Lupo JM, Chen MH, et al. Differentiation of glioblastoma multiforme and single brain metastasis by peak height and percentage of signal intensity recovery derived from dynamic susceptibility-weighted contrast-enhanced perfusion MR imaging. AJNR Am J Neuroradiol 2007;28(6): 1078–84.

61. Maeda M, Itoh S, Kimura H, et al. Vascularity of meningiomas and neuromas: assessment with dynamic susceptibility-contrasst MRF imaging. Am J Roentgenol 1994;163(1):181–6.

62. Miyati T, Banno T, Mase M, et al. Dual dynamic contrast-enhanced MR imaging. J Magn Reson Imaging 1997;7(1):230–5.

63. Long DM. Vascular ultrastructure in human meningiomas and schwannomas. J Neurosurg 1973; 38(4):409–19.

64. Hakyemez B, Yildirim N, Erdogan C, et al. Meningiomas with conventional MRI findings resembling intraaxial tumors: can perfusion-weighted MRI be helpful in differentiation? Neuroradiology 2006; 48(10):695–702.

65. Yang S, Law M, Zagzag D, et al. Dynamic contrast-enhanced perfusion MR imaging measurements of endothelial permeability: differentiation between atypical and typical meningiomas. AJNR Am J Neuroradiol 2003;24(8):1554–9.

66. Zhang H, Rodiger LA, Shen T, et al. Perfusion MR imaging for differentiation of benign and malignant meningiomas. Neuroradiology 2008;50(6):525–30.

67. Aronen HJ, Pardo FS, Kennedy DN, et al. High microvascular blood volume is associated with high glucose uptake and tumor angiogenesis in human gliomas. Clin Cancer Res 2000;6(6): 2189–200.

68. Aronen HJ, Gazit IE, Louis DN, et al. Cerebral blood volume maps of gliomas: comparison with tumor grade and histologic findings. Radiology 1994;191(1):41–51.

69. Aronen HJ, Glass J, Pardo FS, et al. Echo-planar MR cerebral blood volume mapping of gliomas. Clinical utility. Acta Radiol 1995;36(5):520–8.

70. Knopp EA, Cha S, Johnson G, et al. Glial neoplasms: dynamic contrast-enhanced T2*-weighted MR imaging. Radiology 1999;211(3): 791–8.

71. Law M, Yang S, Wang H, et al. Glioma grading: sensitivity, specificity, and predictive values of perfusion MR imaging and proton MR spectroscopic imaging compared with conventional MR imaging. AJNR Am J Neuroradiol 2003;24(10): 1989–98.

72. Ludemann L, Grieger W, Wurm R, et al. Comparison of dynamic contrast-enhanced MRI with WHO tumor grading for gliomas. Eur Radiol 2001; 11(7):1231–41.

73. Provenzale JM, Wang GR, Brenner T, et al. Comparison of permeability in high-grade and low-grade brain tumors using dynamic susceptibility contrast MR imaging. AJR Am J Roentgenol 2002;178(3):711–6.

74. Ding B, Ling HW, Chen KM, et al. Comparison of cerebral blood volume and permeability in preoperative grading of intracranial glioma using CT

perfusion imaging. Neuroradiology 2006;48(10): 773–81.

75. Ellika SK, Jain R, Patel SC, et al. Role of perfusion CT in glioma grading and comparison with conventional MR imaging features. AJNR Am J Neuroradiol 2007;28(10):1981–7.

76. Di Costanzo A, Scarabino T, Trojsi F, et al. Multiparametric 3T MR approach to the assessment of cerebral gliomas: tumor extent and malignancy. Neuroradiology 2006;48(9):622–31.

77. Patankar TF, Haroon HA, Mills SJ, et al. Is volume transfer coefficient (K(trans)) related to histologic grade in human gliomas? AJNR Am J Neuroradiol 2005;26(10):2455–65.

78. Law M, Yang S, Babb JS, et al. Comparison of cerebral blood volume and vascular permeability from dynamic susceptibility contrast-enhanced perfusion MR imaging with glioma grade. AJNR Am J Neuroradiol 2004;25(5): 746–55.

79. Jain R, Ellika SK, Scarpace L, et al. Quantitative estimation of permeability surface-area product in astroglial brain tumors using perfusion CT and correlation with histopathologic grade. AJNR Am J Neuroradiol 2008;29(4):694–700.

80. Warmuth C, Gunther M, Zimmer C. Quantification of blood flow in brain tumors: comparison of arterial spin labeling and dynamic susceptibility-weighted contrast-enhanced MR imaging. Radiology 2003; 228(2):523–32.

81. Brown GG, Clark C, Liu TT. Measurement of cerebral perfusion with arterial spin labeling: part 2. Applications. J Int Neuropsychol Soc 2007;13(3): 526–38.

82. Kimura H, Takeuchi H, Koshimoto Y, et al. Perfusion imaging of meningioma by using continuous arterial spin-labeling: comparison with dynamic susceptibility-weighted contrast-enhanced MR images and histopathologic features. AJNR Am J Neuroradiol 2006;27(1):85–93.

83. Sugahara T, Korogi Y, Kochi M, et al. Correlation of MR imaging-determined cerebral blood volume maps with histologic and angiographic determination of vascularity of gliomas. AJR Am J Roentgenol 1998;171(6):1479–86.

84. Roberts HC, Roberts TP, Brasch RC, et al. Quantitative measurement of microvascular permeability in human brain tumors achieved using dynamic contrast-enhanced MR imaging: correlation with histologic grade. AJNR Am J Neuroradiol 2000; 21(5):891–9.

85. Roberts HC, Roberts TP, Bollen AW, et al. Correlation of microvascular permeability derived from dynamic contrast-enhanced MR imaging with histologic grade and tumor labeling index: a study in human brain tumors. Acad Radiol 2001;8(5): 384–91.

86. Maeda M, Itoh S, Kimura H, et al. Tumor vascularity in the brain: evaluation with dynamic susceptibility-contrast MR imaging. Radiology 1993; 189(1):233–8.

87. Pathak AP, Schmainda KM, Ward BD, et al. MR-derived cerebral blood volume maps: issues regarding histological validation and assessment of tumor angiogenesis. Magn Reson Med 2001; 46(4):735–47.

88. Sadeghi N, Salmon I, Tang BN, et al. Correlation between dynamic susceptibility contrast perfusion MRI and methionine metabolism in brain gliomas: preliminary results. J Magn Reson Imaging 2006; 24(5):989–94.

89. Roux FX, Nataf F. Cerebral oligodendrogliomas in adults and children. Current data and perspectives. Neurochirurgie 2005;51(3–4 Pt 2):410–4.

90. Cairncross JG, Ueki K, Zlatescu MC, et al. Specific genetic predictors of chemotherapeutic response and survival in patients with anaplastic oligodendrogliomas. J Natl Cancer Inst 1998; 90(19):1473–9.

91. Xu M, See SJ, Ng WH, et al. Comparison of magnetic resonance spectroscopy and perfusion-weighted imaging in presurgical grading of oligodendroglial tumors. Neurosurgery 2005;56(5): 919–26 [discussion: 26].

92. White ML, Zhang Y, Kirby P, et al. Can tumor contrast enhancement be used as a criterion for differentiating tumor grades of oligodendrogliomas? AJNR Am J Neuroradiol 2005;26(4):784–90.

93. Lev MH, Ozsunar Y, Henson JW, et al. Glial tumor grading and outcome prediction using dynamic spin-echo MR susceptibility mapping compared with conventional contrast-enhanced MR: confounding effect of elevated rCBV of oligodendrogliomas [corrected]. AJNR Am J Neuroradiol 2004;25(2):214–21.

94. Jenkinson MD, Smith TS, Joyce KA, et al. Cerebral blood volume, genotype and chemosensitivity in oligodendroglial tumours. Neuroradiology 2006; 48(10):703–13.

95. Law M, Brodsky JE, Babb J, et al. High cerebral blood volume in human gliomas predicts deletion of chromosome 1p: preliminary results of molecular studies in gliomas with elevated perfusion. J Magn Reson Imaging 2007;25(6):1113–9.

96. Whitmore RG, Krejza J, Kapoor GS, et al. Prediction of oligodendroglial tumor subtype and grade using perfusion weighted magnetic resonance imaging. J Neurosurg 2007;107(3):600–9.

97. Caseiras GB, Chheang S, Babb J, et al. Relative cerebral blood volume measurements of low-grade gliomas predict patient outcome in a multi-institution setting. Eur J Radiol 2010;73(2):215–20.

98. Law M, Young RJ, Babb JS, et al. Gliomas: predicting time to progression or survival with cerebral

blood volume measurements at dynamic susceptibility-weighted contrast-enhanced perfusion MR imaging. Radiology 2008;247(2):490–8.

99. Danchaivijitr N, Waldman AD, Tozer DJ, et al. Low-grade gliomas: do changes in rCBV measurements at longitudinal perfusion-weighted MR imaging predict malignant transformation? Radiology 2008;247(1):170–8.

100. Wong ET, Jackson EF, Hess KR, et al. Correlation between dynamic MRI and outcome in patients with malignant gliomas. Neurology 1998;50(3): 777–81.

101. Hawighorst H, Knopp MV, Debus J, et al. Pharmacokinetic MRI for assessment of malignant glioma response to stereotactic radiotherapy: initial results. J Magn Reson Imaging 1998;8(4):783–8.

102. Cao Y, Tsien CI, Nagesh V, et al. Survival prediction in high-grade gliomas by MRI perfusion before and during early stage of RT [corrected]. Int J Radiat Oncol Biol Phys 2006;64(3):876–85.

103. Chaskis C, Stadnik T, Michotte A, et al. Prognostic value of perfusion-weighted imaging in brain glioma: a prospective study. Acta Neurochir (Wien) 2006;148(3):277–85 [discussion: 85].

104. Mills SJ, Patankar TA, Haroon HA, et al. Do cerebral blood volume and contrast transfer coefficient predict prognosis in human glioma? AJNR Am J Neuroradiol 2006;27(4):853–8.

105. Leimgruber A, Ostermann S, Yeon EJ, et al. Perfusion and diffusion MRI of glioblastoma progression in a four-year prospective temozolomide clinical trial. Int J Radiat Oncol Biol Phys 2006; 64(3):869–75.

106. Galban CJ, Chenevert TL, Meyer CR, et al. The parametric response map is an imaging biomarker for early cancer treatment outcome. Nat Med 2009; 15(5):572–6.

107. Hamstra DA, Chenevert TL, Moffat BA, et al. Evaluation of the functional diffusion map as an early biomarker of time-to-progression and overall survival in high-grade glioma. Proc Natl Acad Sci U S A 2005;102(46):16759–64.

108. Hamstra DA, Galban CJ, Meyer CR, et al. Functional diffusion map as an early imaging biomarker for high-grade glioma: correlation with conventional radiologic response and overall survival. J Clin Oncol 2008;26(20):3387–94.

109. Tsien C, Galban CJ, Chenevert TL, et al. Parametric response map as an imaging biomarker to distinguish progression from pseudoprogression in high-grade glioma. J Clin Oncol 2010;28(13): 2293–9.

110. Narayana A, Golfinos JG, Fischer I, et al. Feasibility of using bevacizumab with radiation therapy and temozolomide in newly diagnosed high-grade

glioma. Int J Radiat Oncol Biol Phys 2008;72(2): 383–9.

111. Batchelor TT, Sorensen AG, di Tomaso E, et al. AZD2171, a pan-VEGF receptor tyrosine kinase inhibitor, normalizes tumor vasculature and alleviates edema in glioblastoma patients. Cancer Cell 2007;11(1):83–95.

112. Quarles CC, Schmainda KM. Assessment of the morphological and functional effects of the antiangiogenic agent SU11657 on 9L gliosarcoma vasculature using dynamic susceptibility contrast MRI. Magn Reson Med 2007;57(4):680–7.

113. O'Connor JPB, Jackson A, Parker GJM, et al. DCE-MRI biomarkers in the clinical evaluation of antiangiogenic and avascular disupting agents. Br J Cancer 2007;96:189–95.

114. Cha S, Knopp EA, Johnson G, et al. Dynamic contrast-enhanced T2-weighted MR imaging of recurrent malignant gliomas treated with thalidomide and carboplatin. AJNR Am J Neuroradiol 2000;21(5):881–90.

115. Laperriere N, Zuraw L, Cairncross G. Radiotherapy for newly diagnosed malignant glioma in adults: a systematic review. Radiother Oncol 2002;64(3): 259–73.

116. Alavi JB, Alavi A, Chawluk J, et al. Positron emission tomography in patients with glioma. A predictor of prognosis. Cancer 1988;62(6): 1074–8.

117. Rosen BR, Belliveau JW, Aronen HJ, et al. Susceptibility contrast imaging of cerebral blood volume: human experience. Magn Reson Med 1991;22(2): 293–9.

118. Boxerman J, Hamberg L, Rosen B, et al. MR contrast due to intravascular magnetic susceptibility perturbations. Magn Reson Med 1995;34: 555–66.

119. Reinhold HS, Endrich B. Tumour microcirculation as a target for hyperthermia. Int J Hyperthermia 1986;2(2):111–37.

120. Hu LS, Baxter LC, Smith KA, et al. Relative cerebral blood volume values to differentiate high-grade glioma recurrence from posttreatment radiation effect: direct correlation between image-guided tissue histopathology and localized dynamic susceptibility-weighted contrast-enhanced perfusion MR imaging measurements. AJNR Am J Neuroradiol 2009;30(3):552–8.

121. Gobbel GT, Seilhan TM, Fike JR. Cerebrovascular response after interstitial irradiation. Radiat Res 1992;130(2):236–40.

122. Hein PA, Eskey CJ, Dunn JF, et al. Diffusion-weighted imaging in the follow-up of treated high-grade gliomas: tumor recurrence versus radiation injury. AJNR Am J Neuroradiol 2004;25(2):201–9.

Future Potential of MRI-Guided Focused Ultrasound Brain Surgery

Rivka R. Colen, MD*, Ferenc A. Jolesz, MD

KEYWORDS

- MRgFUS • Brain tumor • Focused ultrasound
- Image-guided therapy

Magnetic resonance image-guided focused ultrasound surgery (MRgFUS) of the brain is expected to revolutionize central nervous system (CNS) therapy and, in general, to change current treatment paradigms.[1,2] The potential clinical applications include but are not limited to the treatment of benign and malignant brain tumors,[3] vascular malformations,[4] and ischemic or hemorrhagic stroke,[5] as well as the nonablative targeted delivery of therapeutic drugs,[6,7] genes,[8] and antibodies.[9] The integration of magnetic resonance imaging (MRI) guidance with advanced phased-array ultrasound technology has allowed this new therapeutic modality to emerge as a viable noninvasive alternative to current invasive and minimally invasive treatments. The development of MRgFUS therapy delivery systems with large numbers of phased-array transducer elements has permitted complete, noninvasive transcranial delivery of ultrasound waves through the intact bony skull, termed transcranial MRgFUS (TcMRgFUS).[10,11]

Multiple recent articles elaborate on MRgFUS' historical progression by detailing the step-wise advancement of focused ultrasound (FUS) technology to MRgFUS' current state.[12,13] Since the discovery of the piezoelectric effect (the production of acoustic energy when electric current is applied to a piezoelectric crystals) by Pierre and Jacques Curie in 1880, its subsequent incorporation into acoustic systems in 1918, and the first demonstration of its therapeutic effects in the brain by Lynn and colleagues[14] in 1942, FUS has

visibly materialized into the present-day therapeutic instrument. Investigated by Heimburger,[15] FUS for brain tumor thermal ablation began with a single-element FUS transducer without image guidance and required a relatively large craniotomy to fit the transducer. In the early development of FUS, Lars Leksell, the acknowledged pioneer of radiosurgery, became an early advocate of FUS' role in neurosurgical applications. However, Leksell abandoned FUS as a potential lesioning device because of its need for a craniotomy to create an acoustic window, which made it invasive. He rather focused on targeted ionizing radiation, an effort that resulted in the development of the gamma knife in 1967. The early failure of FUS brain applications was due to the inability to focus through the intact bony skull that necessitated a craniotomy and the lack of an imaging modality to accurately and reliably visualize brain tumors and monitor temperature elevation and tissue changes.

However, these fundamental technical challenges for the most part have been successfully identified and commensurately addressed today. The focusing through the skull has been resolved by correcting phase aberrations caused by unequal bone thickness. The correction method uses skull thickness measurements computed from computed tomography (CT) and entails focusing through a large number of phased arrays that are arranged in a helmet surrounding the skull.[10,11,16] The development of MRI in the

Department of Radiology, Brigham and Women's Hospital, Harvard Medical School, 75 Francis Street, Boston, MA 02115, USA
* Corresponding author.
E-mail address: rrcolen@partners.org

Neuroimag Clin N Am 20 (2010) 355–366
doi:10.1016/j.nic.2010.05.003
1052-5149/10/$ – see front matter © 2010 Elsevier Inc. All rights reserved.

1980s and MRI thermometry in the early 1990s[17,18] were significant in the advancement of MRgFUS. MRI as a noninvasive imaging modality has made possible the essential anatomic and functional roadmap. It unquestionably provides accurate preoperative definition and delineation of the target lesion and preoperative planning ability, intraoperative monitoring of ultrasound-induced thermal changes through magnetic resonance thermometry (temperature-sensitive maps), and postoperative validation of treatment success. In the early 1990s, the collaboration of researchers at the Brigham and Women's Hospital (BWH) with General Electric (GE Health care, Milwaukee, Wisconsin) and Insightec (Haifa, Israel) resulted in the integration of FUS and MRI into a single image-guided therapy delivery system, MRgFUS.[19,20] This development marks an important milestone for FUS as a therapeutic instrument for soft tissue tumors in general and intracranial tumors in particular. These developments have allowed FUS to re-emerge as a potential therapeutic instrument for the treatment of brain tumors and other CNS diseases. Therefore, when compared with related interventional procedures, MRgFUS of the brain has indisputably had to overcome disproportionate and challenging obstacles.

Inspired by the results of MRgFUS for the treatment of fibroadenomas,[21] clinical trials were initiated in breast cancer[22] and later for uterine fibroids. That last endeavor of MRgFUS ablation of uterine fibroids subsequently received approval by the US Food and Drug Administration (FDA).[23] Consequently, this technology has been released to the surgical arena for further clinical applications and clinical trials in noncranial diseases such as cancers of the prostate,[24] liver,[25] and bone.[26]

MILESTONES FOR TRANSCRANIAL DELIVERY OF FUS

In the last decade, a progression has occurred from the use of a single-element FUS transducer with and without MRI guidance that required a craniectomy or craniotomy as an acoustic window[15,27] to an integrated multielement phased-array ultrasound with MRI guidance.[28] Most recently, however, the completion of a noninvasive TcMRgFUS system[3] demonstrates a positive step toward resolution of an important limitation in transcranial delivery of FUS: the intact bony skull. Unlike air- and gas-containing cavities, the bony skull is not an absolute barrier to the transmission of acoustic waves and acoustic energy deposition.[29] Bone remains a relatively impenetrable acoustic barrier because of its high acoustic attenuation

coefficient that proportionally reflects its thickness and density.[10] Therefore, in the absence of an acoustic window provided by a craniotomy, the intact osseous skull creates two major challenges when performing transcranial FUS:

1. Defocusing due to the inhomogenous thickness and density of the skull that results in phase distortions and aberrations that, in turn, inhibit the establishment of a focal point of convergence, the consequence of which is inaccurate targeting and noncontrolled energy deposition
2. Heating of the skull and near-field soft tissues caused by the absorptive properties of bone with a proportional decrease in acoustic energy that reaches the deeply located lesions.

The current phased-array configuration addresses these challenges from defocusing by permitting adjustments of the phases of each element to correct for skull-induced phase aberration. Bone's high acoustic attenuation coefficient causes scatter and energy absorption.[30] Irregular bone thickness and inhomogeneous density further augment these latter artifacts and cause severe aberrations and phase distortions that result in defocusing. Preprocedural CT scans provide the information necessary to allow phased-array transducers to correct and compensate for inhomogenous skull thickness and density[10] via transcranial focusing[16,31] and acoustic modeling.[10,11,31,32] With the advent of the first prototype integrated MRgFUS brain system developed by Insightec, overheating of the skull and the near field tissues can be addressed by two methods:

1. A helmet-type, hemispherically configured phased-array transducer that spatially spreads the transducer elements and consequently distributes heating across a larger surface area, while it simultaneously deposits sufficient thermal energy at the focal point of convergence (the target lesion)
2. A cold water cap containing circulating degassed water chilled to about 15°C that is placed between the patient's head and transducer to provide an active cooling system for the scalp and the skull (Fig. 1).[11]

PRINCIPLES OF MRgFUS

MRgFUS combines and integrates a therapeutic and imaging modality, the FUS device, and MRI, respectively, into a single image-guided therapy delivery system. FUS, the therapeutic instrument, causes direct ultrasound-induced nonthermal (nonablative) and thermal (ablative) changes in

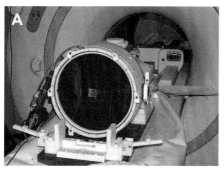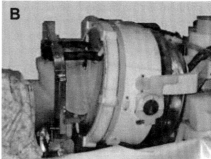

Fig. 1. Transcranial treatment system (Exablate 4000, Insightec, Haifa, Israel). *(A)* The helmet-type, hemispherically configured phased array transducer results in spatial spreading of the transducer elements and consequently distributes heating across a larger surface area. *(B)* This is placed over the patient's head. A degassed cold-water cap is placed between the patient's head and the transducer.

the target tissue. As an ablative modality, FUS' effects on tissue are caused by thermal heating. As a nonablative tool, FUS can reversibly disrupt the BBB, resulting in an increase in cerebrovascular capillary permeability and a consequent increase in the flux of relatively larger, nonlipophilic, and high molecular weight molecules that otherwise would not cross the BBB.[33] Other nonthermal effects include an increase in cell membrane permeability for use in gene therapy[8,34] and neuromodulation.[35]

Ultrasound penetrates through tissues without depositing any significant amount of energy. The focusing of ultrasound beams results in a concentration of energy at the focal point. At a given absorption coefficient corresponding to the specific tissue, in thermal ablations, the generation of thermal energy is maximal at the point of convergence where the summation of the acoustic intensity is highest. Overlapping sonications are delivered to the target tissues, generating heat at the focal point that exceeds a 60°C thermal coagulation threshold. FUS induces thermal coagulative necrosis of approximately 1 to 3 mm in diameter (perpendicular to the beam) and about twice as long in length (parallel to the beam).[11] Given the small focal point per sonication, multiple strategies are employed in an effort to increase the focal point size and decrease overall treatment time. Strategies to increase the ablation volume include "cavitation-enhanced ablation" and treating multiple sites simultaneously.

Before delivering the sufficient treatment doses, subthreshold, noncoagulative low-power sonications are delivered to identify the location of the focus and to provide correct targeting of the preselected location or lesion. Magnetic resonance thermometry confirms the focal point on the target lesion by detecting only short and small temperature elevations below 60°C at a time when there

are no tissue changes. After this targeting confirmation, high-power focused sonications (500 to 20,000 W/cm²) of short duration (1 to 60 seconds) are administered. Because of the relatively long cooling time (over minutes) between sonications, the overall treatment time is lengthy. Cooling is necessary to avoid the summation of heat effects, which, without cooling, can result in larger tissue volumes than the focal volume. Unlike probe-delivered thermal ablations with wide gradients, FUS has steep thermal gradients. Short sonication times prevent substantial cooling effects from blood flow and perfusion and simultaneously reduce heat build-up. To monitor and control energy deposition in a closed-loop treatment imaging system, magnetic resonance temperature-sensitive maps are obtained during and between each sonication[36] for immediate feedback that allows real-time dosimetry.

In thermal ablative therapy, FUS-induced thermal energy is exploited to cause tissue coagulative necrosis. Above 57°C to 60°C over a few seconds, irreversible cell damage invariably occurs secondary to protein denaturing. The thermal ablation is nonselective and, therefore, both neoplastic and normal tissues are destroyed. Given the nonselective, heat-induced cell death, this treatment signals the need for a reliable and sensitive imaging method for monitoring tissue changes. As it can accurately detect temperature changes of less than 2°C to 3°C, magnetic resonance temperature-sensitive imaging (magnetic resonance thermometry) fulfills these criteria.[37,38]

This all-or-none ablative effect of FUS irrespective of tissue type resembles surgical treatment. However, unlike surgery where the overlying tissue in the surgical path is destroyed, in FUS, the nonablated surrounding parenchyma is preserved. On the other hand, hyperthermia, similar to FUS, uses heat to cause its ablative effects on tissue. Unlike FUS, however, hyperthermia distributes relatively lower temperatures (43°C) over a longer period of time (30 to 60 minutes), thereby causing selective cell death of malignant cells as opposed to nontumoral cells that may survive the treatment.[39] Other types of thermal ablative tool are the percutaneous heat-conducting probes, such as those used in radiofrequency ablation and laser therapy, that are obviously more invasive than FUS.[40] Unlike FUS, which has a steep temperature gradient, heat-conducting probes cause a shallow temperature gradient when the heat is dissipated as it travels from the single-source probe. Probe-delivered thermal ablations, therefore, require long tissue exposures to increase the ablative volume and to reach sufficient thermal energy to cause cell death within the entire target volume. Additionally, unlike FUS, the probe ablation zone extends in each direction equally (spherically) and, therefore, cannot be tailored to fit the complex shape of a target volume. Underscoring its significance in thermal ablations, regardless of the ablative source, spatial monitoring and temporal monitoring of thermal heating are of utmost importance to avoid under- or overtreatment.

The nonthermal, nonablative effects of FUS are caused by multiple complex mechanisms, the most important being cavitation. Cavitation, defined as acoustically induced interactions from microscopic gas bubbles in the medium,[41,42] results in the following: bubble oscillation, acoustic streaming, mechanical (acoustic radiation) forces, and inertial (transient) cavitation (Fig. 2).[34,43-45] Of these, inertial cavitation is believed to be responsible for most of the nonthermal biologic effects. In general, microbubbles are cavities filled with gas or vapor. More specifically, according to Minneart's[46] theory, a bubble is a spherical gas-filled structure in a liquid of constant hydrostatic pressure. Microbubbles can be seeded and induced by the ultrasound itself and generated within the native sonicated tissue or preformed microbubbles (clinically used ultrasound imaging contrast agents) that can be intravenously administered, the latter termed microbubble-enhanced therapeutic ultrasound.[47,48] Preformed microbubbles are made from human serum albumin shells filled with perfluorocarbon gas perflutren (mean bubble diameter, 2.0 to 4.5 μm).

On interaction with an ultrasound beam and in response to a sound field, microbubbles, whether generated internally or administered iatrogenically, can cause any of the four previously mentioned biologic effects. Ultrasound bio-effects are either linear, stable, predictable, and controlled, or nonlinear, unstable, unpredictable, and uncontrolled, respectively. At low acoustic power, microbubbles oscillate and grow in size via rectified diffusion.[42,49] Known as stable cavitation, this growth and oscillation contribute to nonthermal effects (the most important among them is disruption of the BBB) secondary to shear stresses on the cells caused by bubble oscillation, microstreaming, and radiation forces.[41,42] Microstreaming, also termed acoustic streaming, refers to eddying circulation motions of fluid around the bubble. Radiation forces cause the bubble to move in the direction of the wave propagation, exerting mechanical force on and deformation of the endothelium perpendicular to the direction of the blood flow and length of the vessel.[50] The shear stresses, resulting from bubble oscillation, microstreaming, and radiation forces, cause localized stretching of the cell membrane and stimulation of the endothelial cells via activation of stretch-sensitive ion channels, thereby inducing its

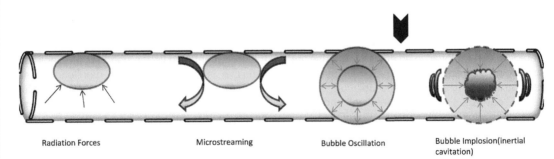

Radiation Forces   Microstreaming   Bubble Oscillation   Bubble Implosion(inertial cavitation)

Fig. 2. Cavitation. Radiation forces exert mechanical force on and deform the endothelium perpendicular to the direction of the blood flow and length of the vessel. Microstreaming is due to eddying circular currents of fluid around the bubble. Focused ultrasound also causes oscillation and the rapid growth of bubbles, that, on implosion unpredictably release stored energy in the form of shock waves. Shear stresses, resulting from bubble oscillation, microstreaming, radiation forces, and shock waves from bubble implosion cause localized stretching of cells and disruption of the endothelial tight junction (arrowhead) resulting in blood–brain barrier disruption.

biologic effects on the BBB. At high acoustic pressures, however, FUS causes oscillation and the rapid growth of bubbles, which, on implosion, unpredictably release stored energy in the form of shock waves.[41,51] This violent collapse, also known as inertial cavitation, produces high-velocity jets[52] and free radicals.[53] The resulting biologic effects disrupt the cell membrane and endothelial tight junctions, allowing uncontrolled deposition of thermal heat. Nonlinear effects on heating can lead to hemorrhage and unwanted tissue destruction outside the focal area.[54] The effects of cavitation, however, can be exploited in both thermal ablations and nonthermal treatments. In thermal ablations, cavitation-enhanced ablation causes the tissue to heat more rapidly to create a large volume of thermal ablation of a larger volume within relatively short treatment times. This latter method has been used in uterine fibroids. Both innate and preformed microbubbles allow BBB disruption (BBBD), to occur at lower energy levels. By acting as cavitation nucleation sites, preformed microbubbles further enhance the local ultrasound effects by dramatically lowering the ultrasound energy required to obtain the same amount of BBBD or tissue damage. Therefore, with the introduction of preformed contrast microbubble agents,[45,47,55] the aforementioned adverse effects of uncontrolled heating, including hemorrhage and unwanted tissue destruction, will decrease.[43]

Pretreatment Planning and Localization

Preprocedural planning is of utmost importance and involves the definition of the anatomy of the target lesion and adjacent structures, determination of the procedural approach, and calculation of a feasible trajectory for the delivery of sonications. MRI remains the imaging method of choice in all stages of an MRgFUS procedure, including preprocedural planning, intraprocedural monitoring, and postprocedural treatment validation, as it offers exquisite three-dimensional anatomic tissue characterization and functional mapping. Recently, at the Brigham and Women's Hospital, the recommended MRI protocols have been released for all stages of an MRgFUS procedure.[56] In the pretreatment stage, aside from the conventional MRI sequences, functional and advanced imaging techniques such as functional MRI (fMRI), perfusion imaging, and tractography are recommended. fMRI and tractography are important for functional assessment and preoperative planning, particularly in those patients in whom the tumor is adjacent or involving eloquent cortex and important white matter tracts,

respectively. In addition to diffusion-weighted imaging, magnetic resonance perfusion imaging can be used to establish baseline and subsequently for magnetic resonance biomarkers to assess treatment response, especially in those patients whose radiological picture can be confounded on the administration of adjuvant chemotherapy and radiation.

Intraprocedure Targeting and Monitoring

Once the transcranial apparatus, consisting of the hemispherical phased-array transducer and underlying cranial cooling system, is secured and the patient is in positioned in the MRI suite, an immediate pretreatment MRI is obtained for retargeting the preselected lesion and re-evaluating the perilesional parenchyma. Both magnetic resonance thermometry and conventional and advanced MRI techniques are pivotal.

MRI thermometry remains the imaging modality of choice for intraprocedural monitoring and establishing treatment conclusion. Using proton resonance frequency shifts,[57] magnetic resonance thermometry detects with great precision minute changes in temperature caused by focused sonications,[36] and it can be used as a surrogate for tissue viability.[58] At the onset of the procedure, magnetic resonance thermometry confirms the correct focal point on the target lesion by detecting noncoagulative tissue changes caused by low-power sonications. Subsequently, magnetic resonance temperature-sensitive measurements are obtained during and between each high-power therapeutic sonication. Therefore, MRI thermometry, unlike other imaging modalities, allows for a controlled energy deposition by providing immediate real-time dosimetry and permitting real-time intra-procedural closed-loop feedback of thermal ablative procedures.

Conventional and, depending on the situation and tumor type, advanced MRI sequences obtained intraoperatively provide real-time updates on the progress and extent of tumor ablation. MRI sequences have been put forth by the Brigham and Women's Hospital, and they are tailored to confer the least amount of intraprocedural acquisition time.[56] As such, the acquisition of postcontrast T1 weighted imaging in enhancing high-grade tumors and fluid-attenuated inversion recovery (FLAIR) sequences in both high- and low-grade tumors/gliomas is used to determine the extent of ablation. This evaluation is important, as the subtotal removal remains one of the single most important independent predictors of tumor recurrence and, therefore, poor prognosis.

Postprocedure Validation

Once the desired therapeutic endpoint is achieved, postcontrast MRI is acquired for treatment validation and to establish a post-treatment baseline MRI. In thermal ablations, a focal region of nonenhancement reflects a positive response to ultrasound-induced thermal ablation and corresponds to tissue necrosis and blocked capillaries.[36] In nonthermal therapy such as with disruption of the BBB,[59] enhancement of the sonicated area reflects increased permeability, confirming a positive response to therapy. MRI also can be used to document postprocedure perilesional edema that progressively resolves after 48 to 74 hours.[60]

CLINICAL APPLICATIONS
Thermal Ablations

Given that the goal of ideal tumor surgery is complete removal of the entire tissue volume of the target lesion with functional and structural preservation of the surrounding tissue, including sparing of the tissue in the surgical path, an invasive or even minimally invasive surgical procedure is only an approximation to the ideal surgery. The ideal therapeutic modality, MRgFUS, is noninvasive and targeted at the point of acoustic convergence, thereby sparing the overlying tissue and depositing sufficient thermal energy to ablate the even deep-seated lesions.

Currently, in clinical trials, MRgFUS' role in brain tumors includes thermal ablation of primary malignant CNS neoplasms only (**Fig. 3**).[3,28] Of note, certain primary brain tumors, particularly gliomas, invade the normal brain and, therefore, they cannot be completely removed or ablated without associated injury of normal tissue and related functional damage. In most of these patients, tumor debulking to decrease tumor volume can be considered a satisfactory outcome. Benign tumors and metastases, on the other hand, demonstrate more confined and often well-defined borders, in which case complete destruction of tumor volume would be deemed adequate treatment. However, whether in gross total or total removal, MRgFUS unmistakably maintains anatomic and functional preservation of the surrounding brain parenchyma. Furthermore, in the case of debulking surgery, specifically in glioblastoma, where recurrence will invariably occur, FUS allows for unlimited retreatment sessions, an option not present in surgery or radiation therapy.

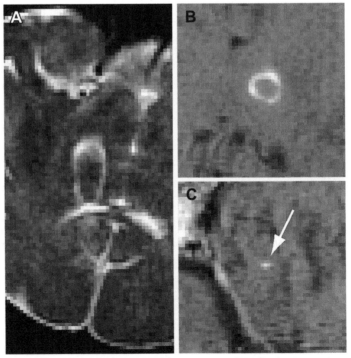

Fig. 3. Thermal lesions produced in the primate brain through a craniotomy. *A* and *B* show a large thalamic lesion. (*A*) T2 weighted image along the direction of the ultrasound beam. (*B*) Contrast-enhanced T1 weighted image in the focal plane where the center of the lesion is nonenhancing. (*C*) Shows contrast-enhanced T1 weighted image of a small lesion produced in the hippocampus.

FUS may have more applications in benign tumors that are either completely treatable or that can be rendered limited through their shrinkage in their ability to cause functional deficits. MRgFUS will, therefore, most likely be applied in the future for treatment of benign tumors. Furthermore, given MRI's ability to temperature monitor and achieve a sharp thermal gradient, it is anticipated that MRgFUS treatment of tumors adjacent to nerves (ie, optic and other cranial nerves) can be achieved.

Given that FUS has been shown to play a part in the treatment of certain functional neurologic disorders such as movement disorders, epilepsy, or pain,[61,62] FUS might also have a major role in functional neurosurgery. As such, the FUS research team from Zurich, Switzerland, recently published encouraging results of a clinical trial on treating chronic neuropathic pain using MRgFUS-induced thalamotomy that confirm FUS' role in functional neurosurgery.[62] Sonication sites can be pretested functionally before an irreversible lesion is made, rendering FUS useful for pain control and the treatment of spastic diseases.[63] However, although an improvement over stereotactic surgery, to compete with the current deep brain stimulation and transcranial magnetic stimulation (TMS) and replace the current neurosurgical approach, MRgFUS will require real-time functional localization ability. Given ultrasound's ability to temporarily block nerve conduction[35] and also activate (stimulate) the brain, FUS may have a future as a tool for non invasive functional testing and mapping, similar to the currently investigated modality, TMS.

Nonthermal Effects

Effective therapy using larger molecules remains a challenge in the brain, because larger molecules do not penetrate the BBB. In brain tumors, contrary to general belief and gross misconception, the BBB remains partially intact with some permeability and leakage seen in the tumor center (the region of necrosis) and barrier integrity maintained in the well-vascularized actively proliferating tumor edge (the area of active enhancement seen on MRI).[64]

The BBB is formed by a single continuous layer of endothelial cells cemented together by tight junctions, the basal lamina, and glial cell processes.[65] When intact, the BBB effectively excludes more than 98% of large-molecular neurotherapeutic drugs.[66] In addition to their size, molecules' charge and lipid solubility determine penetration potential across the BBB. As such, ionized water-soluble molecules of greater than 180 Da do not cross the BBB,[67] while lipophilic agents with a molecular mass less than 400 to 500 Da can cross the BBB in pharmacologic significant amounts.[68]

In an attempt to increase the delivery of drugs across the BBB, multiple concerted efforts have been undertaken including the development and modification of drugs that can penetrate the BBB and the development of methods to mechanically disrupt the BBB. Among the former efforts, numerous lipophilic agents and water-soluble drugs with high affinities for carriers that penetrate the BBB have been investigated, and existing ones have been modified.[68] However, unlike multiple diseases, such as affective disorders and epilepsy, that consistently respond to small-molecular lipophilic drugs, brain tumors, autism, and neurodegenerative processes, such as Alzheimer disease and Huntington disease are not effectively treated with such; therefore, treatment remains limited. Most of the clinical experience has been in mechanical disruption of the BBB using intra-arterial infusion of hyper osmotic solutions, such as mannitol, that are currently under investigation and in clinical trials[69,70] and that cause the endothelial cells to shrink, resulting in loosening of the tight junctions and increased permeability of the BBB. Although reversible and usually lasting 5 hours,[70] BBBD is diffuse within the parenchymal territory, perfused by the injected vessel, and requires invasive intra-arterial catheterization. Direct parenchymal injections of drugs and implanted delivery systems into the resection cavity are also under investigation.[67,71] However, although localized and targeted to the lesion, these are invasive and require opening of the skull that can destroy the overlying nontargeted trajectorial parenchyma, and thus, increase the risk of complications.

Finally, although noninvasive, the development and modification of drugs to increase drug permeability across the BBB comes at a significant economic cost, with a delay in translation into clinical practice. Furthermore, development is tailored to fit a specific investigated drug. Hyperosmotic BBBD and direct parenchymal injections are invasive and, in the former, also diffusely deliver in the arterial territory of the injected artery. Therefore, the ideal targeted drug delivery system remains one that is generic and not tailored to a specific drug; additionally, it should be non-invasive, targeted and localized, and cause transient effects. Of the aforementioned, MRgFUS is the only method that consistently fulfills all criteria. Therefore, although research focuses have slanted toward thermal ablation of brain tumors, nonthermal nonablative BBBD in brain tumor treatment for delivery of therapeutic agents and chemotherapy has not been far behind.[21] In 1955, Barnard and colleagues[72] led the first study of ultrasound-induced BBBD. A year later, similar research was conducted by the Bakay[73] and Lele[74] group, describing the biologic effects of FUS on sonicated brain tissue. Recent studies performed at the authors' institution demonstrate and continue to confirm the ability of MRgFUS to produce selective, targeted, reversible BBBD, and therefore, increase BBB permeability.[33,51] Currently, preclinical trials are underway at the Brigham and Women's Hospital for delivering chemotherapy in brain tumors.[6,7]

The ability of MRgFUS to reversibly disrupt the BBB and increase its permeability can potentially transform and replace current nonselective drug delivery methods that cause systemic toxicity, which is an important limiting factor in chemotherapy today. Ultrasound's capacity to increase BBB permeability enables the targeted delivery of chemotherapeutic drugs into the region of interest that otherwise would not enter the desired site due to almost complete BBB impermeability (Fig. 4).[7,55] BBBD can occur when preformed microbubbles are delivered via intravenous administration. However, the chemotherapeutic drugs also can be encapsulated in bubbles or liposomes and attached to nanoparticles before administration.[75,76] At the moment of bubble rupture, the encapsulated drug is released locally in the sonicated region. Furthermore, MRI can subsequently confirm BBBD when the enhancement of the sonicated region is identified. The ability to deliver a dose of chemotherapy to a target region using a noninvasive opening of the BBB, compounded with the capacity to confirm treatment using contrast MRI, makes for an unparalleled combination. Studies are investigating the ability of large molecular drugs, such as trastuzumab (Herceptin) in CNS breast cancer metastasis, and doxorubicin, to pass through the BBB after sonication, with the hope that these protocols can be successfully used in the future to treat primary and secondary CNS malignancies.[6,7] Due to the noninvasiveness of the procedure and the potential to enhance the therapeutic delivery of drugs, this technique has the potential to translate into clinical practice in patients with CNS malignancies.

There are numerous non-neoplastic applications for MRgFUS, such as targeted delivery of genes,[8,77,78] antibodies,[9] and diagnostic and therapeutic agents for Parkinson disease and Alzheimer disease.[9,79] In the treatment of Alzheimer disease, recent animal model studies[9,79] have demonstrated promising results in diagnostic and therapeutic strategies that focus on detection and decreasing protein aggregates. Furthermore, the coupling of thermal effects of FUS on thrombolytic drugs increases thrombolysis, thereby improving the effectiveness of therapy in acute stroke patients.[5] This benefit, however, comes with an increase in the risk of cavitation-induced hemorrhage in ischemic stroke that can be reduced by using FUS-induced closure of the hemorrhaging vessels to generate hemostasis,[80,81] which is an FUS effect that can be exploited for the treatment of vascular malformations.[4]

ADVANTAGES AND LIMITATIONS

MRgFUS offers clear, unambiguous advantages over other current treatment modalities (surgery, radiation therapy, and probe-delivered thermal

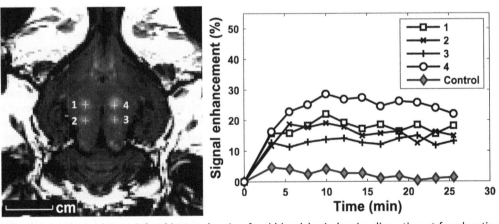

Fig. 4. Contrast-enhanced T1 weighted image showing focal blood–brain barrier disruption at four locations in the rabbit brain with different ultrasound exposures. The plot on the right shows the enhancement at these locations and for a nontargeted region.

ablations), as it is noninvasive (incisionless, scarless, bloodless). Therefore, complications such as bleeding and infection are minimized, and collateral damage to nontarget tissue is almost nonexistent. Unlike the other noninvasive alternative, radiation therapy, MRgFUS does not deliver ionizing radiation to either patient or physician. Furthermore, in radiation therapy and radiation surgery like use of the gamma knife, the radiation dose is statistically set based on accumulated prior experience, and, because their toxic cumulative effects, lend themselves to only a single treatment session (irrelevant of the treatment success). On the other hand, FUS is nontoxic, allowing for unlimited treatments in a single session and unlimited repeated sessions over a period of time, which is a feature of particular importance when a tumor recurs. Unlike surgery and radiotherapy, magnetic resonance thermometry in FUS therapy permits accurate real-time noninvasive intraprocedural monitoring, and conventional MRI provides outstanding anatomic definition of the target site. MRI thermometry remains the sole modality available to evaluate thermal tissue effects and to determine a therapeutic endpoint, and, therefore, treatment success.[37,38] The ability to repeat unlimited treatment sessions coupled with the presence of real-time intraprocedural feedback provides risk-free personalized treatment, especially when confronted with geometrically asymmetric or noncircular target lesions, when such feedback prevents under- or overtreatment. Secondary tumor formation, caused by radiosurgery and radiotherapy, does not occur with FUS therapy. Furthermore, because the thermal gradients of FUS are much narrower than the dose curves in radiotherapy, FUS is more precise and causes less thermal damage to adjacent tissues.

Still, both technical and natural impediments remain, and ongoing research is striving to eliminate or at least decrease these limitations to a certain extent. A particular focus of research is the reduction of lengthy treatment sessions. Addressing the previously mentioned limitation will reduce the complexity of the procedure so that it requires less manpower. Such an advance may ease MRgFUS' way into standard clinical practice so that it becomes an integral part of the therapeutic paradigm for treating brain tumors.

THE FUTURE

Although many challenges remain to be addressed, MRgFUS has emerged as a noninvasive alternative therapy that provides unparalleled treatment control. Inspired by recent advances in transcranial FUS delivery, there has been a marked interest in both thermal and nonthermal effects of TcMRgFUS. Although once considered idealistic and visionary, TcMRgFUS' recent milestones and technological advancements, as evidenced by the latest upsurge in research interest and the results of the first clinical trials, lend unmistakable credence to the potential of this now realistic and pragmatic technology. The ability of MRgFUS to selectively ablate a target lesion while maintaining structural and functional viability of the surrounding tissue redefines brain tumor treatment. Furthermore, MRgFUS' capacity to cause transient, selective, and reversible disruption of the BBB for focal targeted delivery of therapeutic agents into the CNS will revolutionize the way chemotherapeutic CNS drugs are delivered and enhanced.

Insightec and SuperSonic Imagine (Aix-en-Provence, France) are developing an MRgFUS system for the treatment of brain tumors. So far, four patients have been treated at the Brigham and Women's Hospital using Insightec's Exablate transcranial treatment system (Exablate 3000 and 4000). The initial results of this phase 1 clinical trial have just been published by McDannold and colleagues[3] and describe the thermal ablation using TcMRgFUS in three patients. Additionally, thalamotomy, using MRgFUS thermal ablation, was performed in 10 patients in Zurich, Switzerland, for the treatment of intractable pain, and these results also were published recently.[62] The release of MRgFUS for BBBD for the commencement of clinical trials is eminent, and preclinical research is underway for the targeted delivery of chemotherapeutic drugs that normally do not cross the BBB.[6,7] With its benefits far overshadowing its remaining challenges, this integrated noninvasive therapy delivery system is anticipated to radically shift treatment paradigms in neurosurgery and the clinical neurosciences.

REFERENCES

1. Jolesz FA. MRI-guided focused ultrasound surgery. Annu Rev Med 2009;60:417–30.
2. Jolesz FA, McDannold N. Current status and future potential of MRI-guided focused ultrasound surgery. J Magn Reson Imaging 2008;27(2):391–9.
3. McDannold N, Clement GT, Black P, et al. Transcranial magnetic resonance imaging–guided focused ultrasound surgery of brain tumors: initial findings in 3 patients. Neurosurgery 2010;66(2):323–32 [discussion: 332].
4. Vaezy S, Martin R, Yaziji H, et al. Hemostasis of punctured blood vessels using high-intensity focused ultrasound. Ultrasound Med Biol 1998; 24(6):903–10.

5. Medel R, Crowley RW, McKisic MS, et al. Sono-thrombolysis: an emerging modality for the management of stroke. Neurosurgery 2009;65(5):979–93 [discussion: 993].

6. Treat LH, McDannold N, Vykhodtseva N, et al. Targeted delivery of doxorubicin to the rat brain at therapeutic levels using MRI-guided focused ultrasound. Int J Cancer 2007;121(4):901–7.

7. Kinoshita M, McDannold N, Jolesz FA, et al. Noninvasive localized delivery of Herceptin to the mouse brain by MRI-guided focused ultrasound-induced blood–brain barrier disruption PNAS. Proc Natl Acad Sci U S A 2006;103(31):11719–23.

8. Frenkel V. Ultrasound-mediated delivery of drugs and genes to solid tumors. Adv Drug Deliv Rev 2008;60(10):1193–208.

9. Kinoshita M, McDannold N, Jolesz FA, et al. Targeted delivery of antibodies through the blood–brain barrier by MRI-guided focused ultrasound. Biochem Biophys Res Commun 2006;340(4):1085–90.

10. Hynynen K, Jolesz FA. Demonstration of potential noninvasive ultrasound brain therapy through an intact skull. Ultrasound Med Biol 1998;24(2):275–83.

11. Hynynen K, McDannold N, Clement G, et al. Preclinical testing of a phased array ultrasound system for MRI-guided noninvasive surgery of the brain—a primate study. Eur J Radiol 2006;59(2):149–56.

12. Colen RR, Jolesz FA. MRI-guided focused ultrasound: introduction and history. In: Hall W, Nimsky C, Truwit C, editors. Intraoperative MR-guided neurosurgery. Thieme; 2010. Chapter 24, p. 233–40.

13. Jagannathan J, Sanghvi NT, Crum LA, et al. High-intensity focused ultrasound surgery of the brain: part 1—a historical perspective with modern applications. Neurosurgery 2009;64(2):201–11.

14. Lynn JG, Zwemer RL, Chick AJ. The biological application of focused ultrasonic waves. Science 1942;96(2483):119–20.

15. Heimburger RF. Ultrasound augmentation of central nervous system tumor therapy. Indiana Med 1985;78(6):469–76.

16. Hynynen K, Clement GT, McDannold N, et al. 500-Element ultrasound phased array system for noninvasive focal surgery of the brain: a preliminary rabbit study with ex vivo human skulls. Magn Reson Med 2004;52(1):100–7.

17. Jolesz FA, Bleier AR, Jakab P, et al. MR imaging of laser-tissue interactions. Radiology 1988;168(1):249–53.

18. Bleier AR, Jolesz FA, Cohen MS, et al. Real-time magnetic resonance imaging of laser heat deposition in tissue. Magn Reson Med 1991;21(1):132–7.

19. Cline HE, Schenck JF, Watkins RD, et al. Magnetic resonance-guided thermal surgery. Magn Reson Med 1993;30(1):98–106.

20. Cline HE, Hynynen K, Hardy CJ, et al. MR temperature mapping of focused ultrasound surgery. Magn Reson Med 1994;31:628–36.

21. Hynynen K, Pomeroy O, Smith DN, et al. MR imaging-guided focused ultrasound surgery of fibroadenomas in the breast: a feasibility study. Radiology 2001;219(1):176–85.

22. Gianfelice D, Khiat A, Amara M, et al. MR imaging-guided focused US ablation of breast cancer: histopathologic assessment of effectiveness—initial experience. Radiology 2003;227(3):849–55.

23. Tempany CM, Stewart EA, McDannold N, et al. MR imaging-guided focused ultrasound surgery of uterine leiomyomas: a feasibility study. Radiology 2003;226(3):897–905.

24. Uchida T, Ohkusa H, Yamashita H, et al. Five years experience of transrectal high-intensity focused ultrasound using the Sonablate device in the treatment of localized prostate cancer. Int J Urol 2006;13(3):228–33.

25. Fischer K, Gedroyc W, Jolesz FA. Focused ultrasound as a local therapy for liver cancer. Cancer J 2010;16:118–24.

26. Catane R, Beck A, Inbar Y, et al. MR-guided focused ultrasound surgery (MRgFUS) for the palliation of pain in patients with bone metastases—preliminary clinical experience. Ann Oncol 2007;18(1):163–7.

27. Fry WJ, Fry FJ. Fundamental neurological research and human neurosurgery using intense ultrasound. IRE Trans Med Electron 1960;ME-7:166–81.

28. Ram Z, Cohen ZR, Harnof S, et al. Magnetic resonance imaging-guided, high-intensity focused ultrasound for brain tumor therapy. Neurosurgery 2006;59(5):949–55 [discussion: 955–6].

29. Connor CW, Hynynen K. Patterns of thermal deposition in the skull during transcranial focused ultrasound surgery. IEEE Trans Biomed Eng 2004;51(10):1693–706.

30. Fry FJ, Barger JE. Acoustical properties of the human skull. J Acoust Soc Am 1978;63(5):1576–90.

31. Clement GT, Sun J, Giesecke T, et al. A hemisphere array for noninvasive ultrasound brain therapy and surgery. Phys Med Biol 2000;45(12):3707–19.

32. Clement GT, White PJ, King RL, et al. A magnetic resonance imaging–compatible, large-scale array for trans-skull ultrasound surgery and therapy. J Ultrasound Med 2005;24:1117–25.

33. Hynynen K, McDannold N, Vykhodtseva N, et al. Focal disruption of the blood–brain barrier due to 260-kHz ultrasound bursts: a method for molecular imaging and targeted drug delivery. J Neurosurg 2006;105(3):445–54.

34. Deng CX, Sieling F, Pan H, et al. Ultrasound-induced cell membrane porosity. Ultrasound Med Biol 2004;30(4):519–26.

35. Colucci V, Strichartz G, Jolesz F, et al. Focused ultrasound effects on nerve action potential in vitro. Ultrasound Med Biol 2009;35(10):1737–47.

36. McDannold N, King R, Jolesz FA, et al. Usefulness of MR imaging-derived thermometry and dosimetry in determining the threshold for tissue damage induced by thermal surgery in rabbits. Radiology 2000;216(2):517–23.

37. Hynynen K, Vykhodtseva N, Chung AH, et al. Thermal effects of focused ultrasound on the brain: determination with MR imaging. Radiology 1997;204:247–53.

38. Vykhodtseva N, Sorrentino V, Jolesz FA, et al. MRI detection of the thermal effects of focused ultrasound on the brain. Ultrasound Med Biol 2000;26(5):871–80.

39. Diederich CJ, Hynynen K. Ultrasound technology for hyperthermia. Ultrasound Med Biol 1999;25(6):871–87.

40. Wood BJ, Ramkaransingh JR, Fojo T, et al. Percutaneous tumor ablation with radiofrequency. Cancer 2002;94(2):443–51.

41. Nyborg WL. Mechanisms for nonthermal effects of sound. J Acoust Soc Am 1968;44(5):1302–9.

42. Nyborg WL. Biological effects of ultrasound: development of safety guidelines. Part II: general review. Ultrasound Med Biol 2001;27(3):301–33.

43. Hynynen K, McDannold N, Vykhodtseva N, et al. Noninvasive MR imaging-guided focal opening of the blood–brain barrier in rabbits. Radiology 2001;220(3):640–6.

44. Mitragotri S. Healing sound: the use of ultrasound in drug delivery and other therapeutic applications. Nat Rev Drug Discov 2005;4(3):255–60.

45. Sheikov N, McDannold N, Vykhodtseva N, et al. Cellular mechanisms of the blood–brain barrier opening induced by ultrasound in presence of microbubbles. Ultrasound Med Biol 2004;30:979–89.

46. Minnaert M. On musical air bubbles and sounds of running water. Phil Mag 1933;16:235–48.

47. Hynynen K, McDannold N, Martin H, et al. The threshold for brain damage in rabbits induced by bursts of ultrasound in the presence of an ultrasound contrast agent (Optison). Ultrasound Med Biol 2003;29(3):473–81.

48. McDannold NJ, Vykhodtseva NI, Hynynen K. Microbubble contrast agent with focused ultrasound to create brain lesions at low power levels: MR imaging and histologic study in rabbits. Radiology 2006;241(1):95–106.

49. Nyborg WL. Biological effects of ultrasound: development of safety guidelines. Part I: personal histories. Ultrasound Med Biol 2000;26(6):911–64.

50. Leighton TG. The acoustic bubble. San Diego (CA): Academic Press; 1994.

51. Vykhodtseva N, McDannold N, Hynynen K. Progress and problems in the application of focused ultrasound for blood–brain barrier disruption. Ultrasonics 2008;48(4):279–96.

52. Brujan EA, Ikeda T, Matsumoto Y. Jet formation and shock wave emission during collapse of ultrasound-induced cavitation bubbles and their role in the therapeutic applications of high-intensity focused ultrasound. Phys Med Biol 2005;50(20):4797–809.

53. Riesz P, Kondo T. Free radical formation induced by ultrasound and its biological implications. Free Radic Biol Med 1992;13(3):247–70.

54. Vykhodtseva NI, Hynynen K, Damianou C. Histologic effects of high intensity pulsed ultrasound exposure with subharmonic emission in rabbit brain in vivo. Ultrasound Med Biol 1995;21(7):969–79.

55. Sheikov N, McDannold N, Sharma S, et al. Effect of focused ultrasound applied with an ultrasound contrast agent on the tight junctional integrity of the brain microvascular endothelium. Ultrasound Med Biol 2008;34(7):1093–104.

56. Colen RR, Jolesz FA. MRgFUS and intraoperative MR imaging protocols. Brigham and Women's Hospital Institutional Policy 2010.

57. McDannold NJ, Jolesz FA. Magnetic resonance image-guided thermal ablations. Top Magn Reson Imaging 2000;11(3):191–202.

58. Chen L, Bouley DM, Harris BT, et al. MRI study of immediate cell viability in focused ultrasound lesions in the rabbit brain. J Magn Reson Imaging 2001;13(1):23–30.

59. McDannold N, Vykhodtseva N, Hynynen K. Effects of acoustic parameters and ultrasound contrast agent dose on focused-ultrasound induced blood–brain barrier disruption. Ultrasound Med Biol 2008;34(6):930–7.

60. Morocz IA, Hynynen K, Gudbjartsson H, et al. Brain edema development after MRI-guided focused ultrasound treatment. J Magn Reson Imaging 1998;8(1):136–42.

61. Meyers R, Fry WJ, Fry FJ, et al. Early experiences with ultrasonic irradiation of the pallidofugal and nigral complexes in hyperkinetic and hypertonic disorders. J Neurosurg 1959;16(1):32–54.

62. Martin E, Jeanmonod D, Morel A, et al. High-intensity focused ultrasound for noninvasive functional neurosurgery. Ann Neurol 2009;66(6):858–61.

63. Foley JL, Little JW, Starr FL 3rd, et al. Image-guided HIFU neurolysis of peripheral nerves to treat spasticity and pain. Ultrasound Med Biol 2004;30(9):1199–207.

64. Neuwelt EA. Mechanisms of disease: the blood–brain barrier. Neurosurgery 2004;54(1):131–40 [discussion: 141–2].

65. Rubin LL, Staddon JM. The cell biology of the blood–brain barrier. Annu Rev Neurosci 1999;22:11–28.

66. Pardridge WM. The blood–brain barrier: bottleneck in brain drug development. NeuroRx 2005;2(1):3–14.

67. Kroll RA, Neuwelt EA. Outwitting the blood–brain barrier for therapeutic purposes: osmotic

opening and other means. Neurosurgery 1998; 42(5):1083–99 [discussion: 1099–100].

68. Pardridge WM. Blood–brain barrier drug targeting: the future of brain drug development. Mol Interv 2003;3(2):90–105, 151.

69. Guillaume DJ, Doolittle ND, Gahramanov S, et al. Intra-arterial chemotherapy with osmotic blood-brain barrier disruption for aggressive oligo-dendroglial tumors: results of a phase I study. Neurosurgery 2010;66(1):48–58 [discussion: 58].

70. Doolittle ND, Miner ME, Hall WA, et al. Safety and efficacy of a multicenter study using intraarterial chemotherapy in conjunction with osmotic opening of the blood–brain barrier for the treatment of patients with malignant brain tumors. Cancer 2000;88(3):637–47.

71. Guerin C, Olivi A, Weingart JD, et al. Recent advances in brain tumor therapy: local intracerebral drug delivery by polymers. Invest New Drugs 2004;22(1):27–37.

72. Barnard JW, Fry WJ, Fry FJ, et al. Effects of high intensity ultrasound on the central nervous system of the cat. J Comp Neurol 1955;103(3):459–84.

73. Bakay L, Ballantine HT Jr, Hueter TF, et al. Ultrasonically produced changes in the blood–brain barrier. AMA Arch Neurol Psychiatry 1956;76(5):457–67.

74. Lele PP. A simple method for production of trackless focal lesions with focused ultrasound: physical factors. J Physiol 1962;160:494–512.

75. Bednarski MD, Lee JW, Callstrom MR, et al. In vivo target-specific delivery of macromolecular agents with MR-guided focused ultrasound. Radiology 1997;204(1):263–8.

76. Unger EC, Porter T, Culp W, et al. Therapeutic applications of lipid-coated microbubbles. Adv Drug Deliv Rev 2004;56(9):1291–314.

77. Ferrara K, Pollard R, Borden M. Ultrasound microbubble contrast agents: fundamentals and application to gene and drug delivery. Annu Rev Biomed Eng 2007;9:415–47.

78. Moonen CT. Spatio-temporal control of gene expression and cancer treatment using magnetic resonance imaging-guided focused ultrasound. Clin Cancer Res 2007;13(12):3482–9.

79. Raymond SB, Treat LH, Dewey JD, et al. Ultrasound enhanced delivery of molecular imaging and therapeutic agents in Alzheimer's disease mouse models. PLoS One 2008;3(5):e2175.

80. Hynynen K, Colucci V, Chung AH, et al. Noninvasive arterial occlusion using MRI-guided focused ultrasound. Ultrasound Med Biol 1996; 22:1071–7.

81. Zderic V, Brayman AA, Sharar SR, et al. Microbubble-enhanced hemorrhage control using high-intensity focused ultrasound. Ultrasonics 2006;45: 113–20.

Liposomal Contrast Agents in Brain Tumor Imaging

Ketan B. Ghaghada, PhD[a], Rivka R. Colen, MD[b],
Catherine R. Hawley, BS[c], Neil Patel, BS[d],
Srinivasan Mukundan Jr, MD, PhD[e,f,*]

KEYWORDS

- Brain tumor • Nanomedicine • Liposome • Nanoparticle
- Imaging • Contrast agent

Nanomedicine, the application of nanotechnology in the diagnosis and treatment of diseases, is expected to have a major impact on central nervous system–related pathologies.[1,2] Nanotechnology involves the manipulation and engineering of molecules and molecular constructs at the nanoscale (1–100 nm). Nanomedicine can provide solutions to a variety of problems related to diagnosis and treatment.[3] In the imaging field, the development of nanoparticle contrast agents has allowed for cellular and molecular imaging, monitoring of drug delivery to tumors, and efficient surgical removal of solid tumors.[4,5] In the therapeutic field, nanoparticles have been shown to increase the bioavailability of poorly water soluble drugs; prevent in vivo degradation of therapeutic molecules, including genetic materials; reduce side effects; and enhance the efficacy of conventional anticancer drugs as well as increase the specificity of delivery of drugs to diseased sites.[6]

Liposomes, one of the most extensively studied nanoparticles, have been investigated for use as a platform technology for the delivery of therapeutic molecules and imaging agents. Liposomal nanocarriers encapsulating cytotoxic molecules, such as doxorubicin, daunorubicin, and cytarabine, have been clinically investigated for treatment of brain tumors.[7–10] Liposomes have also been tested clinically for delivery of gene therapy products.[11] In preclinical studies using brain tumor models, liposomes have been used for delivery of agents for neutron-capture therapy,[12] increasing the specificity of cytotoxic agents by molecular targeting of tumors cells,[13–15] as well as convection-enhanced delivery (CED) of drugs.[16]

Liposomes have also received considerable attention for use as a nanoparticle-based MR imaging contrast agent.[17,18] In comparison to conventional small molecule contrast agents, liposomes provide a unique nanoparticle platform because they confer specific desirable properties with respect to pharmacokinetics, target specificity, therapy monitoring, and signal amplification in contrast agents. MR imaging–based liposomal contrast agents have been preclinically tested

Disclosures: Dr Ghaghada and Dr Mukundan are stockholders in Marval Biosciences Inc, a start-up company developing nanoparticle contrast agents for use in x-ray and CT imaging.

[a] School of Health Information Sciences, The University of Texas Health Science Center at Houston, 7000 Fannin Street, Suite 600, Houston, TX 77030, USA

[b] Department of Radiology, Brigham and Women's Hospital, 75 Francis Street, Boston, MA 02115, USA

[c] Vanderbilt University School of Medicine, 215 Light Hall, Box #377, Nashville, TN 37232, USA

[d] University of Illinois College of Medicine, 103 South McCullough Street, Apartment B, Urbana, IL 61801, USA

[e] Division of Neuroradiology, Department of Radiology, Brigham and Women's Hospital, 75 Francis Street, Boston, MA 02115, USA

[f] Department of Radiology, Harvard Medical School, Boston, MA, USA

* Corresponding author. Division of Neuroradiology, Department of Radiology, Brigham and Women's Hospital, 75 Francis Street, Boston, MA 02115.

E-mail address: smukundan@partners.org

Neuroimag Clin N Am 20 (2010) 367–378

doi:10.1016/j.nic.2010.05.001

and shown to be successful for MR microangiography of the neurovasculature[19] as well as monitoring CED of drugs to brain tumors.[20] This article reports the advances made in the use of liposomes for brain tumor imaging, beginning with a description of various nanoparticle platforms available for use as contrast agents, then describing the design and functional properties of liposomes that make them versatile nanocarriers. Finally, the development of MR imaging–based liposomal contrast agents and their use in brain tumors is described.

CLASSES OF NANOPARTICLES USED AS CONTRAST AGENTS

Many nanoparticles have been used as contrast agents. The majority of these nanoparticles can be classified within one of the following categories: lipid-based, polymeric, iron oxide, and metal-based nanoparticles.

Lipid-based Nanoparticles

Lipid-based nanoparticles can be subdivided into three categories: liposomes, micelles, and lipid-coated perfluorocarbon (PFC) nanoparticles. A detailed discussion about liposomes is provided later.

Micelles are self-assembled nanoparticles, typically 10 to 50 nm in size, consisting of amphiphilic molecules with a hydrophobic core and a hydrophilic shell. The lipid molecules are typically conjugated to a hydrophilic polymer, such as polyethylene glycol (PEG), to provide long circulation properties to the micellar structures. The hydrophobic core of micelles has been used for delivery of poorly water-soluble therapeutic molecules to solid tumors.[21] Nontargeted and ligand-targeted micelles have been developed for treatment of cancers.[22] For the development of contrast agents, imaging moieties conjugated to amphiphilic molecules have been incorporated into micelles.[23]

PFC nanoparticles are approximately 250 nm in size and consist of a lipid monolayer surrounding a hydrophobic core of liquid PFC.[24] Imaging agents, drug molecules, and targeting ligands can be incorporated into the lipid monolayer. In addition to their role in standard proton-based MR imaging, the ability to encapsulate fluorine atoms within the internal core allows for ^{19}F-based MR imaging.[25] PFC nanoparticles have been used extensively as molecular imaging contrast agents and multifunctional nanoparticles in cardiovascular and cancer applications.[26]

Polymeric Nanoparticles

Polymeric nanoparticles are fabricated using biodegradable polymers, such as polylactic acid, poly(lactic-co-glycolic acid), polylysine, and PEG-based copolymers. Depending on the type of polymer backbone and fabrication process, polymeric nanoparticles can be prepared in a variety of sizes, ranging from 10 nm to 1000 nm. Dendrimers are highly branched, multigenerational nanoparticles consisting of exterior end groups that can be functionalized with imaging moieties,[27–30] therapeutic molecules,[31,32] or specific ligands[33,34] for tumor targeting. These are spherical in shape and their size increases with the addition of each polymer shell layer. The ability to precisely control the size and functionality of dendrimers makes them one of the most extensively studied nanoparticle platforms.[35] Several dendrimer platforms, including polyamidoamine dendrimers, have been investigated for use as contrast agents and for delivery of therapeutics to brain tumors.[36–39] In addition to dendrimers, polymeric nanoparticles and micelles prepared using other polymers have been investigated for use as nanotherapeutics[40,41] and imaging agents[42–45] in a variety of cancers, including brain tumors.[46,47]

Iron Oxide Nanoparticles

Iron oxide nanoparticles have been extensively investigated as MR imaging contrast agents for more than two decades.[48] They are the only nanoparticle-based contrast agent approved for use in humans.[49] These nanoparticles consist of an iron oxide core surrounded with an outer coating of hydrophilic polymers, typically dextran, for particle stability.[50,51] Two types of iron oxide nanoparticles have been developed. Ultrasmall superparamagnetic iron oxide particles (USPIOs) are smaller than 50 nm in size, whereas superparamagnetic iron oxide particles (SPIOs) range between 50 and 200 nm.[52] SPIOs have high T2 relaxivities ($r_2 > 60$ $mM^{-1} \cdot sec^{-1}$) and are primarily used in T2-weighted imaging.[53] USPIOs have low T2 relaxivities compared with SPIOs and have been investigated for use as blood pool contrast agents.[54,55] Unlike conventional gadolinium (Gd)-based contrast agents, iron oxide nanoparticles have a blood half-life of more than 18 hours. The presence of dextran on the surface of iron oxide nanoparticles facilitates their uptake by lymphocytes. As a result, these nanoparticles have been investigated in inflammatory-related diseases, lymph-node staging, and cancer imaging.[56,57] In brain tumors, iron oxide nanoparticles have been used in dynamic contrast-enhanced MR imaging[58,59] and imaging of the neovasculature[60–62] as well as evaluating therapeutic response to antiangiogenic therapy.[59] The high-contrast sensitivity of MR imaging combined with efficient cellular uptake of iron oxide nanoparticles has been used for in vivo MR imaging–based tracking of tumor cells, stem cells,[63,64] and inflammatory cells.[65,66]

Metal-based Nanoparticles

Two of the most commonly used metal-based nanoparticles are metal nanoshells and quantum dots. Metal nanoshells are composed of a silica core surrounded by a thin metal shell.[67] The most common of these nanoparticles are gold nanoshells consisting of an ultrathin coating of gold. The nanoparticles can be fabricated to absorb or scatter light, depending on the relative dimensions of the core size and shell thickness.[68,69] Consequently, gold nanoshells have been used as contrast agents in optical imaging.[70,71] Furthermore, the ability of these nanoparticles to absorb light in the near-infrared (700–1000 nm wavelength) spectrum has facilitated their use in photothermal therapy.[72–74] Gold nanoshells have also been investigated for thermal ablation of brain tumors in the canine model.[75] Recently, these nanoparticles entered clinical trials for treatment of refractory head and neck cancer.[76] Quantum dots are based on semiconductor compounds consisting of a cadmium-based core surrounded by an inert layer of metallic shell.[77,78] Similar to gold nanoshells, quantum dots have excellent optical properties that are dependent on particle size. The tunable optical properties of these agents have primarily been used in preclinical optical imaging for a variety of cancer applications, including cellular and molecular imaging of tumors,[79–81] and in surgical operations.[82]

LIPOSOMES

Liposomes have been used as a platform technology for delivery of drugs[83,84] and encapsulation of small molecule contrast agents.[18,85,86] Liposomes are spherical vesicles made of lipid bilayer, thus resembling tiny cells. The lipid bilayer also serves to separate the internal aqueous core of the liposome from the external medium. Systemically administered liposomes, with diameters ranging between 50 and 400 nm, are much larger than conventional drugs and contrast agents, which are typically subnanometer in size.

DESIGN AND FUNCTIONAL PROPERTIES OF LIPOSOMES

The size distribution of liposomes depends on their method of fabrication. Two of the most commonly used methods for fabricating liposomes are (1) high-pressure extrusion and (2) sonication.[87]

The high-pressure extrusion process is the most widely used method for fabricating liposomes, with sizes ranging from 50 to 400 nm in diameter. This method demonstrates a high degree of consistency and reproducibility. Liposomes can have a single bilayer (unilamellar) or multiple bilayers (multilamellar), depending on the method of fabrication and particle size (Fig. 1). Liposomes with multiple bilayers are referred to as multilamellar vesicles (MLVs). Unilamellar liposomes, however, are divided into two classes on the basis of size. Liposomes under 100 nm are considered small unilamellar vesicles (SUVs), whereas those larger than 100 nm are considered large unilamellar vesicles (LUVs). MLVs generally have a broad particle size distribution compared with SUVs. The sonication process is primarily used for fabrication of SUVs, typically 30 to 50 nm in diameter.

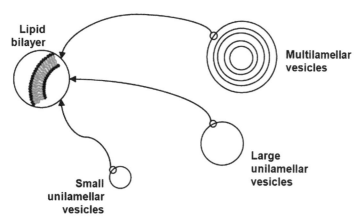

Fig. 1. Classification of liposomes. Depending on the particle size and lamellarity, liposomes can be classified into SUVs, LUVs, and MLVs.

Liposomes provide several desirable properties in vivo that can be exploited for use in specific imaging applications. For instance, long circulating liposomes have been used as blood-pool contrast agents for MR imaging and CT applications.[86,88] Ligand-targeted liposomes have been used as molecular imaging contrast agents in MR imaging applications.[89] Multifunctional nanoparticles, developed by coencapsulating an imaging moiety and a therapeutic agent within the same liposome, have been used in image-guided drug delivery.[90,91] The fabrication of such constructs is facilitated by the characteristics of liposomes, described as follows.

Clearance Route

Small molecule contrast agents are typically cleared via the kidneys. In comparison, liposomes, which are generally larger than 50 nm, have an alternate clearance pathway. Liposomes are primarily cleared by the phagocytic cells of the liver and spleen, referred to as the reticuloendothelial system (RES). Thus, in the context of imaging agents, liposomal contrast agents result in a change in the clearance route from being renal based to RES based.

Pharmacokinetics

The in vivo pharmacokinetics of liposomes is dictated by their surface characteristics (**Fig. 2**). The clearance of conventional liposomes is initiated by binding of opsonins on the surface of liposomes followed by a cascade of events, which results in their recognition by the RES.[92] Conventional liposomes have a moderate in vivo half life, typically on the order of minutes to few hours. The half-life of liposomes also depends on their size with particles larger than 200 nm

demonstrating shorter half-life compared with smaller particles.[93] Their half-life can be prolonged to several hours by decorating the liposomal surface with biocompatible hydrophilic polymers.[94,95] The most common polymer used in the development of long circulating liposomes is PEG. Pegylated liposomes, also known as stealth liposomes, are able to evade the RES by preventing opsonization, thereby increasing blood half-life to approximately 18 hours.[96] Similar to conventional liposomes, the blood circulation times of pegylated liposomes is also dependent on particle size.

Payload Encapsulation

The central hydrophilic core of a liposome can be used as a nanocarrier to encapsulate a payload, such as a therapeutic or a contrast agent. This construct has been used in several clinically available chemotherapeutic products, such as doxorubicin-encapsulated pegylated liposomes (Doxil), amphotericin-B liposomes (AmBisome), daunorubicin-encapsulated liposomes (DaunoXome), and doxorubicin-encapsulated liposomes (Myocet). In addition to drugs, liposomes have been used to encapsulate iodine and Gd-based small molecule contrast agents.[85,86,97,98] In some cases, the liposomal core has also been used to carry both a therapeutic and a contrast agent, thus allowing for monitoring the delivery of therapeutic agents. This is exemplified by their use in CED of drugs to brain tumors.[99] The hydrophobic bilayer has also been used to carry therapeutic or imaging agents.[100,101] The encapsulation of chemotherapeutic agents within the liposome offers improved safety and patient tolerance combined with reduced side effects and equivalent or improved therapeutic efficacy.[102–104]

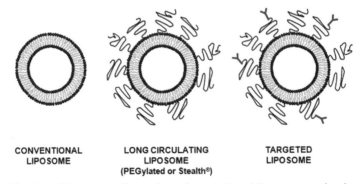

CONVENTIONAL
LIPOSOME

LONG CIRCULATING
LIPOSOME
(PEGylated or Stealth®)

TARGETED
LIPOSOME

Fig. 2. Surface modification of liposomes. The surface of conventional liposome can be decorated with PEG for long blood circulation property or with ligands attached to the distal end of PEG for targeting to cell-surface receptors on specific cells.

Targeting to Tumors

Two different mechanisms, passive and active, have been used for targeting liposomes to tumors. Passive targeting takes advantage of the lack continuous lining of endothelial cells and the presence of large pores on luminal surface of tumor blood vessels.[105] Liposomes are able to extravasate through the leaky tumor vasculature and accumulate within the interstitial space of tumor tissue by a process known as the enhanced permeation and retention effect.[106,107] Their accumulation results in an increase in deposition of chemotherapeutic drug within the tumor tissue, thus improving therapeutic efficacy.[104] The extravasation and accumulation of liposomes within tumors is also size dependent, with larger size liposomes ($\geq$400 nm) showing significantly reduced tumor uptake compared with smaller size liposomes.[108]

Active targeting involves molecular recognition of tumor cells. Ligands ranging from small molecules to monoclonal antibodies have been conjugated to the distal end of PEG chains to facilitate binding of liposomes to cell-surface receptors. Ligand-targeted liposomes delivered via the systemic route can achieve molecular recognition by targeting tumor cells located in the interstitial environment or endothelial cells present on angiogenic blood vessels. Systemically administered liposomes, however, deliver low amount of drug to the tumor cells due to limited transport within the tumor interstitium. Ligand-targeted liposomes have been demonstrated to increase the specificity of delivery of chemotherapeutics by targeting tumor cells that overexpress surface receptors, such as folate receptor, epidermal growth factor receptor (EGFR), and transferrin receptor, among others.[13,15,109,110] In addition to single ligand targeting, liposomes bearing multiple-type ligands that simultaneously target different receptors coexpressed on tumor cells have been investigated.[111]

One final modification that can be used in tumor targeting involves triggered release of liposome-encapsulated contents. The bilayer of liposomes can be modulated depending on the microenvironment to increase the release of the payload.[112–114] Hyperthermia-mediated delivery of chemotherapeutics from temperature-sensitive liposomal formulation is currently in clinical trials for the treatment of patients with locally recurrent breast cancer.[76]

MR IMAGING–BASED LIPOSOMAL CONTRAST AGENTS

For more than two decades, liposomes have been used as MR imaging–based nanoparticle contrast agents.[17,115,116] The usefulness of liposomal contrast agents has been demonstrated in small animal models. For the development of T1-based liposomal contrast agents, three different constructs have been used: (1) core-encapsulated Gd (CE-Gd) liposomes,[97,98,117] (2) surface-conjugated Gd (SC-Gd) liposomes,[118,119] and (3) dual-Gd liposomes (**Fig. 3**).[115] In CE-Gd liposomes, small molecule conventional Gd chelates are encapsulated within the core of the liposome. In SC-Gd liposomes, the Gd chelates are conjugated on the surface of the lipid bilayer. Dual-Gd liposomes comprise two pools of Gd: core encapsulated and surface conjugated. For MR angiography applications, long circulating liposomal-Gd contrast agents provide uniform signal intensity and stable enhancement over an extended period of imaging.[88]

The T1 relaxivity of liposomal-Gd contrast agents is determined by interactions between the Gd atoms and the bulk water molecules. The encapsulation of Gd chelates within the interior core of the liposomes results in lower T1 relaxivities for CE-Gd compared with conventional contrast agents.[98] The low T1 relaxivity of CE-Gd

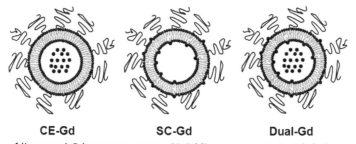

CE-Gd   **SC-Gd**   **Dual-Gd**

Fig. 3. Classification of liposomal-Gd contrast agents. CE-Gd liposomes contain Gd chelates encapsulated within the interior core of the liposome. SC-Gd liposomes contain Gd chelates conjugated on the internal and external surfaces of the liposome bilayer. Dual-Gd liposomes consist of two Gd pools: core encapsulated and surface conjugated. The stars indicate Gd chelates. All of the liposomal constructs have a surface coating of PEG that provides long blood circulation half-life.

is a result of slow transport of water molecules across the lipid bilayer, rendering external bulk water relatively inaccessible to the relaxing influence of the encapsulated Gd atom. The T1 relaxivity of CE-Gd agents can, however, be increased by decreasing particle size. In spite of reduced T1 relaxivity, the advantages of CE-Gd liposomes have been demonstrated in preclinical imaging studies.[120,121] In a rat model, conventional contrast agents demonstrated rapid extravasation from normal vasculature into the surrounding extravascular space.[120] Consequently, higher background signal and low vessel conspicuity were obtained, limiting visualization of the spinal microvasculature. Alternatively, CE-Gd liposomes demonstrated low background signal and higher vessel conspicuity because of negligible extravasation from the vascular compartment. As a result, CE-Gd agent demonstrated visualization of spinal vasculature, including the artery of Adamkiewicz and the venous plexus.[120] The superior imaging characteristics of CE-Gd agents have also enabled excellent visualization of the mouse cardiovascular structures, including the coronary arteries.[121] The uniform and steady signal enhancement provided by long circulating CE-Gd agent enabled accurate and repeated quantitative assessment of cardiac function for mouse phenotyping.[122]

SC-Gd agents represent a second-generation liposomal-based MR contrast nanoparticle. Compared with CE-Gd agents, SC-Gd agents show higher T1 relaxivities because the lanthanide center is readily accessible to bulk water. In a mouse model, the higher T1 relaxivity of SC-Gd enabled ultrahigh-resolution imaging of neurovasculature at approximately 50 μm in-plane resolution.[19] Excellent visualization of the circle of Willis and perforating vessels was demonstrated using SC-Gd (Fig. 4). In addition to visualizing the arterial blood supply, SC-Gd agents enabled simultaneous visualization of the venous system.

More recently, a third-generation liposomal-Gd agent, referred to as dual-Gd, was developed.[115] Dual-Gd agents demonstrate high nanoparticle-based T1 relaxivity compared with previous generations of liposomal contrast agents. The development of ligand-bearing dual-Gd constructs could, therefore, serve as a signal amplification vehicle for molecular imaging because they can deliver several thousand Gd moieties to each cell-surface receptor of the targeted cell.

Liposomal nanoparticles have also been investigated for their use in T2-weighted imaging. These agents typically consist of USPIOs that are encapsulated within the core of the liposome.[123] The sequestration of USPIOs within the liposome interior results in a high T2 relaxivity compared with the free USPIOs.

LIPOSOMES IN BRAIN TUMOR IMAGING

Although systemically administered liposomes and other nanoparticles can extravasate and

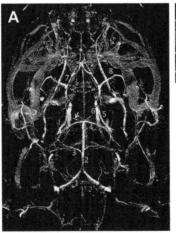
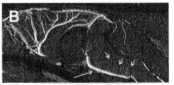
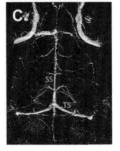

Fig. 4. MR angiography of the mouse brain obtained using SC-Gd liposomal contrast agent. (*A*) Coronal maximum intensity projection image demonstrating detailed visualization of the mouse circle of Willis. The arterial and venous structures are simultaneously visualized. 1, Ventral artery; 2, basilar artery; 3, anterior inferior choroid artery; 4, superior cerebral artery; 5, posterior cerebral artery; 6, internal carotid artery; 7, anterior cerebral artery; 8, middle cerebral artery. Posterior communicating artery is also demonstrated (*arrow*). (*B*) Sagittal maximum intensity projection image demonstrating visualization of the pontine arteries (*short arrows*) originating from the basilar artery (*long arrow*). (*C*) Coronal maximum intensity projection image demonstrating visualization of the superior sagittal (SS) and transverse sinus (TS).

accumulate in tumors through compromised vasculature, their migration within the tumor interstitial space is slow and limited. Small molecules, such as conventional therapeutic and contrast agents, rapidly diffuse in and out of the tumor via brownian motion. Alternatively, macromolecular constructs, such as nanoparticle contrast agents, are diffusion limited, moving slowly or not at all within the tumor interstitium.[124] One approach to overcoming this limitation is the use of CED, a drug delivery system designed at the National Institutes of Health in 1994.[125] In CED, a canula is surgically placed into the targeted lesion via a burr hole and the drug or contrast agent is actively infused. Positive pressure gradients resulting from direct intracerebral infusion cause bulk flow and result in distribution of the agent throughout the target volume. Thus, unlike intraarterial infusion, CED is not limited by diffusivity within the tumor bed. During the initial infusion phase, positive pressure is used to distribute the infusate throughout the prescribed volume. Once pressure equilibrium is achieved, diffusion rather than bulk flow of the agent into the surrounding perimeter occurs.[126] Furthermore, the ability of therapeutic or contrast agents to bypass the blood-brain barrier facilitated by CED allows for distribution beyond the tumor margins, where an intact blood-brain barrier would be expected to limit deposition via vascular infusion.

CED, similar to other techniques, demonstrates some limitations. Firstly, it is invasive, requiring surgical placement of a canula and complicated infusion techniques. Secondly, although canula placement can be tailored to distribute asymmetrically, distribution for the most part is spherical around the point of infusion.

Although it may be possible to overcome this second limitation by infusing a larger amount and distributing the agent over a larger tissue volume beyond the tumor margin, this can result in a third limitation, overtreatment. Unlike other ablative technologies, however, in which there is a sharp zone of transition between the treated and non-treated tissue, CED has a zone of transition in which diffusion peripheral to the actively infused agent occurs, thus potentially treating those tumor cells that have infiltrated beyond the zone.[127,128]

A technical limitation caused by the canula design, which resulted in backflow of the infusate, has been addressed with the development of reflux-free stepped canulas, resulting in a more accurate distribution of nanoparticles.[129]

The coupling of liposomal-encapsulated chemotherapeutic drugs with CED for treatment of brain tumors has been extensively investigated in preclinical models, confirming safety and feasibility.[16,130,131] A major limitation with CED of liposomal therapeutics, however, has been the difficultly in monitoring the delivery and distribution within brain tumors. To circumvent this problem, Saito and colleagues pioneered the use of Gd-encapsulated liposomal agents for MR imaging–based real-time monitoring of convection-enhanced delivery (CED) of therapeutics into brain tumors.[90] Preclinical CED studies conducted in rodents and primates demonstrated that Gd-encapsulated liposomal contrast agents not only predict delivery but also allow for an accurate correlation between the infused and final volume of distribution.[132] To further optimize the CED method for delivery of liposomal therapeutics, studies have been conducted on liposomes coencapsulating both Gd contrast agents and chemotherapeutic molecules.[133] The same group has recently published their preliminary results on CED of coencapsulated liposomal agents in a primate brain.[99] These potentially mark the final phase of preclinical trials before translating into clinical trials.

SUMMARY

The versatile nature of liposomal platforms has proved its usefulness as a multifunctional nanoparticle for brain tumor imaging. The ability to coencapsulate therapeutic molecules and imaging agents within liposomes coupled with surface decoration allows for the targeting of cell-surface receptors overexpressed on brain tumor cells, such as EGFR or EGFRvIII. The latter has the potential to expand the usefulness of CED-based approach in the treatment of brain tumors.[134] In addition to CED-based methods, liposomal-based multifunctional nanoparticles could be delivered systemically for monitoring the efficacy of neoadjuvant brain tumor therapies. The long circulating property of liposomal contrast agents could also be used for measuring nanoparticle-based transvascular permeability in brain tumors as well as accurate fractional blood volume measurements during antiangiogenic therapy.[135] Given the encouraging results from current preclinical studies, it seems that human clinical trials would be expected. Moreover, liposomal applications in brain tumor imaging might surface as an adjuvant modality for diagnosis and targeting of tumors as well as monitoring therapy response.

REFERENCES

1. Bhaskar S, Tian F, Stoeger T, et al. Multifunctional nanocarriers for diagnostics, drug delivery and targeted treatment across blood-brain barrier: perspectives on tracking and neuroimaging. Part Fibre Toxicol 2010;7:3.

2. Leary SP, Liu CY, Yu C, et al. Toward the emergence of nanoneurosurgery: part I—progress in nanoscience, nanotechnology, and the comprehension of events in the mesoscale realm. Neurosurgery 2005;57(4):606–34.

3. Ferrari M. Cancer nanotechnology: opportunities and challenges. Nat Rev Cancer 2005; 5(3):161–71.

4. McCarthy JR, Weissleder R. Multifunctional magnetic nanoparticles for targeted imaging and therapy. Adv Drug Deliv Rev 2008;60(11):1241–51.

5. Leary SP, Liu CY, Apuzzo ML. Toward the emergence of nanoneurosurgery: part II-nanomedicine: diagnostics and imaging at the nanoscale level. Neurosurgery 2006;58(5):805–23.

6. Kateb B, Chiu K, Yamamoto V, et al. Nanoplatforms for constructing new approaches to cancer treatment, imaging, and drug delivery: what should be the policy? Neuroimage 2010. [Epub ahead of print]. DOI:10.1016/j.neuroimage.2010.01.105.

7. Fabel K, Dietrich J, Hau P, et al. Long-term stabilization in patients with malignant glioma after treatment with liposomal doxorubicin. Cancer 2001; 92(7):1936–42.

8. Marina NM, Cochrane D, Harney E, et al. Dose escalation and pharmacokinetics of pegylated liposomal doxorubicin (Doxil) in children with solid tumors: a pediatric oncology group study. Clin Cancer Res 2002;8(2):413–8.

9. Lippens RJ. Liposomal daunorubicin (DaunoXome) in children with recurrent or progressive brain tumors. Pediatr Hematol Oncol 1999;16(2):131–9.

10. Lassaletta A, Lopez-Ibor B, Mateos E, et al. Intrathecal liposomal cytarabine in children under 4 years with malignant brain tumors. J Neurooncol 2009;95(1):65–9.

11. Yoshida J, Mizuno M. Clinical gene therapy for brain tumors. Liposomal delivery of anticancer molecule to glioma. J Neurooncol 2003;65(3): 261–7.

12. Nakamura H. Liposomal boron delivery for neutron capture therapy. Methods Enzymol 2009;465:179–208.

13. Mamot C, Drummond DC, Noble CO, et al. Epidermal growth factor receptor-targeted immunoliposomes significantly enhance the efficacy of multiple anticancer drugs in vivo. Cancer Res 2005;65(24):11631–8.

14. Madhankumar AB, Slagle-Webb B, Wang X, et al. Efficacy of interleukin-13 receptor-targeted liposomal doxorubicin in the intracranial brain tumor model. Mol Cancer Ther 2009;8(3):648–54.

15. Doi A, Kawabata S, Iida K, et al. Tumor-specific targeting of sodium borocaptate (BSH) to malignant glioma by transferrin-PEG liposomes: a modality for boron neutron capture therapy. J Neurooncol 2008;87(3):287–94.

16. Krauze MT, Noble CO, Kawaguchi T, et al. Convection-enhanced delivery of nanoliposomal CPT-11 (irinotecan) and PEGylated liposomal doxorubicin (Doxil) in rodent intracranial brain tumor xenografts. Neuro Oncol 2007;9(4):393–403.

17. Unger EC, Shen DK, Fritz TA. Status of liposomes as MR contrast agents. J Magn Reson Imaging 1993;3(1):195–8.

18. Mulder WJ, Strijkers GJ, van Tilborg GA, et al. Lipid-based nanoparticles for contrast-enhanced MRI and molecular imaging. NMR Biomed 2006; 19(1):142–64.

19. Howles GP, Ghaghada KB, Qi Y, et al. High-resolution magnetic resonance angiography in the mouse using a nanoparticle blood-pool contrast agent. Magn Reson Med 2009;62(6):1447–56.

20. Krauze MT, Forsayeth J, Park JW, et al. Real-time imaging and quantification of brain delivery of liposomes. Pharm Res 2006;23(11):2493–504.

21. Dabholkar RD, Sawant RM, Mongayt DA, et al. Polyethylene glycol-phosphatidylethanolamine conjugate (PEG-PE)-based mixed micelles: some properties, loading with paclitaxel, and modulation of P-glycoprotein-mediated efflux. Int J Pharm 2006;315(1–2):148–57.

22. Torchilin VP. Lipid-core micelles for targeted drug delivery. Curr Drug Deliv 2005;2(4):319–27.

23. Amirbekian V, Lipinski MJ, Briley-Saebo KC, et al. Detecting and assessing macrophages in vivo to evaluate atherosclerosis noninvasively using molecular MRI. Proc Natl Acad Sci U S A 2007; 104(3):961–6.

24. Kaneda MM, Caruthers S, Lanza GM, et al. Perfluorocarbon nanoemulsions for quantitative molecular imaging and targeted therapeutics. Ann Biomed Eng 2009;37(10):1922–33.

25. Lanza GM, Winter PM, Neubauer AM, et al. 1H/19F magnetic resonance molecular imaging with perfluorocarbon nanoparticles. Curr Top Dev Biol 2005;70:57–76.

26. Tran TD, Caruthers SD, Hughes M, et al. Clinical applications of perfluorocarbon nanoparticles for molecular imaging and targeted therapeutics. Int J Nanomedicine 2007;2(4):515–26.

27. Wiener EC, Magnin RL, Gansow OA, et al. Dendrimer-based metal chelates: a new class of magnetic resonance imaging contrast agents. Magn Reson Med 1994;31(1):1–8.

28. Tan M, Wu X, Jeong EK, et al. Peptide-targeted nanoglobular Gd-DOTA monoamide conjugates for magnetic resonance cancer molecular imaging. Biomacromolecules 2010;11(3):754–61.

29. Cheng Z, Thorek DL, Tsourkas A. Gadolinium-conjugated dendrimer nanoclusters as a tumor-targeted T1 magnetic resonance imaging contrast agent. Angew Chem Int Ed Engl 2010; 49(2):346–50.

30. Longmire M, Choyke PL, Kobayashi H. Dendrimer-based contrast agents for molecular imaging. Curr Top Med Chem 2008;8(14):1180–6.

31. Medina SH, El-Sayed ME. Dendrimers as carriers for delivery of chemotherapeutic agents. Chem Rev 2009;109(7):3141–57.

32. Choi YS, Thomas T, Kotlyar A, et al. Synthesis and functional evaluation of DNA-assembled polyamidoamine dendrimer clusters for cancer cell-specific targeting. Chem Biol 2005;12:35–43.

33. Singh P, Gupta U, Asthana A, et al. Folate and folate-PEG-PAMAM dendrimers: synthesis, characterization, and targeted anticancer drug delivery potential in tumor bearing mice. Bioconjug Chem 2008;19(11):2239–52.

34. Boswell CA, Eck PK, Regino CA, et al. Synthesis, characterization, and biological evaluation of integrin alphavbeta3-targeted PAMAM dendrimers. Mol Pharm 2008;5(4):527–39.

35. Tomalia DA, Naylor AM, Goddard WA. Starburst dendrimers: molecular-level control of size, shape, surface chemistry, topology, and flexibility from atoms to macroscopic matter. Angew Chem Int Ed Engl 1990;29:138–75.

36. Yang W, Wu G, Barth RF, et al. Molecular targeting and treatment of composite EGFR and EGFRvIII-positive gliomas using boronated monoclonal antibodies. Clin Cancer Res 2008;14(3):883–91.

37. Sarin H, Kanevsky AS, Wu H, et al. Effective transvascular delivery of nanoparticles across the blood-brain tumor barrier into malignant glioma cells. J Transl Med 2008;6:80.

38. Regino CA, Walbridge S, Bernardo M, et al. A dual CT-MR dendrimer contrast agent as a surrogate marker for convection-enhanced delivery of intracerebral macromolecular therapeutic agents. Contrast Media Mol Imaging 2008;3(1):2–8.

39. Han L, Zhang A, Wang H, et al. Tat-BMPs-PAMAM conjugates enhance therapeutic effect of small interference RNA on U251 glioma cells in vitro and in vivo. Hum Gene Ther 2010;21(4):417–26.

40. Blanco E, Kessinger CW, Sumer BD, et al. Multifunctional micellar nanomedicine for cancer therapy. Exp Biol Med (Maywood) 2009;234(2):123–31.

41. Danson S, Ferry D, Alakhov V, et al. Phase I dose escalation and pharmacokinetic study of pluronic polymer-bound doxorubicin (SP1049C) in patients with advanced cancer. Br J Cancer 2004;90:2085–91.

42. Torchilin VP. Polymeric contrast agents for medical imaging. Curr Pharm Biotechnol 2000;1(2):183–215.

43. Torchilin VP. PEG-based micelles as carriers of contrast agents for different imaging modalities. Adv Drug Deliv Rev 2002;54:235–52.

44. Guthi JS, Yang SG, Huang G, et al. MRI-visible micellar nanomedicine for targeted drug delivery to lung cancer cells. Mol Pharm 2010;7(1):32–40.

45. Torchilin VP, Frank-Kamenetsky MD, Wolf GL. CT visualization of blood pool in rats by using long-circulating, iodine-containing micelles. Acad Radiol 1999;6(1):61–5.

46. Kuroda J, Kuratsu J, Yasunaga M, et al. Antitumor effect of NK012, a 7-ethyl-10-hydroxycamptothecin-incorporating polymeric micelle, on U87MG orthotopic glioblastoma in mice compared with irinotecan hydrochloride in combination with bevacizumab. Clin Cancer Res 2010;16(2):521–9.

47. Inoue T, Yamashita Y, Nishihara M, et al. Therapeutic efficacy of a polymeric micellar doxorubicin infused by convection-enhanced delivery against intracranial 9L brain tumor models. Neuro Oncol 2009;11(2):151–7.

48. Weissleder R, Elizondo G, Wittenberg J, et al. Ultrasmall superparamagnetic iron oxide: characterization of a new class of contrast agents for MR imaging. Radiology 1990;175:489–93.

49. Ros PR, Freeny PC, Harms SE, et al. Hepatic MR imaging with ferumoxides: a multicenter clinical trial of the safety and efficacy in the detection of focal hepatic lesions. Radiology 1995;196:481–8.

50. Laurent S, Forge D, Port M, et al. Magnetic iron oxide nanoparticles: synthesis, stabilization, vectorization, physicochemical characterizations, and biological applications. Chem Rev 2008;108:2064–110.

51. Thorek DL, Chen AK, Czupryna J, et al. Superparamagnetic iron oxide nanoparticle probes for molecular imaging. Ann Biomed Eng 2006;34:23–38.

52. Laurent S, Boutry S, Mahieu I, et al. Iron oxide based MR contrast agents: from chemistry to cell labeling. Curr Med Chem 2009;16(35):4712–27.

53. Wang YX, Hussain SM, Krestin GP. Superparamagnetic iron oxide contrast agents: physicochemical characteristics and applications in MR imaging. Eur Radiol 2001;11:2319–31.

54. Li W, Tutton S, Vu AT, et al. First-pass contrast-enhanced magnetic resonance angiography in humans using ferumoxytol, a novel ultrasmall superparamagnetic iron oxide (USPIO)-based blood pool agent. J Magn Reson Imaging 2005;21(1):46–52.

55. Tombach B, Reimer P, Bremer C, et al. First-pass and equilibrium-MRA of the aortoiliac region with a superparamagnetic iron oxide blood pool MR contrast agent (SH U 555 C): results of a human pilot study. NMR Biomed 2004;17(7):500–6.

56. Lahaye MJ, Engelen SM, Kessels AG, et al. USPIO-enhanced MR imaging for nodal staging in patients with primary rectal cancer: predictive criteria. Radiology 2008;246(3):804–11.

57. Harisinghani MG, Barentsz J, Hahn PF, et al. Noninvasive detection of clinically occult lymph-node metastases in prostate cancer. N Engl J Med 2003;348(25):2491–9.

58. Weinstein JS, Varallyay CG, Dosa E, et al. Superparamagnetic iron oxide nanoparticles: diagnostic magnetic resonance imaging and potential therapeutic applications in neurooncology and central nervous system inflammatory pathologies, a review. J Cereb Blood Flow Metab 2010;30(1):15–35.

59. Varallyay CG, Muldoon LL, Gahramanov S, et al. Dynamic MRI using iron oxide nanoparticles to assess early vascular effects of antiangiogenic versus corticosteroid treatment in a glioma model. J Cereb Blood Flow Metab 2009;29:853–60.

60. Neuwelt EA, Várallyay CG, Manninger S, et al. The potential of ferumoxytol nanoparticle magnetic resonance imaging, perfusion, and angiography in central nervous system malignancy: a pilot study. Neurosurgery 2007;60(4):601–11.

61. Christoforidis GA, Yang M, Kontzialis MS, et al. High resolution ultra high field magnetic resonance imaging of glioma microvascularity and hypoxia using ultra-small particles of iron oxide. Invest Radiol 2009;44(7):375–83.

62. Gambarota G, Leenders W, Maass C, et al. Characterisation of tumour vasculature in mouse brain by USPIO contrast-enhanced MRI. Br J Cancer 2008;98(11):1784–9.

63. Wu X, Hu J, Zhou L, et al. In vivo tracking of superparamagnetic iron oxide nanoparticle-labeled mesenchymal stem cell tropism to malignant gliomas using magnetic resonance imaging. Laboratory investigation. J Neurosurg 2008; 108(2):320–9.

64. Thu MS, Najbauer J, Kendall SE, et al. Iron labeling and pre-clinical MRI visualization of therapeutic human neural stem cells in a murine glioma model. PLoS One 2009;4(9):e7218.

65. Valable S, Barbier EL, Bernaudin M, et al. In vivo MRI tracking of exogenous monocytes/macrophages targeting brain tumors in a rat model of glioma. Neuroimage 2008;40(2):973–83.

66. Fleige G, Nolte C, Synowitz M, et al. Magnetic labeling of activated microglia in experimental gliomas. Neoplasia 2001;3(6):489–99.

67. Hirsch LR, Gobin AM, Lowery AR, et al. Metal nanoshells. Ann Biomed Eng 2006;34(1):15–22.

68. Loo C, Hirsch L, Lee MH, et al. Gold nanoshell bioconjugates for molecular imaging in living cells. Opt Lett 2005;30:1012–4.

69. West JL, Halas NJ. Engineered nanomaterials for biophotonics applications: improving sensing, imaging, and therapeutics. Annu Rev Biomed Eng 2003;5:285–92.

70. Lin AW, Lewinski NA, West JL, et al. Optically tunable nanoparticle contrast agents for early cancer detection: model-based analysis of gold nanoshells. J Biomed Opt 2005;10(6):064035.

71. Talley CE, Jackson JB, Oubre C, et al. Surface-enhanced raman scattering from individual au nanoparticles and nanoparticle dimer substrates. Nano Lett 2005;5(8):1569–74.

72. Loo C, Lowery A, Halas N, et al. Immunotargeted nanoshells for integrated cancer imaging and therapy. Nano Lett 2005;5(4):709–11.

73. Hirsch LR, Stafford RJ, Bankson JA, et al. Nanoshell-mediated near-infrared thermal therapy of tumors under magnetic resonance guidance. Proc Natl Acad Sci U S A 2003;100(23):13549–54.

74. O'Neal DP, Hirsch LR, Halas NJ, et al. Photothermal tumor ablation in mice using near infrared-absorbing nanoparticles. Cancer Lett 2004;209(2):171–6.

75. Schwartz JA, Shetty AM, Price RE, et al. Feasibility study of particle-assisted laser ablation of brain tumors in orthotopic canine model. Cancer Res 2009;69(4):1659–67.

76. Available at: http://www.clinicaltrials.gov. Accessed March 20, 2010.

77. Reiss P, Protière M, Li L. Core/Shell semiconductor nanocrystals. Small 2009;5(2):154–68.

78. Arya H, Kaul Z, Wadhwa R, et al. Quantum dots in bio-imaging: revolution by the small. Biochem Biophys Res Commun 2005;329(4):1173–7.

79. Smith AM, Duan H, Mohs AM, et al. Bioconjugated quantum dots for in vivo molecular and cellular imaging. Adv Drug Deliv Rev 2008;60(11):1226–40.

80. Jackson H, Muhammad O, Daneshvar H, et al. Quantum dots are phagocytized by macrophages and colocalize with experimental gliomas. Neurosurgery 2007;60(3):524–9.

81. Popescu MA, Toms SA. In vivo optical imaging using quantum dots for the management of brain tumors. Expert Rev Mol Diagn 2006;6(6):879–90.

82. Khalessi AA, Liu CY, Apuzzo ML. Neurosurgery and quantum dots: part I—state of the art. Neurosurgery 2009;64(6):1015–27.

83. Lasic DD, Papahadjopoulos D. Liposomes revisited. Science 1995;267(5202):1275–6.

84. Lasic D, Martin F. Stealth liposomes. Boca Raton (FL): CRC; 1995.

85. Seltzer SE, Blau M, Herman LW, et al. Contrast material-carrying liposomes: biodistribution, clearance, and imaging characteristics. Radiology 1995;194(3):775–81.

86. Mukundan S, Ghaghada KB, Badea CT, et al. A liposomal nanoscale contrast agent for preclinical CT in mice. AJR Am J Roentgenol 2006; 186(2):300–7.

87. Lasic DD. Preparation of liposomes. In: Lasic D, Martin F, editors. Liposomes: from physics to applications. Amsterdam (The Netherlands): Elsevier; 1993. p. 63–98.

88. Ayyagari AL, Zhang X, Ghaghada KB, et al. Long circulating liposomal-based contrast agents for 3D magnetic resonance imaging. Magn Reson Med 2006;55(5):1023–9.

89. Mulder WJ, Strijkers GJ, Habets JW, et al. MR molecular imaging and fluorescence microscopy for identification of activated tumor endothelium using a bimodal lipidic nanoparticle. FASEB J 2005;19(14):2008–10.

90. Saito R, Bringas JR, McKnight TR, et al. Distribution of liposomes into brain and rat brain tumor models by convection-enhanced delivery monitored with magnetic resonance imaging. Cancer Res 2004; 64(7):2572–9.

91. Karathanasis E, Chan L, Balusu SR, et al. Multi-functional nanocarriers for mammographic quantification of tumor dosing and prognosis of breast cancer therapy. Biomaterials 2008;29(36):4815–22.

92. Yan X, Scherphof GL, Kamps JA. Liposome opsonization. J Liposome Res 2005;15(1–2):109–39.

93. Senior JH. Fate and behavior of liposomes in vivo: a review of controlling factors. Crit Rev Ther Drug Carrier Syst 1987;3:123–93.

94. Klibanov AL, Maruyama K, Torchilin VP, et al. Amphipathic polyethyleneglycols effectively prolong the circulation time of liposomes. FEBS Lett 1990;268:235–7.

95. Allen TM, Hansen C, Martin F, et al. Liposomes containing synthetic lipid derivatives of poly(ethylene glycol) show prolonged circulation half-lives in vivo. Biochim Biophys Acta 1991;1066:29–36.

96. Woodle MC, Newman MS, Cohen JA. Sterically stabilized liposomes: physical and biological properties. J Drug Target 1994;2(5):397–403.

97. Tilcock C, Unger E, Cullis P, et al. Liposomal Gd-DTPA: preparation and characterization of relaxivity. Radiology 1989;171(1):77–80.

98. Ghaghada KB, Hawley C, Kawaji K, et al. T1 relaxivity of core-encapsulated gadolinium liposomal contrast agents—effect of liposome size and internal gadolinium concentration. Acad Radiol 2008;15(10):1259–63.

99. Grahn AY, Bankiewicz KS, Dugich-Djordjevic M, et al. Non-PEGylated liposomes for convection-enhanced delivery of topotecan and gadodiamide in malignant glioma: initial experience. J Neurooncol 2009;95(2):185–97.

100. Adler-Moore J, Proffitt RT. AmBisome: liposomal formulation, structure, mechanism of action and pre-clinical experience. J Antimicrob Chemother 2002;49(Suppl 1):21–30.

101. Mulder WJ, van der Schaft DW, Hautvast PA, et al. Early in vivo assessment of angiostatic therapy efficacy by molecular MRI. FASEB J 2007;21(2):378–83.

102. Muggia FM, Hainsworth JD, Jeffers S, et al. Phase II study of liposomal doxorubicin in refractory ovarian cancer: antitumor activity and toxicity modification by liposomal encapsulation. J Clin Oncol 1997;15:987–93.

103. Orlowski RZ, Nagler A, Sonneveld P, et al. Randomized phase III study of pegylated liposomal doxorubicin plus bortezomib compared with bortezomib alone in relapsed or refractory multiple myeloma: combination therapy improves time to progression. J Clin Oncol 2007;25:3892–901.

104. Alberts DS, Muggia FM, Carmichael J, et al. Efficacy and safety of liposomal anthracyclines in phase I/II clinical trials. Semin Oncol 2004;31(6 Suppl 13):53–90.

105. McDonald DM, Choyke PL. Imaging of angiogenesis: from microscope to clinic. Nat Med 2003; 9(6):713–25.

106. Maeda H, Wu J, Sawa T, et al. Tumor vascular permeability and the EPR effect in macromolecular therapeutics: a review. J Control Release 2000; 65(1–2):271–84.

107. Jain RK. Delivery of molecular and cellular medicine to solid tumors. Adv Drug Deliv Rev 2001; 46(1–3):149–68.

108. Ishida O, Maruyama K, Sasaki K, et al. Size-dependent extravasation and interstitial localization of polyethyleneglycol liposomes in solid tumor-bearing mice. Int J Pharm 1999;190(1):49–56.

109. McNeeley KM, Karathanasis E, Annapragada AV, et al. Masking and triggered unmasking of targeting ligands on nanocarriers to improve drug delivery to brain tumors. Biomaterials 2009;30(23–24):3986–95.

110. Madhankumar AB, Slagle-Webb B, Mintz A, et al. Interleukin-13 receptor-targeted nanovesicles are a potential therapy for glioblastoma multiforme. Mol Cancer Ther 2006;5(12):3162–9.

111. Saul JM, Annapragada AV, Bellamkonda RV. A dual-ligand approach for enhancing targeting selectivity of therapeutic nanocarriers. J Control Release 2006;114(3):277–87.

112. Ponce AM, Vujaskovic Z, Yuan F, et al. Hyperthermia mediated liposomal drug delivery. Int J Hyperthermia 2006;22(3):205–13.

113. Kale AA, Torchilin VP. Environment-responsive multifunctional liposomes. Methods Mol Biol 2010; 605:213–42.

114. Momekova D, Rangelov S, Lambov N. Long-circulating, pH-sensitive liposomes. Methods Mol Biol 2010;605:527–44.

115. Ghaghada KB, Ravoori M, Gnanasabapathy D, et al. New dual mode gadolinium nanoparticle contrast agent for magnetic resonance imaging. PLoS One 2009;4(10):e7628.

116. Terreno E, Delli Castelli D, Violante E, et al. Osmotically shrunken LIPOCEST agents: an innovative class of magnetic resonance imaging contrast

media based on chemical exchange saturation transfer. Chemistry 2009;15(6):1440–8.

117. Fossheim SL, Colet JM, Månsson S, et al. Paramagnetic liposomes as magnetic resonance imaging contrast agents. Assessment of contrast efficacy in various liver models. Invest Radiol 1998;33(11):810–21.

118. Tilcock C, Ahkong QF, Koenig SH, et al. The design of liposomal paramagnetic MR agents: effect of vesicle size upon the relaxivity of surface-incorporated lipophilic chelates. Magn Reson Med 1992;27(1):44–51.

119. Mulder WJ, Strijkers GJ, Griffioen AW, et al. A liposomal system for contrast-enhanced magnetic resonance imaging of molecular targets. Bioconjug Chem 2004;15(4):799–806.

120. Ghaghada KB, Bockhorst KHJ, Mukundan S, et al. High resolution vascular imaging of the rat spine using liposomal blood pool MR agent. AJNR Am J Neuroradiol 2007;28(1):48–53.

121. Buckholz E, Ghaghada KB, Qi Y, et al. Four-dimensional MR microscopy of the mouse heart using radial acquisition and liposomal gadolinium contrast agent. Magn Reson Med 2008;60(1):111–8.

122. Buckholz E, Ghaghada KB, Qi Y, et al. Cardiovascular phenotyping of the mouse heart using a 4D radial acquisition and liposomal Gd-DTPA-BMA. Magn Reson Med 2010;63(4):979–87.

123. Bulte JW, De Cuyper M. Magnetoliposomes as contrast agents. Methods Enzymol 2003;373:175–98.

124. Jain RK. Transport of molecules, particles, and cells in solid tumors. Annu Rev Biomed Eng 1999;1:241–63.

125. Bobo RH, Laske DW, Akbasak A, et al. Convection-enhanced delivery of macromolecules in the brain. Proc Natl Acad Sci U S A 1994;91(6):2076–80.

126. Morrison PF, Laske DW, Bobo H, et al. High-flow microinfusion: tissue penetration and pharmacodynamics. Am J Physiol 1994;266(1 Pt 2):R292–305.

127. Kaiser MG, Parsa AT, Fine RL, et al. Tissue distribution and antitumor activity of topotecan delivered by intracerebral clysis in a rat glioma model. Neurosurgery 2000;47(6):1391–8.

128. Ferguson S, Lesniak MS. Convection enhanced drug delivery of novel therapeutic agents to malignant brain tumors. Curr Drug Deliv 2007;4(2):169–80.

129. Krauze MT, Saito R, Noble C, et al. Reflux-free cannula for convection-enhanced high-speed delivery of therapeutic agents. J Neurosurg 2005;103(5):923–9.

130. Mamot C, Nguyen JB, Pourdehnad M, et al. Extensive distribution of liposomes in rodent brains and brain tumors following convection-enhanced delivery. J Neurooncol 2004;68(1):1–9.

131. Kikuchi T, Saito R, Sugiyama S, et al. Convection-enhanced delivery of polyethylene glycol-coated liposomal doxorubicin: characterization and efficacy in rat intracranial glioma models. J Neurosurg 2008;109(5):867–73.

132. Saito R, Krauze MT, Bringas JR, et al. Gadolinium-loaded liposomes allow for real-time magnetic resonance imaging of convection-enhanced delivery in the primate brain. Exp Neurol 2005;196(2):381–9.

133. Dickinson PJ, LeCouteur RA, Higgins RJ, et al. Canine model of convection-enhanced delivery of liposomes containing CPT-11 monitored with real-time magnetic resonance imaging: laboratory investigation. J Neurosurg 2008;108(5):989–98.

134. Mamot C, Drummond DC, Greiser U, et al. Epidermal growth factor receptor (EGFR)-targeted immunoliposomes mediate specific and efficient drug delivery to EGFR- and EGFRvIII-overexpressing tumor cells. Cancer Res 2003;63(12):3154–61.

135. Persigehl T, Bieker R, Matuszewski L, et al. Antiangiogenic tumor treatment: early noninvasive monitoring with USPIO-enhanced MR imaging in mice. Radiology 2007;244(2):449–56.

Imaging of Brain Tumors: Functional Magnetic Resonance Imaging and Diffusion Tensor Imaging

Ajay Gupta, MD[a], Akash Shah, MD[a],
Robert J. Young, MD[a,b,c],*, Andrei I. Holodny, MD[a,b,c]

KEYWORDS

- DT imaging • fMR imaging • Brain • Tumor

Brain tumor resection is an integral part of the treatment of patients with brain tumors, as most outcomes are believed to improve after gross total resection (a notable exception is central nervous system lymphoma). The goal of surgery is to maximize tumor resection and avoid adjacent eloquent brain structures, because their inadvertent injury can cause profound neurologic deficits. Magnetic resonance (MR) imaging is a noninvasive test used to evaluate and plan therapy for patients with brain tumors. Conventional MR imaging scans provide purely anatomic information (eg, how big the tumor is and what it is doing to the adjacent brain). Rather than simply showing structural changes, advanced MR imaging techniques investigating biophysiologic processes can be used to map the functional parts of the brain responsible for specific activities. The eloquent brain can be identified using functional MR (fMR) imaging for the gray matter and diffusion tensor (DT) imaging for the white matter. fMR imaging and DT imaging are especially important for patients with tumors near the important motor and language centers of the brain, where the normal anatomic references may be distorted by the tumor and associated edema. fMR imaging is a commonly used technique for identifying the eloquent gray matter, whereas DT imaging is a relatively new and still immature technique for showing the white matter. This article explains fMR imaging and DT imaging techniques and illustrates their clinical applications and limitations.

PART I: FMR IMAGING
Theoretic Basis

Blood oxygenation level-dependent (BOLD) fMR imaging uses deoxyhemoglobin as an endogenous contrast agent to measure the hemodynamic response to neuronal activity through the concept of neurovascular coupling.[1–4] Neuronal activity causes increased local oxygen consumption, which in turn causes a marked increase in the cerebral blood flow that overcompensates for the resultant increase in cerebral metabolic rate. This overcompensation leads to an increase in the fraction of local venous blood that is oxygenated. The susceptibility difference between the local ratio of diamagnetic oxyhemoglobin to paramagnetic deoxyhemoglobin leads to the more rapid dephasing of transverse magnetization. This process is captured as a slight increase in the BOLD signal

[a] Neuroradiology Service, Department of Radiology, Memorial Sloan-Kettering Cancer Center, 1275 York Avenue, New York, NY 10065, USA
[b] Department of Radiology, New York Presbyterian Hospital / Weill Cornell Medical College, New York, NY, USA
[c] Brain Tumor Center, Memorial Sloan-Kettering Cancer Center, 1275 York Avenue, New York, NY 10065, USA
* Corresponding author. Neuroradiology Service, Department of Radiology, Memorial Sloan-Kettering Cancer Center, 1275 York Avenue, MRI-1156, New York, NY 10065.
E-mail address: youngr@mskcc.org

Neuroimag Clin N Am 20 (2010) 379–400
doi:10.1016/j.nic.2010.04.004
1052-5149/10/$ – see front matter © 2010 Elsevier Inc. All rights reserved.

by highly sensitive T2∗ imaging techniques, thereby allowing the indirect noninvasive investigation of functional brain activity.

fMR Imaging Acquisition

T2∗ gradient-echo (GE) sequences that lack the refocusing pulse of routine spin-echo (SE) sequences are used to magnify the local magnetic field inhomogeneities and increase the sensitivity of fMR imaging to small changes in hemoglobin composition. Analyzing the time course of the BOLD signal within each imaging voxel gives an estimate of the magnitude of the local hemodynamic response function. Because changes in the imaging target occur on the order of seconds, the area of interest is scanned multiple times usually using echo planar imaging (EPI), with each acquisition taking 2 to 4 seconds. The high temporal resolution requires decreased spatial resolution, although fMR imaging data overlays on the routine anatomic images can overcome this limitation.[4,5]

Because GE EPI sequences are more heavily T2∗-weighted, they are preferred to SE EPI sequences in fMR imaging. In addition, SE EPI sequences are not sensitive to contributions from venous blood, resulting in a smaller signal that is more difficult to discern from background noise. SE EPI can be advantageous in certain settings: (1) SE BOLD images originate from the capillaries, which are closer to the focus of neuronal activity, whereas GE BOLD images originate too from capillaries but also from venules, which are slightly removed from the neuronal focus; and (2) the lower T2∗ weighting renders less susceptibility artifact from adjacent metal and air-bone interfaces, such as when imaging near the paranasal sinuses, skull base, or postoperative sites.[5,6]

fMR Imaging Paradigms

Task designs that elicit neuronal activity, known as paradigms, are used to produce fMR imaging maps of cerebral function. Paradigms can either be event-related (stimulus presentation followed by a period of rest) or block-design (repeated periods of alternating stimulus and rest presentation). Event-related paradigms better mirror the hemodynamic response and eliminate the stimulus predictability seen with block-design paradigms, but their limitations include long acquisition times, low statistical power, and complicated statistical signal analyses. For these reasons, block-design paradigms are the most common type used in clinical practice. After image acquisition, the time course of the task is plotted against the time course of BOLD signal changes within each voxel to assess whether there is significant association between the signal changes and the functional task. Block-design paradigms are able to detect subtle BOLD signal changes across time and able to reduce artifacts from physiologic variations in signal by performing correlations with the timing of tasks.[5–8]

Relevant anatomy

Language and motor paradigms are most commonly used in clinical practice. The left hemisphere is almost always language dominant in right-handed individuals and usually dominant or codominant in left-handed individuals.[9–11] Productive speech function resides primarily in Broca's area in the posterior inferior frontal gyrus. Receptive speech function resides primarily in Wernicke's area in the posterior superior temporal gyrus. Because of significant variations in anatomic specialization between individuals, these functions can be better described as residing in the frontal and temporoparietal regions, respectively. Lesions in dominant frontal speech areas can cause an agrammatic aphasia characterized by halting, labored speech. Lesions in dominant temporoparietal areas can cause a receptive aphasia characterized by poor speech comprehension and repetition. Multiple other areas are involved in secondary speech functions, including the middle frontal gyrus, middle and inferior temporal gyri, supramarginal gyrus, and angular gyrus.

Motor function is organized topographically within the precentral gyrus in a pattern referred to as the homunculus (Fig. 1). From medial to lateral, portions of the precentral gyrus are responsible for the leg, trunk, hand, and face motor activity; the hand localizes to the omega portion. This somatotopic functional organization makes it important to select appropriately directed paradigms that use motor tasks based on lesion proximity to specific regions of the motor homunculus. The supplementary motor area (SMA) in the superior frontal gyrus is also involved in motor planning. Lesions in this region can result in paresis or muteness (Fig. 2).[12]

fMR imaging paradigms

Appropriate paradigm selection requires clinical evaluation of the patient's deficit(s) and inspection of the anatomic images to determine the proximity of the lesion to eloquent cortex. Several factors must be considered, including the patient's handedness and clinical ability. Language tasks are designed to primarily assess productive and receptive function. Tasks that assess productive

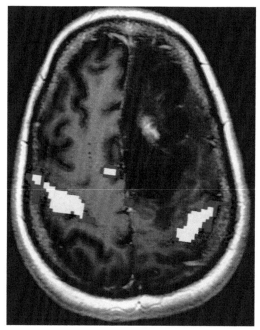

Fig. 1. Motor hand task, fMR imaging overlaid on contrast T1-weighted image. Activated voxels localize to the precentral gyri, with mild posterior displacement of the left precentral gyrus by the frontal lobe glioblastoma.

function are termed fluency tasks, requiring the patient to generate words in response to a cue. Examples include phonemic fluency tasks, in which a patient generates words starting with

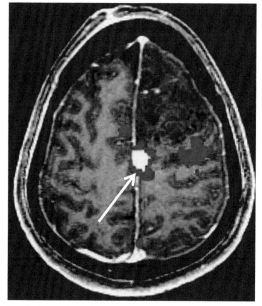

Fig. 2. SMA, fMR imaging overlaid on a contrast T1-weighted image. Activated voxels from a phonemic fluency task localize the SMA (*arrow*) to the posterior medial margin of the frontal lobe glioblastoma.

a specific letter, and semantic fluency tasks, in which a patient generates words of a specific category (**Fig. 3**).[13,14] Receptive tasks generally assess language comprehension and include tasks that involve reading, listening to words, naming, identifying synonyms, and filling in sentences with the appropriate words.[14–16] Fluency and receptive tasks can activate frontal and temporoparietal language regions to varying degrees. Temporoparietal regions in particular are difficult to target with specific tasks, partly because of a wider distribution of receptive language function.[17] It has been suggested that activations in these regions may be transient, and nonperiodic sampling during interstimulus intervals can capture greater signal in these areas.[18]

Because of the potential of head motion with motor tasks and the difficulty of completing certain motor tasks in a supine position, most motor tasks suitable for fMR imaging are limited to a few areas of the body. Among tasks used in motor paradigms are finger tapping, tongue motion, and passive hand and foot stimulation. Finger tapping tasks using the sequential tapping of adjacent fingers have the added advantage of activating premotor planning areas. Finger tapping tasks can be substituted with fist opening and closing in patients with distal limb weakness. Because of the large fraction of the somatotopic motor map devoted to the tongue, even minimal tongue motion can generate large fMR imaging signals. For the paretic patient, paradigm testing an alternate location along the motor cortex or passive sensory function paradigms may enable proper identification of the motor cortex (**Fig. 4**). These passive tasks often activate the motor cortex as well as the sensory cortex through reciprocal neuron connections.

Paradigm preparation and monitoring
Task familiarity before imaging is important to ensure accurate fMR imaging responses. Practice versions of tasks using stimuli that are similar to the real test stimuli can be useful in training the patient, although presentation of actual test stimuli can result in sensitization and should be avoided. Accuracy is also improved by detailed instructions and reassurance during task performance. Patient monitoring is important to ensure accurate and reliable fMR imaging results. Monitoring motor tasks is easy through methods such as video monitoring or using squeeze balls that monitor motor response.[19] Forced choice paradigms, in which the patient must make a choice to complete the task using button boxes, can be an effective method to improve patient performance. Silent language

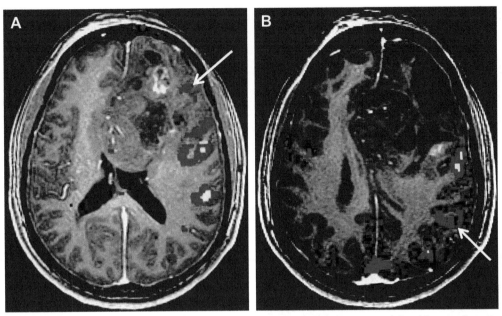

Fig. 3. Semantic fluency language task, fMR imaging overlaid on a contrast T1-weighted image. Broca's area (*arrow, A*) is inferiorly displaced by an anaplastic oligodendroglioma in the frontal lobe. Wernicke's area (*arrow, B*) is not affected.

tasks are advantageous because of the lack of head motion, but monitoring patient performance can be difficult. The use of motion correction algorithms may facilitate vocal speech paradigms, which are easier to monitor and may present more accurate representations of speech production and comprehension.[7,20] Baseline tasks for the rest period should be chosen carefully, with the goal of maximizing the contrast of neural response between rest and activity periods. Depending on the target location, a nonstimulating task such as fixation on a cross or an opposing task can be chosen. For example, a baseline task of passively viewing nonsense objects has been shown to improve detection of signal in Broca's area with sentence generation tasks.[21]

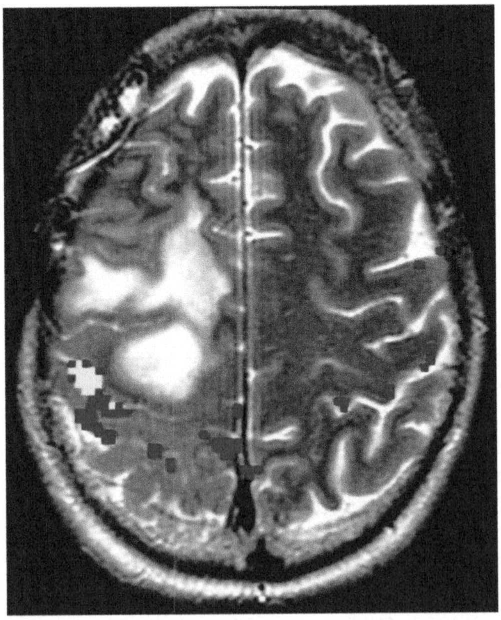

Other Techniques for Functional Mapping

Direct electrical cortical stimulation (ECS) is considered the gold standard for functional mapping. Direct stimulation can evoke positive responses, such as the stimulation of motor cortex activating muscular contraction, or inhibitory responses, such as the stimulation of Broca's area leading to a disruption of speech. Electrocorticography (ECoG) is an intraoperative technique that uses cortical surface electrodes to detect somatosensory evoked potentials (SSEP) that arise from electrical stimulation of nerves. For example, electrical current delivered to the median nerve can be used to identify the central sulcus, by analyzing the resultant SSEP distribution arising from signals being transmitted to the motor and sensory cortex. Other common techniques for functional mapping are summarized in **Table 1**.

Fig. 4. Sensory hand and foot stimulation task, fMR imaging overlaid on T2-weighted image. The sensory task causes activation of motor and sensory voxels in the precentral and postcentral gyri, respectively; the hyperintense anaplastic astrocytoma extends directly into the precentral gyrus.

Table 1
Functional testing

	fMR Imaging	DECS	Wada (ISAP)	PET/CT	MEG/MSI	TMS	fTDC
Mechanism	Hemodynamic response (indirect)	Electrical stimulation (direct)	Anesthesic deactivation (indirect)	Hemodynamic response (indirect)	Magnetic flux (direct)	Electrical interference (direct)	Hemodynamic response (indirect)
Expressive language	Yes	Yes	Yes	Yes	No	Yes	Yes
Receptive language	Yes	Yes	Yes	Yes	Yes	No	Yes
Memory	Yes	Yes	Yes	Yes	Yes	No	No
Motor	Yes	Yes	No	Yes	Yes	Yes	Yes
Invasive	No	Yes	Yes	Minimal[b]	No	No	No
Radiation	No	No	Yes	Yes	No	No	No
Spatial resolution	Good	Excellent	Poor[a]	Poor	Excellent	Excellent	Poor[a]
Temporal resolution	Good	Excellent	Poor	Poor	Excellent	Excellent	Good
Bilateral testing	Yes	No	Yes	Yes	Yes	Yes	Yes
Availability	Good	Good	Limited	Good	Poor	Poor	Poor
Risks	Minimal	Medium	Medium	Minimal	Minimal	Small	Minimal

Abbreviations: DECS, direct electrical cortical stimulation; fTDC, functional transcranial Doppler sonography; ISAP, intracarotid sodium amobarbital procedure; MEG, magnetoencephalography; MSI, magnetic source imaging; TMS, transcranial magnetic stimulation.
[a] Lateralization to the dominant hemisphere only, not within a hemisphere.
[b] Requires intravenous injection of radioisotope.

Clinical Applications of fMR Imaging for Tumor Imaging

fMR imaging is most commonly performed for preoperative planning. The results can help guide decisions on whether to offer surgery, assessment of the risk and prognosis, planning of the surgical approach, and maximize tumor resection. fMR imaging is important in preoperative mapping because of the potential distortion of normal anatomic relationships adjacent to the tumor. The fMR imaging data are often stereotactically coregistered to anatomic data from computed tomography or MR imaging images and imported into the neurosurgical navigational software, to provide an interactive roadmap during surgery.

fMR imaging mapping of motor function

Because of the relatively invariable somatotopic organization of motor and somatosensory function, functional mapping of these systems is more reliable than language mapping. Localization of the somatosensory and motor cortex surrounding the central sulcus is important in tumors at the frontoparietal junction, because of concern of paralysis from injury of motor cortex or descending tracts. ECoG and ECS can be used to identify the central sulcus during surgery. In contrast, fMR imaging can provide useful information before surgery that could then be used to modify the surgical planning, guide ECS mapping, and predict the risk of motor and/or sensory functional loss. fMR imaging mapping of the central sulcus has proved resistant to potentially limiting artifacts from head motion, patient anxiety, and abnormal vasculature. Coactivation of the somatosensory and motor cortices with motor and sensory paradigms can occasionally make differentiation of the 2 cortices difficult. Using anatomic landmarks, for example the omega portion of the central sulcus delineating hand motor representation, and the fact that the posterior portion of gray matter in the precentral and postcentral gyrus activates with fMR imaging tasks, can help differentiate these cortices. fMR imaging mapping also aids in identifying the foot and leg motor cortex, which are difficult to identify by ECS mapping because of their deep location adjacent to the interhemispheric fissure (**Fig. 5**).[22]

fMR imaging mapping of language function

The anatomic localization of the language cortex is less predictable than that of the highly organized motor cortex. Variability may occur in the expected patterns of language dominance, particularly in left-handed persons, and in the distribution of language function, particularly for receptive or temporoparietal language functions.[17]

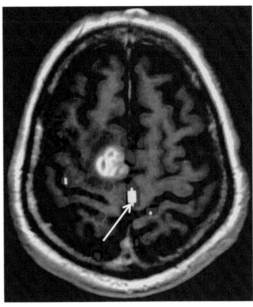

Fig. 5. Foot motor task, fMR imaging overlaid on a contrast T1-weighted image. The enhancing melanoma metastasis is located anterior to the foot portion of the homunculus (*arrow*), and posterior to the motor-related SMA.

Because anatomic predictors cannot solely determine whether a particular language region is affected by tumor, functional imaging is of paramount importance in localizing language function and laterality. fMR imaging is the most common functional imaging modality used in this regard.

Hemispheric language dominance is related to the degree of handedness; only a small fraction of strong right-handed individuals show right language dominance, and nearly one-third of strong left-handed individuals show left language dominance. Cortical reorganization in brain tumor patients may also increase the incidence of atypical dominance.[23] These inconsistencies illustrate the importance of functional mapping in lieu of anatomic predictions. fMR imaging mapping of these eloquent regions may enable the neurosurgeon to offer surgery for tumors believed to be inoperable based on anatomic imaging alone.

Until recently, the Wada test has been the gold standard of determining language dominance in preoperative patients. Its role has been supplanted by fMR imaging, which is more widely available, noninvasise and can be used to assess language dominance and localization of function. Studies comparing the efficacy of fMR imaging and Wada in determining language dominance have shown good concordance, with greater correlations achieved by combining 4 separate language tasks.[24,25] When dominance is atypical or bilateral, fMR imaging and Wada may lead to suboptimal results. A disadvantage to fMR imaging is activation of portions of the brain nonessential for language function during language tasks, which may blur the distinction between nonessential and essential language areas. Using a threshold to exclude these nonessential areas may improve the diagnostic quality, but may also lead to false-negative and false-positive results in assessing hemispheric dominance.[26]

Localization of language function is inherently difficult because of distribution across multiple gyri and marked variability between patients. Despite the widespread distribution of activity, only a few centers of function seem to be essential for language production and comprehension. Lesions close to the lateral precentral gyrus, which is responsible for tongue and facial motion, Broca's area or the inferior frontal gyrus, and Wernicke's area in the superior and middle temporal gyri are of greatest concern. ECS is an important correlative measure to determine language essentiality; some frontal sites that are active on fMR imaging maps do not show the speech disruption expected with intraoperative stimulation.[27–30] Studies assessing the correlation of intraoperative stimulation and fMR imaging have found mixed results.[27,30] fMR imaging activity does not signify that an area is crucial for function, limiting the ability of fMR imaging to target essential functional areas. In contrast, the inhibitory effects of direct cortical stimulation are suited to identifying essential areas. The combination of 3 tasks may increase the ability of fMR imaging to detect critical language areas, providing an alternative for patients who cannot undergo intraoperative stimulation.[30] Interpreting ECS results of Wernicke's or temporoparietal speech areas has proved more difficult, as changes in speech pattern on electrical stimulation can be subtle. In addition, it is difficult to design fMR imaging paradigms that specifically target Wernicke's area; most language comprehension tasks also activate Broca's area to some extent. Some tasks that have shown better results include auditory responsive naming, sentence comprehension, and sentence completion tasks.

Silent language tasks that may be advantageous because of lack of head motion have been noted to favor anterior aspects of the frontal language system and limit precentral gyrus activation.[29] These silent tasks do not seem to fully portray the language production system, as fMR imaging maps based on silent tasks do not correlate so well with intraoperative stimulation. Vocal speech paradigms or the inclusion of tongue movement paradigms can be helpful in this regard.

Although most fMR imaging paradigms target functionality of the 2 major language functions, productive and receptive, damage to secondary language areas such as the SMA can have debilitating effects, including mutism and verbal working memory deficits.[31–34] The degree of lateralization of the SMA has been shown to correlate with degree of postoperative aphasia.[22,33]

Pitfalls of fMR Imaging

Neurovascular uncoupling describes the dissociation of vascular activity from sites of neuronal activation caused by damaged or abnormal vasculature, which may result in decreased or absent BOLD fMR imaging activity (**Fig. 6**). The BOLD signal is comprised of 3 components: true neuronal activity, susceptibility artifacts that can create false-positive signals, and neurovascular uncoupling effects that can create false-negative signals on the fMR imaging map. Holodny and colleagues[35] first described neurovascular uncoupling in a patient with glioblastoma involving the left precentral gyrus, with muted fMR imaging activation of the left motor cortex. This decrease in signal can simulate opposite hemisphere dominance or cortical reorganization.[36] The leading hypothesis for this type of phenomenon is the presence of abnormal tumor vasculature, which

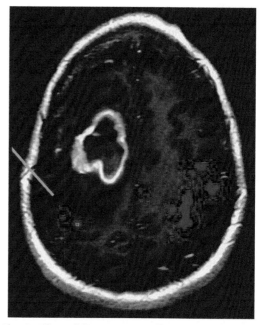

Fig. 6. Bilateral finger tapping fMR imaging overlaid onto a contrast-enhanced T1-weighted image. The decreased activation in the right precentral gyrus (*green line*) is likely due to decreased neuronal response, in the presence of abnormal vasculature from the glioblastoma in the adjacent frontal lobe.

has a diminished ability to respond to neuronal activity with appropriately increased blood flow.[35,37] The baseline blood flow may already be maximally or near maximally increased by direct tumor infiltration, cerebrovascular inflammation, or neovascularity, and thereby minimize any potential increases caused by neuronal activity.[36] Abnormal neovasculature can be analyzed using relative cerebral volume measurements; factors such as tumor volume, peritumoral edema, and edema within the eloquent gyrus are not believed to be associated with neurovascular uncoupling.[38] Despite these limitations, the primary and motor sensory areas can be identified in most preoperative patients. When interpreting preoperative fMR imaging maps for language laterality, however, the possibility of muted fMR imaging signal in the expected language dominant hemisphere must be considered.

Brain plasticity or cortical reorganization refers to the transfer of function to a different area of the brain, often to the opposite hemisphere, in the setting of the growth of a brain tumor. In right-handed patients with extensive left hemisphere tumors, fMR imaging can be crucial in identifying whether language function has transferred to the opposite hemisphere. Several cases have been reported in which expressive or productive language function is transferred to the opposite hemisphere in the presence of tumor.[39,40] Recognition of this potential reorganization, rather than reliance on anatomic landmarks alone, may make surgery a feasible option for some brain tumors that are otherwise considered inoperable.

Because BOLD fMR imaging relies on T2* weighting to produce images, anything that produces large magnetic susceptibility differences can be a significant source of artifact, including metal, recent surgery, and air-bone interfaces. These effects may be reduced by acquiring a field map to correct for inhomogeneities, decreasing the EPI readout times (increasing the bandwidth), decreasing the time to echo, or decreasing the slice thickness. Also, because BOLD fMR imaging signals originate from veins and capillaries, it is important to compare the fMR imaging images with high-resolution MR images to exclude the possibility of a large draining vein creating a false-positive fMR imaging signal. As opposed to the microvasculature, the relationship between large draining veins and site of neuronal activation is unknown.[41–43] Contrast-enhanced T1 imaging can help in differentiating the macrovasculature from the microvasculature. When planning the fMR imaging paradigms, recognition of large draining veins near the tumor or eloquent brain in interest may lead to the use of SE sequences rather than GE sequences to decrease these T2* effects.[44]

Head motion can be a significant source of artifact in fMR imaging. Artifact arises when voxels with higher T2* signal intensity move into neighboring voxels with lower signal intensity. Tumors associated with marked vascularity, extracellular methemoglobin, and surrounding edema show high T2* signal intensity. Motion artifact can lead to false-positive signals in these areas, with a high T2* gradient blurring across neighboring voxels. Motion artifacts occur more often in patients with paresis, as the motion of more proximal muscles increases head motion. Appropriate paradigm selection may help decrease head motion (eg, by selecting tasks that use sensory stimulation, passive movements, or motor imagery). Although avoiding motion artifact is most effective, postprocessing techniques such as time course analysis can help differentiate motion artifact from real activation. In time course analysis, MR signal changes from motion artifact that abruptly peak are discarded, whereas signal changes from neuronal activation that shows a delay before a peak are included in the analysis.[41]

PART II: DT IMAGING
Theoretic Basis

Diffusion imaging
Diffusion imaging examines the motion of water molecules, which is normally random or Brownian in the unimpeded, isotropic state.[45] The brain has natural barriers to the motion of water molecules such as intracellular organelles, macromolecules, and cell membranes that result in anisotropic diffusion. Routine diffusion-weighted imaging (DWI) can be used to calculate the apparent diffusion coefficient (ADC), which is a measure of the magnitude of water diffusion. DT imaging takes advantage of the preferential diffusion of water in brain tissue, which is decreased perpendicular to the myelin sheaths and cell membranes of white matter axons.[46–48] The diffusion tensor is a mathematical model of water diffusion that reflects the anisotropy (directional dependence) and orientation of the local white matter fibers. The most commonly derived DT imaging metrics are mean diffusivity (MD) and fractional anisotropy (FA). MD is the mean of the 3 eigenvalues, or a directionally averaged measure of the magnitude of water diffusion. Analogous to the ADC, MD is related to the integrity of the brain tissue. FA is a measure of diffusion anisotropy that is derived from the standard deviation of the 3 eigenvalues, and ranges

from 0 (isotropic with zero net direction) to 1 (maximal anisotropy that occurs along the primary eigenvector).

Image Acquisition and Postprocessing

Standard DWI is performed with single-shot EPI, which is inherently motion sensitive sequences.[49] Unlike standard DWI, the motion-probing gradients are performed in multiple ($\geq$6) directions for DT imaging.[50] The optimal number of noncollinear gradients is uncertain, with different groups routinely acquiring DT imaging in 6 to 55 directions. Although more than 100 directions are possible, the increased imaging time necessary to acquire greater numbers of directions limits their clinical usefulness. The signal-to-noise ratio can be improved by increasing the number of repetitions, or by increasing the number of applied gradients, although both will also increase the required scan time.

The FA map is a graphical representation of the standard deviation of eigenvalues, in which the signal brightness correlates with the degree of anisotropy for that voxel. By also incorporating data about the primary orientation of each voxel, directionally encoded color FA maps can be generated. The standard color convention shows transverse fibers in red (x-axis), anteroposterior fibers in green (y-axis), and craniocaudal fibers in blue (z-axis). With knowledge of the normal brain anatomy, experienced users can identify specific white matter tracts on the color FA maps.

Qualitative DT imaging measurements are usually obtained using region-of-interest (ROI) analysis. The ROI method is dependent on operator experience, and may be difficult to perform and reproduce in areas of brain tumors with tissue compression and edema. Although there is no standard for analysis, proposed alternatives to the ROI method such as histogram and voxel-based analyses may improve the accuracy and reproducibility of the DT imaging measurements.[51–53]

DT imaging tractography programs can be used to calculate the connectivity of different voxels. There are 2 main theories for fiber tracking: deterministic and probabilistic.[47] In the deterministic method, fibers are assigned by continuous tracking (FACT) of user-defined voxels.[54] In the probabilistic method, there is the additional quantification of the probability of connection between 2 points. This latter method tends to disperse trajectories more widely and may depict a greater portion of the white matter tracts.[50] Probabilistic tractography may be more useful in areas of lower anisotropy, such as in small tracts, through crossing fibers, and in gray matter (**Fig. 7**).[55] Using tractography to first localize the tracts in question, then placing ROIs based on the mapped tracts may decrease some of the site selection biases of ROI measurements.

Using the fMR imaging-activated voxels to draw the seed (and end) ROIs on DT imaging maps may more accurately define functionally related white matter tracts than using DT imaging alone.[56–58]

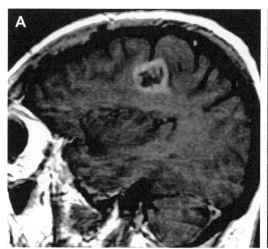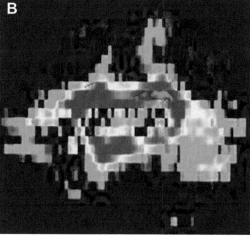

Fig. 7. FACT and probabilistic tractography of the arcuate fasciculus, using fMR imaging activated voxels in Broca's and Wernicke's areas. (*A*) Sagittal contrast T1-weighted image shows an enhancing glioblastoma in the left frontal parietal junction. (*B*) Sagittal tractography shows robust arcuate fasciculus fibers by the probabilistic method (*red voxels*) compared with the shorter fibers by the FACT method (*green voxels*). (Both constructed using DTI&Fiber Tools; Kreher BW , Hennig J, Il'yasov KA, University Hospital, Freiburg, Germany.)

In particular, fMR imaging-driven tractography may allow more discriminative depiction of corticospinal tract components (eg, hand vs foot fibers) and more accurate tracking through peritumoral abnormalities.[57] The use of combined fMR imaging and DT imaging seems to improve the detection of important functional tracts within 5 mm of the tumor, and lower the rate of regional

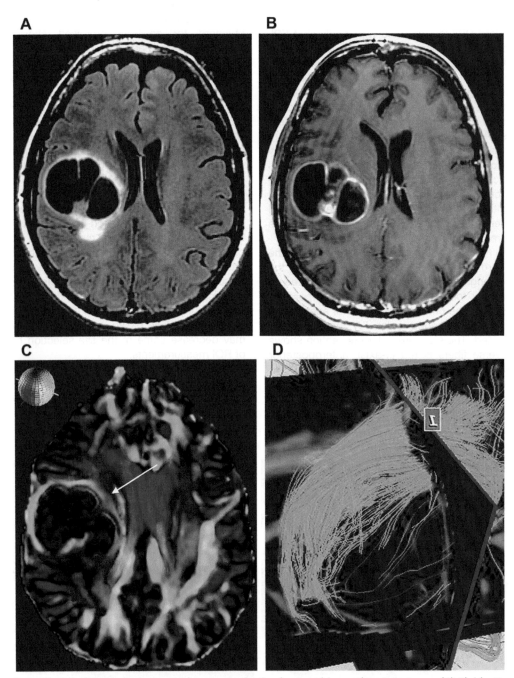

Fig. 8. Corticospinal tract displacement by an anaplastic pleomorphic xanthoastrocytoma. (*A*) Fluid attenuation inversion recovery (FLAIR) and (*B*) contrast T1-weighted images show complex cystic and solid tumor in the right frontal parietal junction at the level of the corona radiata, in the expected region of the corticospinal tract. (*C*) Directionally encoded FA map shows anterior medial displacement of the descending corticospinal tract (*arrow*, coded in blue for superior-inferior direction). (*D*) Tractography confirms the superior and anterior medial displacement. (*Tractography courtesy of* Kyung Peck, PhD, Memorial Sloan-Kettering Cancer Center, New York, NY.)

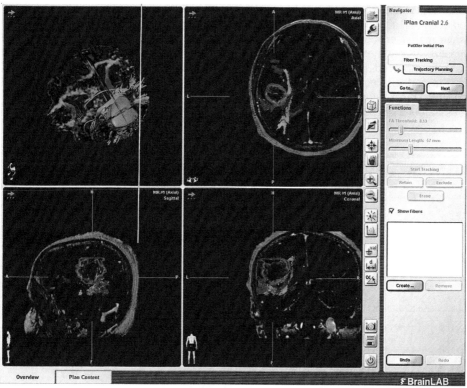

Fig. 9. Tractography seeded from fMR imaging activated voxels in Broca's and Wernicke's areas, screensave from BrainLAB neuronavigational software (clockwise from top left: tractography in three dimensions, and overlaid on axial, coronal, and sagittal contrast T1-weighted images). fMR imaging and DT imaging data show segmented tumor in left parietal lobe (right side of image is left side of patient) causing medial displacement of the arcuate fasciculus fibers. (*Image courtesy of* Nicole Brennan, Memorial Sloan-Kettering Cancer Center, New York, NY.)

surgical complication rate compared with the overall surgical literature.[56]

Clinical Applications of DT Imaging for Tumor Imaging

Neurosurgical planning
DT imaging is the only noninvasive, in vivo method to localize essential white matter tracts. This process is especially important for brain tumor surgery, in which the inadvertent injury to an eloquent white matter tract (eg, the corticospinal tract) can result in catastrophic neurologic deficits. Multiple studies have described the potential roles for DT imaging and tractography in preoperative planning, with both techniques able to identify specific white matter tracts (**Figs. 8** and **9**).[59–64] Although ECS and electrical recording are the standard of care for brain tumors located near eloquent brain, these are highly invasive intraoperative techniques that do not assist in preoperative planning or prognostication. Compared with cortical stimulation, effective white matter stimulation requires greater (deep) exposure and close

proximity to the edge of the resection bed, higher electrical currents, and is less reliable than cortical mapping.

Preoperative tractography can indicate the locations of the important white matter tracts relative to the tumor, and thereby guide the surgical approach and the intraoperative stimulation. Mikuni and colleagues[59] studied patients with tumors near the corticospinal tract and found that preoperative tractography could predict the usefulness of intraoperative stimulation of the motor cortex and subcortical fibers. There was a good correlation between the disruption of motor fibers by the tumor at tractography and the failure of cortical or subcortical stimulation. Given the propensity for stimulation to fail, the investigators suggested that awake brain surgery and evaluation of voluntary muscle movement may be more appropriate than stimulation in such patients. Therefore, tractography may be useful in predicting the value of intraoperative stimulation as well as guiding the stimulation.

Several studies have shown that tractography has a role in assessing the deviation, deformation, infiltration, and/or interruption of white matter tracts adjacent to a brain tumor.[62,63] Some of these white matter changes may be temporary, and normalize after tumor resection (Fig. 10). In patients with improved positions and appearances of the corticospinal tracts after resection of adjacent brain tumors, Laundre and colleagues[62] found a positive correlation with clinical improvements in motor deficits. Tractography may allow more extensive tumor resections by increasing the confidence of resection adjacent to eloquent white matter tracts, and potentially distinguishing between displaced tracts (which should be spared) from disrupted tracts (which perhaps should be included in the resection).[61]

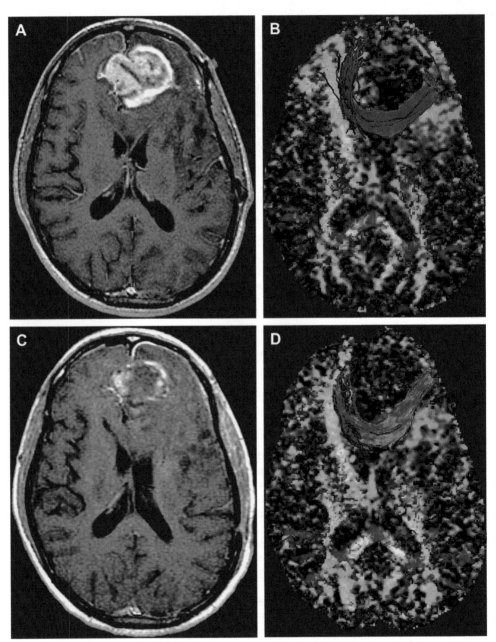

Fig. 10. Tractography changes after surgery, (A, C) Contrast T1-weighted images and (B, D) tractography overlaid on directionally encoded FA maps. The bifrontal enhancing glioblastoma (A) causes splaying and posterior displacement of the genu of the corpus callosum, which has a rounded configuration (B). After subtotal resection (C), there is decreased mass effect on the genu, which now has a more triangular configuration (D).

Differential diagnosis: malignant glioma versus metastasis

The presence of a solitary brain tumor in an adult can pose a clinical dilemma, especially when a systemic cancer is not known or not found after complete medical workup. A malignant glioma and a metastasis may present as an enhancing mass lesion with variable amounts of surrounding peritumoral T2 hyperintensity. The peritumoral abnormality may enable their differentiation: the peritumoral abnormality of malignant gliomas consists of vasogenic edema and microscopic tumor infiltration that often occurs along existing white matter tracts, whereas the peritumoral abnormality of metastases represents pure vasogenic edema and increased interstitial fluid.[65–70] These pathophysiologic differences may result in differences in MD and FA.

Tumoral measurements in malignant gliomas usually show increased MD and decreased FA, as a result of increased extracellular water content and decreased white matter integrity.[71–73] The decrease in FA is usually more marked than seen in metastases, although malignant gliomas may also occasionally show increased FA as a result of increased cellularity with subsequent decreases in extracellular volume and increases in the preferential directionality of water diffusion.[68,74]

Peritumoral measurements in malignant gliomas may reveal less marked increases in MD than in metastases, and more marked decreases in FA.[67] Increases in the peritumoral MD for malignant gliomas, caused by greater influxes of peritumoral water from increased vascular endothelial growth factor and increased vascular permeability, are tempered by the infiltrative rather than expansile growth patterns with the presence of tumor cells in the peritumoral abnormality.[75] Decreases in the peritumoral FA for malignant gliomas also reflect the presence of these infiltrating tumor cells, which may destroy rather than simply displace the white matter tracts. In addition to significantly decreased peritumoral FA, Wang and colleagues[69] also showed significantly decreased pure anisotropic diffusion component q in patients with glioma.[76] This distinction between malignant gliomas and metastases has not been reliably reproduced by other investigators,[67,70,77] leading Lu and colleagues[67] to propose the tumor infiltration index (defined as the expected FA for the corresponding MD minus the observed FA).

Differential diagnosis: glioma grade

The differentiation between high- and low-grade gliomas by conventional MR imaging usually relies on contrast enhancement, although this is an imperfect technique because of the separate contributions of blood-brain barrier disruption and neovascularity. DT imaging may provide complementary information in distinguishing glioma grades.[78–82] Studies using standard DWI suggest that ADC values may be helpful in estimating tumor cellularity and therefore tumor grade.[83–85] Decreasing ADC and MD is believed to indicate increased cellularity and malignancy.[84,85]

Decreasing FA, a measure of diffusion directionality, has been correlated with increasing glioma grade, gross tumor, and cell number (**Fig. 11**).[80,86,87] DT imaging has also been correlated with the Ki-67 labeling index, a marker of proliferative activity associated with tumor invasiveness and prognosis.[88] Goebell and colleagues[78] measured FA values in the tumor center, border, and adjacent normal-appearing white matter (NAWM) of grade II and grade III gliomas, and found that only decreased FA values in the tumor border could distinguish the 2 grades. They concluded that the periphery of low-grade gliomas have relatively more preserved white matter tracts (compared with relative disarrangement of tracts in higher grade gliomas), which may explain the relative changes in FA. Ferda and colleagues[82] graded gliomas using FA measurements alone and found only 81% sensitivity and 87% specificity in discriminating between low- and high-grade gliomas. By integrating tumor enhancement patterns in conjunction with FA measurements, however, they were able to increase the sensitivity and specificity to 100%.

Evaluating glioma margins

The margins of malignant gliomas are nearly impossible to predict by conventional imaging, because of infiltrative growth along white matter tracts that may extend beyond the nonenhancing, T2 hyperintense peritumoral abnormality into the NAWM.[89] DT imaging may be a useful tool in more accurately assessing the nonenhancing glioma margins and white matter invasion (**Fig. 12**).[72,87,90–93]

For example, Provenzale and colleagues[93] showed significantly greater decreases in FA in the NAWM adjacent to a glioma compared with a meningioma, which is an extra-axial tumor not expected to infiltrate along white matter tracts. These investigators also found a trend toward lower FA in the abnormal hyperintense peritumoral white matter in patients with glioma. Stadlbauer and colleagues[87] performed stereotactic biopsies and confirmed that decreasing FA correlated with increasing tumor cell number in the NAWM. As tumor infiltration

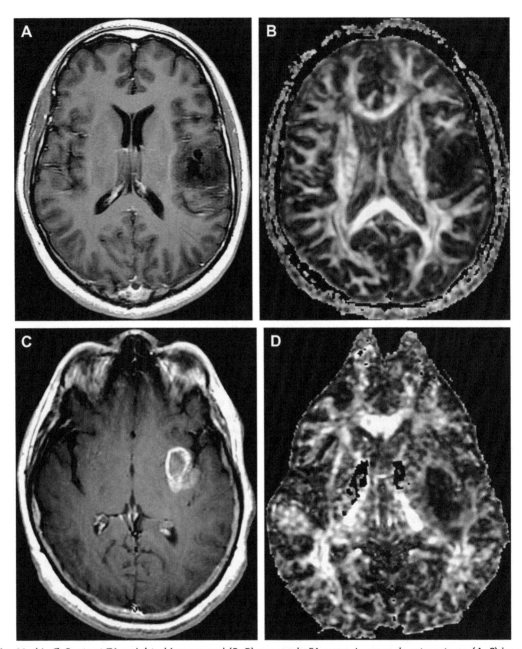

Fig. 11. (*A, C*) Contrast T1-weighted images and (*B, D*) gray-scale FA maps. Low-grade astrocytoma (*A, B*) is seen as a nonenhancing tumor in the left temporal operculum with a minimum FA of 0.041. Glioblastoma (*C, D*) in a different patient reveals a heterogeneously enhancing tumor in the insula with a minimum FA of 0.027. The ill-defined area of decrease anisotropy around both tumors reflects peritumoral edema and/or infiltrating tumor.

increases and causes greater derangement of white matter microarchitecture, a decrease in directionality of diffusion also occurs. Price and colleagues[90] described separate isotropic p and anisotropic q components to define unique diffusion signatures for the displacement versus infiltration of white matter. Despite these promising results, the exact role of DT imaging in defining tumor margins for treatment planning

is uncertain and an active area of investigation; gross total resection refers to removal of all enhancing tumor only.

Radiation therapy planning

Radiation therapy plays an important role in the treatment of patients with brain tumors. Malignant gliomas present a unique problem because of the presence of infiltrating tumor cells in and even

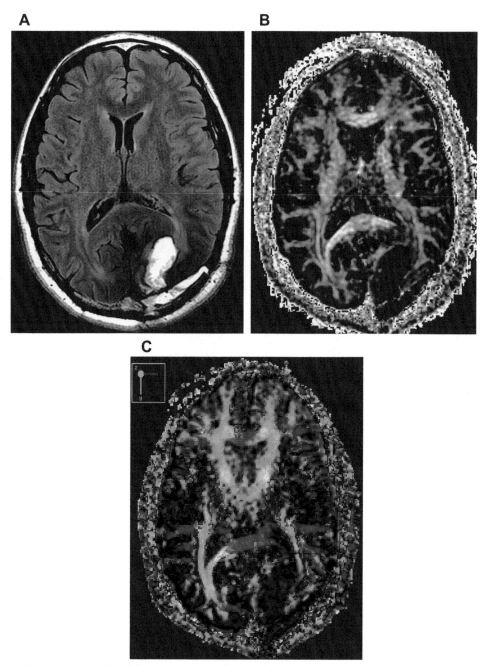

Fig. 12. White matter invasion. (*A*) FLAIR image performed for radiation therapy planning shows postoperative changes from recent gross total resection of a left occipital lobe glioblastoma. (*B*) FA and (*C*) directionally encoded FA maps more clearly show infiltration into the lateral splenium of the corpus callosum.

beyond the peritumoral abnormality. The optimal target for radiation therapy is controversial, with 2 main competing methods currently in use: (1) 46-Gy first phase to the contrast-enhancing abnormality and tumor-associated edema plus a 2-cm margin, followed by additional 14-Gy cone-down second phase to the contrast-enhancing abnormality plus a 2.5-cm margin for a total of 60 Gy; and (2) 60-Gy single phase to the contrast-enhancing abnormality plus 2- to 3-cm margin without explicit inclusion of the tumor-associated edema. Instead of using these isotropic and somewhat arbitrary guidelines, some researchers have proposed using individualized, anisotropic treatment plans that incorporate DT imaging data. By defining an imaging high-risk volume based on DT imaging, Jena and colleagues[94] developed nonuniform plans with decreased planning-target volumes (mean 35%) and mild dose escalations (mean 67 Gy) with equivalent normal tissue complication probabilities. By incorporating tractography data, Krishnan and colleagues[95] showed that tumor progression occurred along paths of preferred water diffusion that connected the primary tumor site and recurrence site. These imaging depictions of the route of glioma progression and site of recurrence are consistent with the known preferential infiltration of tumor along white matter tracts (**Fig. 13**).[89] Confirmation of these early findings in larger, prospective trials may lead to significant modifications to future radiation treatment plans, which will

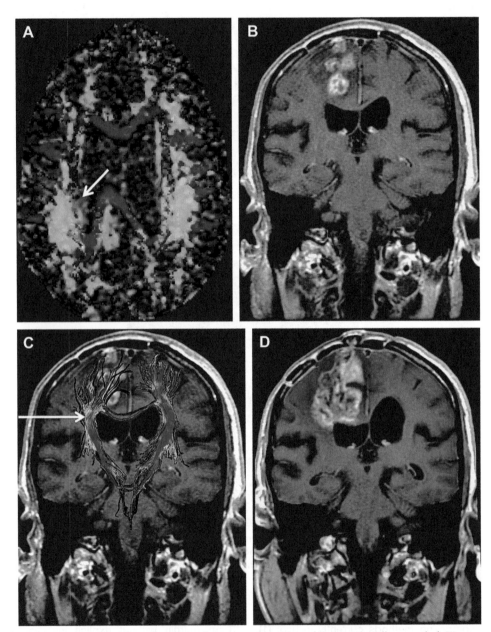

Fig. 13. Tractography suggesting direction of tumor progression. (*A*) Directionally encoded FA map shows decreased anisotropy in the right corticospinal tract (*arrow*) at the level of the corona radiata without abnormal enhancement as seen on (*B*) coronal contrast T1-weighted image. (*C*) Tractography overlaid on coronal contrast T1 image shown in (*B*) reveals decreased fibers in the right corticospinal tract (*arrow*) compared with the normal contralateral tract. (*D*) Contrast T1 image obtained 4 months later shows progression of enhancing tumor along the right corticospinal tract.

incorporate biologic as well as anatomic MR imaging data to improve targeting, escalate dosing, decrease toxicity, and perhaps positively affect patient outcomes.

Treatment response monitoring

DT imaging may play a role in evaluating the efficacy of medications administered during tumor treatment. For instance, steroids such as dexamethasone are a mainstay in reducing peritumoral brain edema. DT imaging may be sensitive to changes in water diffusion parameters in edematous brain after steroid treatment. Sinha and colleagues[96] suggested that patients treated with dexamethasone had significant decreases in MD in the edematous brain (without associated change in FA) at follow-up DT imaging in 48 to 72 hours. These data indicate that steroids reduce

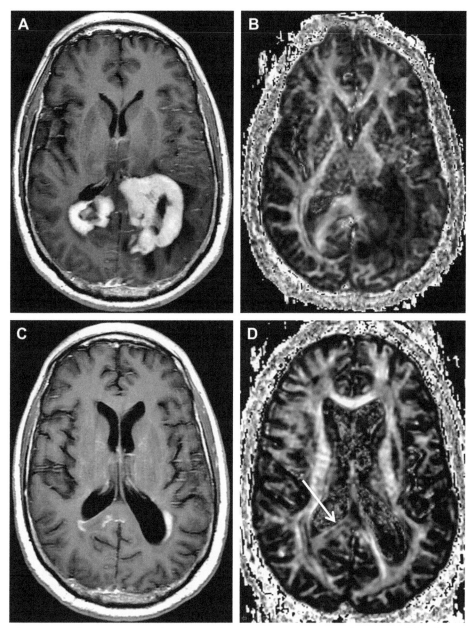

Fig. 14. Primary central nervous system lymphoma. (*A, C*) Contrast T1-weighted images and (*B, D*) gray-scale FA maps. At presentation (*A, B*), there are large bilateral posterior callosal tumors. After 2 months of chemoradiation therapy (*C, D*), only minor residual enhancement remains. The right splenium of the corpus callosum shows post-therapeutic gliosis (*arrow, D*), whereas the left splenium has nearly recovered relative to the normal genu.

the overall extracellular water content and mobility, and that the DT imaging metrics may be valid in evaluating the response of peritumoral edema to other chemotherapeutic agents.

A difficult but common diagnostic dilemma, particularly after combination chemotherapy and radiation therapy, is the new or increasing enhancing mass in treated patients that may represent radiation necrosis or recurrent tumor. Sundgren and colleagues[97] found that patients with radiation injury had significantly lower ADC, $\lambda_{\parallel}$ and $\lambda_{\perp}$ eigenvalues in the enhancing mass and higher FA ratios (relative to the contralateral normal brain) in the NAWM tract. In a recent retrospective review of 208 patients with glioblastoma, we found that diffusion restriction manifesting as low-ADC lesions preceded enhancing tumor by a median of 3.0 months in 23 of 27 (85.2%) patients (Young RJ, unpublished data, 2010). We postulate that restricted diffusion signifying high tumor cellularity or ischemia may become a useful imaging marker for disease progression. The exact role of DT imaging for new mass evaluation is uncertain, as is its role amongst other technologies such as MR imaging perfusion, MR imaging spectroscopy and fluorodeoxyglucose positron emission tomography (PET) scanning. With no clear benefit to any single technique, the most positive correlations may rely on a multiparametric approach that incorporates multiple data streams.

Treatment toxicity

White matter is sensitive to radiation injury.[98,99] The leukoencephalopathy is believed to reflect vascular endothelial and glial injury, and the severity has been correlated with vascular risk factors and advancing age.[100,101] Radiation therapy has been correlated with decreased intelligence quotients and increased cognitive impairment.[102,103] Patchy and confluent T2 hyperintense changes in the white matter on conventional MR imaging often present late and lag behind clinical deterioration. In contrast, DT imaging is able to show early radiation-induced damage. Welzel and colleagues[101] showed decreased FA in the white matter of patients receiving prophylactic cranial irradiation, which occurred as soon as radiation therapy ended and continued to decrease for 6 weeks. Mabbott and colleagues[104] studied 8 children who had been irradiated for medulloblastoma, and found decreased FA and increased ADC correlated with decreased IQ on long-term follow-up. Although these findings need to be corroborated in larger studies, they suggest that DT imaging is a highly sensitive indicator of clinically significant compromise of white matter microstructure that may result in an adverse clinical outcome (**Fig. 14**).

SUMMARY

At Memorial Sloan-Kettering Cancer Center, New York, a large percentage of patients with brain tumor undergo preoperative fMR imaging. We average approximately 4 preoperative fMR imaging cases per week. This large number of studies emphasizes the importance that our neurosurgeons place on acquisition of preoperative fMR imaging. Preoperative and intraoperative identification of essential white matter tracts using DT imaging is becoming routine clinical practice. These techniques have become more commonplace with the introduction of intraoperative MR imaging scanners. We have begun to incorporate the PET markers of malignancy into preoperative MR imaging scans as well as into the operating room to guide tumor resection. It is not unreasonable to assume that essentially all neurosurgical procedures will soon require image guidance. In the future, the surgeon will be able to view not only the anatomy of the tumor to be resected but also the adjacent eloquent cortices and essential white matter tracts as well as the most malignant areas of the tumor that are desirable to resect, all in real time, which can be updated using the intraoperative MR imaging to account for tumor resection and brain shift.

REFERENCES

1. Ogawa S, Lee TM. Magnetic resonance imaging of blood vessels at high fields: in vivo and in vitro measurements and image simulation. Magn Reson Med 1990;16(1):9–18.
2. Ogawa S, Lee TM, Nayak AS, et al. Oxygenation-sensitive contrast in magnetic resonance image of rodent brain at high magnetic fields. Magn Reson Med 1990;14(1):68–78.
3. Buxton RB, Uludag K, Dubowitz DJ, et al. Modeling the hemodynamic response to brain activation. Neuroimage 2004;23(Suppl 1):S220–33.
4. Logothetis NK, Wandell BA. Interpreting the BOLD signal. Annu Rev Physiol 2004;66:735–69.
5. Holodny A, Hou B. Physical principles of BOLD fMRI–what is important for the clinician. In: Holodny A, editor. Functional neuroimaging: a clinical approach. New York: Informa Healthcare; 2008. p. 1–12.
6. Kennan RP, Zhong J, Gore JC. Intravascular susceptibility contrast mechanisms in tissues. Magn Reson Med 1994;31(1):9–21.
7. Petrovich Brennan NM. Preparing the patient for the fMRI study and optimization of paradigm

selection and delivery. In: Holodny A, editor. Functional neuroimaging: a clinical approach. New York: Informa Healthcare; 2008. p. 13–22.

8. Buckner RL. Event-related fMRI and the hemodynamic response. Hum Brain Mapp 1998;6(5–6): 373–7.

9. Knecht S, Deppe M, Drager B, et al. Language lateralization in healthy right-handers. Brain 2000; 123(Pt 1):74–81.

10. Knecht S, Drager B, Deppe M, et al. Handedness and hemispheric language dominance in healthy humans. Brain 2000;123(Pt 12):2512–8.

11. Isaacs KL, Barr WB, Nelson PK, et al. Degree of handedness and cerebral dominance. Neurology 2006;66(12):1855–8.

12. Van Oostende S, Van Hecke P, Sunaert S, et al. FMRI studies of the supplementary motor area and the premotor cortex. Neuroimage 1997;6(3): 181–90.

13. Yetkin FZ, Mueller WM, Morris GL, et al. Functional MR activation correlated with intraoperative cortical mapping. AJNR Am J Neuroradiol 1997;18(7): 1311–5.

14. Lehericy S, Cohen L, Bazin B, et al. Functional MR evaluation of temporal and frontal language dominance compared with the Wada test. Neurology 2000;54(8):1625–33.

15. Gaillard WD, Balsamo L, Xu B, et al. fMRI language task panel improves determination of language dominance. Neurology 2004;63(8):1403–8.

16. Spreer J, Arnold S, Quiske A, et al. Determination of hemisphere dominance for language: comparison of frontal and temporal fMRI activation with intracarotid amytal testing. Neuroradiology 2002; 44(6):467–74.

17. Ojemann GA. Individual variability in cortical localization of language. J Neurosurg 1979; 50(2):164–9.

18. Price CJ, Veltman DJ, Ashburner J, et al. The critical relationship between the timing of stimulus presentation and data acquisition in blocked designs with fMRI. Neuroimage 1999;10(1):36–44.

19. Desmond JE, Sum JM, Wagner AD, et al. Functional MRI measurement of language lateralization in Wada-tested patients. Brain 1995;118(Pt 6): 1411–9.

20. Huang J, Carr TH, Cao Y. Comparing cortical activations for silent and overt speech using event-related fMRI. Hum Brain Mapp 2002;15(1):39–53.

21. Peck KK, Wierenga CE, Moore AB, et al. Comparison of baseline conditions to investigate syntactic production using functional magnetic resonance imaging. Neuroimage 2004;23(1):104–10.

22. Brennan CW, Petrovich Brennan NM. Functional image-guided neurosurgery. In: Holodny A, editor. Functional neuroimaging: a clinical approach. New York: Informa Healthcare; 2008. p. 91–106.

23. Seitz RJ, Huang Y, Knorr U, et al. Large-scale plasticity of the human motor cortex. Neuroreport 1995; 6(5):742–4.

24. Ramsey NF, Sommer IE, Rutten GJ, et al. Combined analysis of language tasks in fMRI improves assessment of hemispheric dominance for language functions in individual subjects. Neuroimage 2001;13(4):719–33.

25. Abou-Khalil B. Methods for determination of language dominance: the Wada test and proposed noninvasive alternatives. Curr Neurol Neurosci Rep 2007;7(6):483–90.

26. Pelletier I, Sauerwein HC, Lepore F, et al. Noninvasive alternatives to the Wada test in the presurgical evaluation of language and memory functions in epilepsy patients. Epileptic Disord 2007;9(2):111–26.

27. Roux FE, Boulanouar K, Lotterie JA, et al. Language functional magnetic resonance imaging in preoperative assessment of language areas: correlation with direct cortical stimulation. Neurosurgery 2003;52(6):1335–45 [discussion: 1345–7].

28. Ruge MI, Victor J, Hosain S, et al. Concordance between functional magnetic resonance imaging and intraoperative language mapping. Stereotact Funct Neurosurg 1999;72(2–4):95–102.

29. Petrovich N, Holodny AI, Tabar V, et al. Discordance between functional magnetic resonance imaging during silent speech tasks and intraoperative speech arrest. J Neurosurg 2005;103(2):267–74.

30. Rutten GJ, Ramsey NF, van Rijen PC, et al. Development of a functional magnetic resonance imaging protocol for intraoperative localization of critical temporoparietal language areas. Ann Neurol 2002;51(3):350–60.

31. Peled R, Harnes B, Borovich B, et al. Speech arrest and supplementary motor area seizures. Neurology 1984;34(1):110–1.

32. Wober C, Holzner F, Wessely P, et al. Speech arrest as first symptom of a tumour in the supplementary motor area. Wien Klin Wochenschr 1992;104(3): 73–5.

33. Krainik A, Lehericy S, Duffau H, et al. Postoperative speech disorder after medial frontal surgery: role of the supplementary motor area. Neurology 2003; 60(4):587–94.

34. Kho KH, Rutten GJ, Leijten FS, et al. Working memory deficits after resection of the dorsolateral prefrontal cortex predicted by functional magnetic resonance imaging and electrocortical stimulation mapping. Case report. J Neurosurg 2007;106(6 Suppl):501–5.

35. Holodny AI, Schulder M, Liu WC, et al. Decreased BOLD functional MR activation of the motor and sensory cortices adjacent to a glioblastoma multiforme: implications for image-guided neurosurgery. AJNR Am J Neuroradiol 1999;20(4):609–12.

36. Ulmer JL, Hacein-Bey L, Mathews VP, et al. Lesion-induced pseudo-dominance at functional magnetic resonance imaging: implications for preoperative assessments. Neurosurgery 2004;55(3):569–79 [discussion: 580–1].

37. Holodny AI, Schulder M, Liu WC, et al. The effect of brain tumors on BOLD functional MR imaging activation in the adjacent motor cortex: implications for image-guided neurosurgery. AJNR Am J Neuroradiol 2000;21(8):1415–22.

38. Holodny A. Cortical plasticity. In: Holodny A, editor. Functional neuroimaging: a clinical approach. New York: Informa Healthcare; 2008. p. 81–90.

39. Petrovich NM, Holodny AI, Brennan CW, et al. Isolated translocation of Wernicke's area to the right hemisphere in a 62-year-man with a temporo-parietal glioma. AJNR Am J Neuroradiol 2004;25(1):130–3.

40. Holodny AI, Schulder M, Ybasco A, et al. Translocation of Broca's area to the contralateral hemisphere as the result of the growth of a left inferior frontal glioma. J Comput Assist Tomogr 2002;26(6):941–3.

41. Krings T, Reinges MH, Erberich S, et al. Functional MRI for presurgical planning: problems, artefacts, and solution strategies. J Neurol Neurosurg Psychiatry 2001;70(6):749–60.

42. Frahm J, Merboldt KD, Hanicke W, et al. Brain or vein–oxygenation or flow? On signal physiology in functional MRI of human brain activation. NMR Biomed 1994;7(1–2):45–53.

43. Lai S, Hopkins AL, Haacke EM, et al. Identification of vascular structures as a major source of signal contrast in high resolution 2D and 3D functional activation imaging of the motor cortex at 1.5T: preliminary results. Magn Reson Med 1993;30(3):387–92.

44. Boxerman JL, Bandettini PA, Kwong KK, et al. The intravascular contribution to fMRI signal change: Monte Carlo modeling and diffusion-weighted studies in vivo. Magn Reson Med 1995;34(1):4–10.

45. Schaefer PW, Grant PE, Gonzalez RG. Diffusion-weighted MR imaging of the brain. Radiology 2000;217(2):331–45.

46. Riad S, Holodny A, Mukherjee SK. Diffusion imaging in brain tumors and treatment response. In: Holodny A, editor. Functional neuroimaging: a clinical approach. New York: Informa Healthcare; 2008. p. 201–16.

47. Mukherjee P, Berman JI, Chung SW, et al. Diffusion tensor MR imaging and fiber tractography: theoretic underpinnings. AJNR Am J Neuroradiol 2008;29(4):632–41.

48. Mukherjee P, Chung SW, Berman JI, et al. Diffusion tensor MR imaging and fiber tractography: technical considerations. AJNR Am J Neuroradiol 2008;29(5):843–52.

49. Young RJ, Knopp EA. Brain MRI: tumor evaluation. J Magn Reson Imaging 2006;24(4):709–24.

50. Nucifora PG, Verma R, Lee SK, et al. Diffusion-tensor MR imaging and tractography: exploring brain microstructure and connectivity. Radiology 2007;245(2):367–84.

51. Della Nave R, Foresti S, Pratesi A, et al. Whole-brain histogram and voxel-based analyses of diffusion tensor imaging in patients with leukoaraiosis: correlation with motor and cognitive impairment. AJNR Am J Neuroradiol 2007;28(7):1313–9.

52. Fushimi Y, Miki Y, Okada T, et al. Fractional anisotropy and mean diffusivity: comparison between 3.0-T and 1.5-T diffusion tensor imaging with parallel imaging using histogram and region of interest analysis. NMR Biomed 2007;20(8):743–8.

53. Stieltjes B, Schluter M, Didinger B, et al. Diffusion tensor imaging in primary brain tumors: reproducible quantitative analysis of corpus callosum infiltration and contralateral involvement using a probabilistic mixture model. Neuroimage 2006;31(2):531–42.

54. Catani M, Howard RJ, Pajevic S, et al. Virtual in vivo interactive dissection of white matter fasciculi in the human brain. Neuroimage 2002;17(1):77–94.

55. Behrens TE, Johansen-Berg H, Woolrich MW, et al. Non-invasive mapping of connections between human thalamus and cortex using diffusion imaging. Nat Neurosci 2003;6(7):750–7.

56. Ulmer JL, Salvan CV, Mueller WM, et al. The role of diffusion tensor imaging in establishing the proximity of tumor borders to functional brain systems: implications for preoperative risk assessments and postoperative outcomes. Technol Cancer Res Treat 2004;3(6):567–76.

57. Smits M, Vernooij MW, Wielopolski PA, et al. Incorporating functional MR imaging into diffusion tensor tractography in the preoperative assessment of the corticospinal tract in patients with brain tumors. AJNR Am J Neuroradiol 2007;28(7):1354–61.

58. Schonberg T, Pianka P, Hendler T, et al. Characterization of displaced white matter by brain tumors using combined DTI and fMRI. Neuroimage 2006;30(4):1100–11.

59. Mikuni N, Okada T, Enatsu R, et al. Clinical significance of preoperative fibre-tracking to preserve the affected pyramidal tracts during resection of brain tumours in patients with preoperative motor weakness. J Neurol Neurosurg Psychiatry 2007;78(7):716–21.

60. Nimsky C, Ganslandt O, Hastreiter P, et al. Preoperative and intraoperative diffusion tensor imaging-based fiber tracking in glioma surgery. Neurosurgery 2005;56(1):130–7 [discussion: 138].

61. Yu CS, Li KC, Xuan Y, et al. Diffusion tensor tractography in patients with cerebral tumors:

a helpful technique for neurosurgical planning and postoperative assessment. Eur J Radiol 2005;56(2):197–204.

62. Laundre BJ, Jellison BJ, Badie B, et al. Diffusion tensor imaging of the corticospinal tract before and after mass resection as correlated with clinical motor findings: preliminary data. AJNR Am J Neuroradiol 2005;26(4):791–6.

63. Lazar M, Alexander AL, Thottakara PJ, et al. White matter reorganization after surgical resection of brain tumors and vascular malformations. AJNR Am J Neuroradiol 2006;27(6):1258–71.

64. Holodny AI, Schwartz TH, Ollenschleger M, et al. Tumor involvement of the corticospinal tract: diffusion magnetic resonance tractography with intraoperative correlation. J Neurosurg 2001; 95(6):1082.

65. Johnson PC, Hunt SJ, Drayer BP. Human cerebral gliomas: correlation of postmortem MR imaging and neuropathologic findings. Radiology 1989; 170(1 Pt 1):211–7.

66. Watanabe M, Tanaka R, Takeda N. Magnetic resonance imaging and histopathology of cerebral gliomas. Neuroradiology 1992;34(6):463–9.

67. Lu S, Ahn D, Johnson G, et al. Diffusion-tensor MR imaging of intracranial neoplasia and associated peritumoral edema: introduction of the tumor infiltration index. Radiology 2004;232(1):221–8.

68. Wang S, Kim S, Chawla S, et al. Differentiation between glioblastomas and solitary brain metastases using diffusion tensor imaging. Neuroimage 2009;44(3):653–60.

69. Wang W, Steward CE, Desmond PM. Diffusion tensor imaging in glioblastoma multiforme and brain metastases: the role of p, q, L, and fractional anisotropy. AJNR Am J Neuroradiol 2009;30(1): 203–8.

70. Tsuchiya K, Fujikawa A, Nakajima M, et al. Differentiation between solitary brain metastasis and high-grade glioma by diffusion tensor imaging. Br J Radiol 2005;78(930):533–7.

71. Wieshmann UC, Clark CA, Symms MR, et al. Reduced anisotropy of water diffusion in structural cerebral abnormalities demonstrated with diffusion tensor imaging. Magn Reson Imaging 1999;17(9): 1269–74.

72. Sinha S, Bastin ME, Whittle IR, et al. Diffusion tensor MR imaging of high-grade cerebral gliomas. AJNR Am J Neuroradiol 2002;23(4):520–7.

73. Brunberg JA, Chenevert TL, McKeever PE, et al. In vivo MR determination of water diffusion coefficients and diffusion anisotropy: correlation with structural alteration in gliomas of the cerebral hemispheres. AJNR Am J Neuroradiol 1995;16(2):361–71.

74. Altman DA, Atkinson DS Jr, Brat DJ. Best cases from the AFIP: glioblastoma multiforme. Radiographics 2007;27(3):883–8.

75. Cha S, Knopp EA, Johnson G, et al. Intracranial mass lesions: dynamic contrast-enhanced susceptibility-weighted echo-planar perfusion MR imaging. Radiology 2002;223(1):11–29.

76. Witwer BP, Moftakhar R, Hasan KM, et al. Diffusion-tensor imaging of white matter tracts in patients with cerebral neoplasm. J Neurosurg 2002;97(3): 568–75.

77. van Westen D, Latt J, Englund E, et al. Tumor extension in high-grade gliomas assessed with diffusion magnetic resonance imaging: values and lesion-to-brain ratios of apparent diffusion coefficient and fractional anisotropy. Acta Radiol 2006;47(3):311–9.

78. Goebell E, Paustenbach S, Vaeterlein O, et al. Low-grade and anaplastic gliomas: differences in architecture evaluated with diffusion-tensor MR imaging. Radiology 2006;239(1):217–22.

79. Tropine A, Vucurevic G, Delani P, et al. Contribution of diffusion tensor imaging to delineation of gliomas and glioblastomas. J Magn Reson Imaging 2004; 20(6):905–12.

80. Inoue T, Ogasawara K, Beppu T, et al. Diffusion tensor imaging for preoperative evaluation of tumor grade in gliomas. Clin Neurol Neurosurg 2005; 107(3):174–80.

81. Yuan W, Holland SK, Jones BV, et al. Characterization of abnormal diffusion properties of supratentorial brain tumors: a preliminary diffusion tensor imaging study. J Neurosurg Pediatr 2008;1(4):263–9.

82. Ferda J, Kastner J, Mukenšnabl P, et al. Diffusion tensor magnetic resonance imaging of glial brain tumors. Eur J Radiol 2009. [Epub ahead of print]. DOI:10.1016/j.ejrad.2009.03.030.

83. Higano S, Yun X, Kumabe T, et al. Malignant astrocytic tumors: clinical importance of apparent diffusion coefficient in prediction of grade and prognosis. Radiology 2006;241(3):839–46.

84. Kitis O, Altay H, Calli C, et al. Minimum apparent diffusion coefficients in the evaluation of brain tumors. Eur J Radiol 2005;55(3):393–400.

85. Bulakbasi N, Guvenc I, Onguru O, et al. The added value of the apparent diffusion coefficient calculation to magnetic resonance imaging in the differentiation and grading of malignant brain tumors. J Comput Assist Tomogr 2004; 28(6):735–46.

86. Price SJ, Jena R, Burnet NG, et al. Improved delineation of glioma margins and regions of infiltration with the use of diffusion tensor imaging: an image-guided biopsy study. AJNR Am J Neuroradiol 2006;27(9):1969–74.

87. Stadlbauer A, Ganslandt O, Buslei R, et al. Gliomas: histopathologic evaluation of changes in directionality and magnitude of water diffusion at diffusion-tensor MR imaging. Radiology 2006; 240(3):803–10.

88. Kinoshita M, Hashimoto N, Goto T, et al. Fractional anisotropy and tumor cell density of the tumor core show positive correlation in diffusion tensor magnetic resonance imaging of malignant brain tumors. Neuroimage 2008;43(1):29–35.

89. DeAngelis LM. Brain tumors. N Engl J Med 2001; 344(2):114–23.

90. Price SJ, Pena A, Burnet NG, et al. Tissue signature characterisation of diffusion tensor abnormalities in cerebral gliomas. Eur Radiol 2004;14(10):1909–17.

91. Roberts TP, Liu F, Kassner A, et al. Fiber density index correlates with reduced fractional anisotropy in white matter of patients with glioblastoma. AJNR Am J Neuroradiol 2005;26(9):2183–6.

92. Price SJ, Burnet NG, Donovan T, et al. Diffusion tensor imaging of brain tumours at 3T: a potential tool for assessing white matter tract invasion? Clin Radiol 2003;58(6):455–62.

93. Provenzale JM, McGraw P, Mhatre P, et al. Peritumoral brain regions in gliomas and meningiomas: investigation with isotropic diffusion-weighted MR imaging and diffusion-tensor MR imaging. Radiology 2004;232(2):451–60.

94. Jena R, Price SJ, Baker C, et al. Diffusion tensor imaging: possible implications for radiotherapy treatment planning of patients with high-grade glioma. Clin Oncol (R Coll Radiol) 2005;17(8):581–90.

95. Krishnan AP, Asher IM, Davis D, et al. Evidence that MR diffusion tensor imaging (tractography) predicts the natural history of regional progression in patients irradiated conformally for primary brain tumors. Int J Radiat Oncol Biol Phys 2008;71(5): 1553–62.

96. Sinha S, Bastin ME, Wardlaw JM, et al. Effects of dexamethasone on peritumoural oedematous brain: a DT-MRI study. J Neurol Neurosurg Psychiatry 2004;75(11):1632–5.

97. Sundgren PC, Fan X, Weybright P, et al. Differentiation of recurrent brain tumor versus radiation injury using diffusion tensor imaging in patients with new contrast-enhancing lesions. Magn Reson Imaging 2006;24(9):1131–42.

98. Valk PE, Dillon WP. Radiation injury of the brain. AJNR Am J Neuroradiol 1991;12(1):45–62.

99. Ball WS Jr, Prenger EC, Ballard ET. Neurotoxicity of radio/chemotherapy in children: pathologic and MR correlation. AJNR Am J Neuroradiol 1992; 13(2):761–76.

100. Miot-Noirault E, Akoka S, Hoffschir D, et al. Potential of T2 relaxation time measurements for early detection of radiation injury to the brain: experimental study in pigs. AJNR Am J Neuroradiol 1996;17(5):907–12.

101. Welzel T, Niethammer A, Mende U, et al. Diffusion tensor imaging screening of radiation-induced changes in the white matter after prophylactic cranial irradiation of patients with small cell lung cancer: first results of a prospective study. AJNR Am J Neuroradiol 2008;29(2):379–83.

102. Maire JP, Coudin B, Guerin J, et al. Neuropsychologic impairment in adults with brain tumors. Am J Clin Oncol 1987;10(2):156–62.

103. Wassenberg MW, Bromberg JE, Witkamp TD, et al. White matter lesions and encephalopathy in patients treated for primary central nervous system lymphoma. J Neurooncol 2001;52(1):73–80.

104. Mabbott DJ, Noseworthy MD, Bouffet E, et al. Diffusion tensor imaging of white matter after cranial radiation in children for medulloblastoma: correlation with IQ. Neuro Oncol 2006;8(3):244–52.

Radiation Oncology in Brain Tumors: Current Approaches and Clinical Trials in Progress

Michael D. Chan, MD[a],*, Stephen B. Tatter, MD, PhD[b],
Glenn Lesser, MD[c], Edward G. Shaw, MD[a]

KEYWORDS

- Glioblastoma • Glioma • Meningioma • CNS lymphoma

Perhaps the most challenging therapeutic dilemma in the use of radiotherapy for brain tumors is the balance between tumor control and the tolerance of the normal tissues. Radiation oncologists have long referred to this issue as the therapeutic ratio. Radiation therapy has been found to improve several clinical endpoints in brain tumors, such as overall survival in glioblastoma, progression-free survival in low-grade glioma, and local control in atypical meningioma. However, radiation therapy has been implicated in significant delayed toxicities such as radiation-induced neurocognitive dysfunction and radionecrosis. A significant amount of the ongoing research on the use of therapeutic radiation in the treatment of brain tumors is being done to improve the therapeutic ratio between therapeutic gain and treatment toxicity. This review examines the current standards of care in common adult brain tumors and addresses current controversies and ongoing trials.

CURRENT TREATMENT PARADIGM IN GLIOBLASTOMA

Radiation therapy has long been the standard adjuvant approach for glioblastoma, and it remains the primary treatment modality in unresectable glioblastoma. A dose-response analysis performed by Walker in the late 1970s on patients treated in the previous Brain Tumor Cooperative Group Trials had established the standard radiation dose to be 60 Gy.[1] This seminal analysis evaluated patients treated at 4 separate dose levels between 45 and 60 Gy and found a statistically significant improvement in survival in the 60-Gy cohort.[1] Since then, several randomized comparisons have been published to support that 60 Gy is biologically superior to lower doses.[2,3]

Given the advantage of escalating radiation dose to 60 Gy, numerous subsequent trials have attempted to further escalate the dose. But the limiting factor has been the ability of the brain to tolerate higher doses of radiotherapy. Because of the dose-volume relationship that predicts for toxicity of radiation therapy, one strategy to further increase dose was to decrease the irradiated volume. The classic treatment portals for glioblastoma encompassed the whole brain. Randomized trials have since shown that partial brain radiotherapy was no different from the previous whole brain portals in outcome.[4] Patterns of failure data have shown that local

[a] Department of Radiation Oncology, Wake Forest University Health Sciences, 1 Medical Center Boulevard, Winston-Salem, NC 27104, USA
[b] Department of Neurosurgery, Wake Forest University Health Sciences, 1 Medical Center Boulevard, Winston-Salem, NC 27104, USA
[c] Department of Internal Medicine (Hematology and Oncology), Wake Forest University Health Sciences, 1 Medical Center Boulevard, Winston-Salem, NC 27104, USA
* Corresponding author.
E-mail address: mchan@wfubmc.edu

Neuroimag Clin N Am 20 (2010) 401–408
doi:10.1016/j.nic.2010.04.005

failure within 2 cm of the enhancing tumor was the predominant mode of recurrence, whether or not the entire brain was treated.[5,6] Strategies to decrease the treatment volume and increase the local radiotherapy dose were, however, unable to improve outcome. Several dose-escalation studies using hyperfractionation in an attempt to improve the therapeutic ratio were similarly unable to improve outcome.[7–9] Moreover, no randomized trial has ever shown an advantage of treating to a higher dose than 60 Gy.[10] A single-institution series from the Massachusetts General Hospital evaluating the ability of proton beam radiotherapy reported the escalation of radiation doses to 90 cobalt Gy equivalent and these doses were able to prevent tumor recurrences within the volume that received 90 Gy.[11] This series marked the first report of the pattern of failure of glioblastoma being changed secondary to higher doses of radiotherapy. This series, however, was marked by high rates of symptomatic radionecrosis, highlighting the tenuous nature of the therapeutic ratio for glioblastoma.[11] The series did suggest that if the 90-Gy dose could be successfully reached, the failure pattern could potentially be altered.

The advent of temozolomide chemotherapy has changed the treatment paradigm for glioblastoma over the past decade. In a trial published by the European Organisation for Research and Treatment of Cancer (EORTC), 2-year overall survival was improved from 10.4% to 26.5%.[12] The update of the trial, which was presented at the American Society for Therapeutic Radiology and Oncology national meeting in 2007, demonstrated that the survival advantage persisted even after 4 years. Since the EORTC trial, the standard postsurgical treatment for newly diagnosed glioblastoma has become concurrent temozolomide (75 mg/m^2) therapy with radiation therapy (60 Gy), followed by 6 monthly cycles of temozolomide (150–200 mg/m^2) therapy.

CURRENT MANAGEMENT CONTROVERSIES

The optimal radiation treatment volume represents one of the major controversies in the radiotherapeutic management of glioblastoma. There are 2 currently accepted paradigms, each with a slightly different philosophy. In the United States, the Radiation Therapy Oncology Group (RTOG) treatment volumes are the accepted standard. The first 46-Gy dose is delivered to the peritumoral edema with a 2-cm margin. The final 14-Gy booster dose is delivered to the enhancing tumor with a 2.5-cm margin. The US treatment standard is based on biopsy data from several single-institution series

that demonstrate tumor involvement extending into the peritumoral edema. Because the volume of the peritumoral edema is often significantly larger than the volume of the enhancing tumor, the treatment volume is reduced at 46 Gy to spare toxicity.[6] In Europe, however, a 2- to 3-cm margin to the enhancing tumor alone is treated to 60 Gy, without any field reduction. The logic behind this treatment philosophy is that 80% of treatment failures occur within 2 to 3 cm of the enhancing volume.[13,14] Furthermore, glioblastoma as a radioresistant tumor is unlikely to be sterilized by a 46-Gy preboost dose when compared with more sensitive tumors in other organ sites such as the breast and gastrointestinal tract. The next EORTC trial will be addressing this issue specifically and stratifying patients depending on the radiotherapy volumes in an attempt to determine if there may be any difference in the failure patterns. Fig. 1 depicts the controversy in treatment-volume delineation for glioblastoma.

A second issue to be addressed in the future of glioblastoma management with radiotherapy is the optimal imaging modalities for radiation-target delineation. At present, the RTOG accepted standard is the use of T2 or fluid-attenuated inversion recovery magnetic resonance imaging (MRI) sequences to identify peritumoral edema. T1 sequence with contrast images is used to identify the enhancing portion of the tumor. Several series have suggested that the use of metabolic imaging such as positron emission tomography, MR diffusion and MR perfusion, and MR spectroscopy may result in different treatment volumes than the traditional MRI sequences.[15,16] Further advances in imaging may ultimately change the paradigm of tumor delineation.

Although the concept of dose escalation has been investigated in the past, several advances in the delivery of radiotherapy and in the development of effective drug therapy have suggested that this question be reconsidered. Previous dose-escalation trials were done before the advent of temozolomide. In solid tumors outside of the central nervous system (CNS), the use of concurrent chemotherapy has been shown to have a synergistic effect on local control. It may be that the addition of concurrent chemotherapy to a dose-escalation approach may allow a decrease in the radiation dose necessary to prevent a failure in the high-dose region. Furthermore, bevacizumab, which is presently being investigated as an up-front antiangiogenesis agent, has been implicated in decreasing the rate of radionecrosis caused by radiotherapy.[17,18] The addition of such an agent in the up-front setting, as is being evaluated in the next RTOG trial, may ultimately

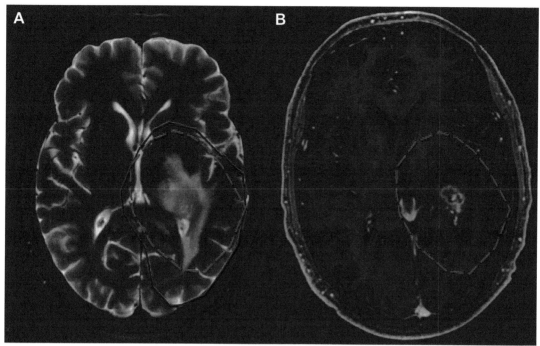

Fig. 1. Volume delineation for glioblastoma. Panel *A* depicts the delineation of treatment volumes by RTOG standards. The edema volume plus margin (*blue*) is treated to 46 Gy. The enhancing tumor plus margin (*red*) is boosted to 60 Gy. Panel *B* depicts the treatment volumes by EORTC standards. A margin is added to the enhancing tumor and this volume is treated to 60 Gy without a field reduction.

allow for higher doses of radiotherapy without the previously seen dose-limiting toxicities. The incorporation of newer treatment modalities such as intensity-modulated radiation therapy (IMRT) and proton beam radiotherapy may allow for better sparing of normal tissues or better-tolerated dose escalation. The tolerance of the brain to radiotherapy is a dose-volume relationship, and with techniques such as proton beam radiotherapy and IMRT, the integral dose may potentially be decreased. The success of dose escalation may ultimately be related to the ability to incorporate the newer imaging techniques to correctly identify tumors on imaging, so that the highest-risk regions for failure can be selectively treated to higher doses.

CURRENT TRIALS

There are 2 major phase III trials underway, regarding the use of adjuvant radiotherapy in the treatment of glioblastoma. The RTOG 0825 trial is investigating the use of bevacizumab in the up-front setting with concurrent temozolomide and radiation therapy. Bevacizumab is a monoclonal antibody against vascular endothelial growth factor. The basis of the RTOG 0825 trial is the high response rates seen in a phase II trial

performed by Duke Medical Center in the salvage setting when bevacizumab was used in combination with irinotecan.[19] The objective response rate was 57%, with 46% of the patients without progression at 6 months. A subsequent randomized phase II trial comparing bevacizumab monotherapy with a combination of bevacizumab and irinotecan revealed that bevacizumab had activity as a single agent.

The second major phase III trial is the EORTC CENTRIC (Cilengitide, Temozolomide, and Radiation Therapy in Treating Patients With Newly Diagnosed Glioblastoma and Methylated Gene Promoter Status) trial that randomizes patients to the standard temozolomide-radiotherapy combination with and without cilengitide. Cilengitide is a selective α_v-integrin inhibitor that has antiangiogenic properties. Two phase II trials have thus far been reported in an abstract form using concurrent cilengitide therapy in the up-front setting with temozolomide therapy and radiotherapy.[20] In the New Approaches to Brain Tumor Therapy (NABTT) 0306 trial presented at American Society of Clinical Oncology (ASCO) 2009, 89 of 112 patients who were enrolled in the trial were alive at 12 months from diagnosis. **Table 1** provides a summary of contemporary trials for glioblastoma.

Table 1
Contemporary trials on adjuvant therapy for glioblastoma

Trial	Adjuvant Therapy	Status
EORTC 26981	60 Gy 60 Gy/TMZ[a] + 5d TMZ[b]	Published in 2005 in the *New England Journal of Medicine*; improved 2-y overall survival with TMZ.
RTOG 0525	60 Gy/TMZ[a] + 5d TMZ[b] 60 Gy/TMZ[a] + 21d TMZ[c]	Closed to accrual; awaiting preliminary analysis
RTOG 0825	60 Gy/TMZ[a] + 5d TMZ[b] 60 Gy/TMZ/bev[d] + 5d TMZ[b]	Open to accrual 2008
EORTC CENTRIC	60 Gy/TMZ[a] 60 Gy/TMZ/CLG[e] + 5d TMZ[b]	Open to accrual 2009

Abbreviations: bev, bevacizumab; CLG, cilengitide; TMZ, temozolomide.
 [a] Temozolomide delivered daily and concurrently with fractionated radiation therapy.
 [b] Temozolomide delivered in a 5-day cycle each month for 6 cycles after radiation therapy.
 [c] Temozolomide delivered in a 21-day cycle each month for 6 cycles after radiation therapy.
 [d] Bevacizumab delivered concurrently with temozolomide and fractionated radiation therapy.
 [e] Cilengitide delivered concurrently with temozolomide and fractionated radiation therapy.

LOW-GRADE GLIOMA
Current Treatment Paradigms in Low-grade Glioma

The value of radiotherapy is considered to be somewhat more controversial in the management of low-grade glioma. This controversy stems from the fact that low-grade glioma has a more prolonged natural history, and as such, patients are more likely to live long enough to suffer from the late effects of radiotherapy. Moreover, the benefit provided by radiotherapy is limited to a benefit in progression-free survival. A randomized trial published by the EORTC evaluated the role of up-front radiotherapy versus observation in low-grade glioma.[21] Patients who had gross surgical resection, subtotal resection, and no resection at all participated in this trial. In this trial, radiotherapy improved progression-free survival at 5 years (55% vs 35%), but both the arms had equivalent overall survival. Also, 2 randomized dose-escalation trials have been published and have found no benefit to dose escalation for radiotherapy in the treatment of low-grade glioma.[22,23] Recent randomized trials are described in **Table 2**.

It has become clear that the benefit of up-front radiotherapy in patients with low-grade glioma may be related to the risk of the tumor to relapse early. The more recent approach to the management of low-grade glioma has been a risk-based approach. With such a management approach for low-grade glioma, identification of the prognostic factors becomes vital. The dominant prognostic factor for low-grade glioma is age.[24] Patients who are younger than 40 years have a longer median survival than patients who are older than 40 years (8.5 vs 4.9 years). Patients with an oligodendroglioma component of their tumor similarly have an improved survival over their counterparts with pure astrocytomas. Extent of resection has been found to be prognostic on several single-institution series as well as subgroup analyses.[25]

The RTOG 98-04 trial was a 3-arm trial that has been presented in an abstract form at ASCO in 2008 and has applied the concept of risk-stratified treatment. In this trial, low-risk patients underwent observation until the time of progression. Low-risk patients were defined as patients who were younger than 40 years with a complete resection. Higher-risk patients were randomized to radiation therapy with or without 6 cycles of adjuvant procarbazine, CCNU, and vincristine (PCV) chemotherapy. Results of the trial revealed that even low-risk low-grade glioma had a poor progression-free survival in half of the patients, with disease recurrence at 5 years. In the randomized arms, the addition of PCV chemotherapy appeared to have a small benefit in progression-free survival, but this benefit was tempered by greater hematologic toxicity.

Current Trials

The RTOG 0424 trial is an ongoing phase II trial in which high-risk low-grade gliomas are being treated with concurrent radiotherapy and temozolomide. This trial represents a paradigm shift with the use of up-front concurrent chemoradiotherapy for high-risk low-grade gliomas. Although the approach is aggressive by conventional standards, to be eligible for this trial, patients must have 3 independent factors in the high-risk categorization. These include age older than 40 years,

Trial	Adjuvant Therapy	5-y PFS (%)	5-y OS (%)
Table 2 Contemporary trials on adjuvant therapy for low-grade glioma			
EORTC 22844	45 Gy	47	58
	59.4 Gy	50	59
NCCTG	50.4 Gy		72
	64.8 Gy		64
EORTC 22845	Observation	35	66
	54 Gy	55	68
RTOG 9802	Observation (nonrandomized low-risk arm)	93	
	54 Gy	72	63
	54 Gy + PCV	84	72
RTOG 0424	54 Gy/TMZ[a] (nonrandomized)		

Abbreviations: OS, overall survival; PCV, procarbazine, CCNU, vincristine; PFS, progression-free survival; TMZ, temozolomide.

[a] Temozolomide delivered daily and concurrently with fractionated radiation therapy.

tumor diameter greater than 6 cm, tumor that crosses the midline, histologic characteristics of astrocytoma, or neurologic deficit. This trial continues the risk-stratification strategy in the treatment of low-grade glioma by attempting to increase the aggressiveness of up-front therapy in the highest-risk population.

PRIMARY CNS LYMPHOMA
Current Treatment Paradigms for Primary CNS Lymphoma

Because of the relative rarity of primary CNS lymphoma, the predominance of the clinical evidence is based on phase II trials or single-institution series. Primary CNS lymphoma has traditionally been managed with definitive whole brain radiotherapy, because its distant brain failure pattern makes partial brain radiotherapy suboptimal. The outcomes with whole brain irradiation had been generally poor with median survival times of approximately 1 year.[26] The advent of high-dose methotrexate-based chemotherapy has changed the treatment paradigm for primary CNS lymphoma over the past 2 decades and outcomes have been significantly improved over radiotherapy alone. The RTOG 9310 trial was an important trial in that it revealed a profound survival advantage of high-dose methotrexate-based chemoradiation over the conventional treatment with radiotherapy alone.[27] However, for patients older than 60 years, there was a significant rate of severe delayed neurocognitive toxicity. Results of the RTOG 9310 trial have now been replicated in several further phase II trials.[28,29] An NABTT phase II trial has also shown that single-agent high-dose methotrexate

is an effective treatment approach with a tolerable toxicity profile.[30]

With more effective systemic therapy available, the role of radiotherapy in primary CNS lymphoma has been called into question. Although there have been several attempts to use a combined chemoradiotherapy approach, such a combined modality approach has the potential of being severely neurotoxic. Several radiotherapy-containing protocols have attempted to de-escalate the radiotherapy dose depending on the response to chemotherapy. Rituximab (Rituxan) has also been added to treatment regimens in an attempt to decrease radiation doses.[31] A nonrandomized comparison of patients from Memorial Sloan-Kettering Cancer Center suggested that deferring whole brain radiotherapy in younger patients may compromise long-term disease control.[32] Although the role of radiotherapy in primary CNS lymphoma is unclear at present, the population older than 60 years likely should have radiotherapy deferred until time of salvage. Moreover, radiotherapy alone should be reserved for patients with insufficient renal function or performance status to tolerate high-dose methotrexate.

Current Trials

The RTOG has recently closed a phase I/II trial evaluating the efficacy of the combination of preirradiation rituximab, temozolomide, and high-dose methotrexate. In this trial, radiotherapy was delivered in a hyperfractionated approach with 1.2-Gy fractions delivered twice daily to a total dose of 36 Gy after completion of chemotherapy. This approach is based on the ability of high-dose methotrexate-based combination chemotherapy to decrease the sufficient tumoricidal radiation dose, thus lessening the likelihood of late neurotoxicity. The addition of rituximab to combination chemotherapy in systemic non-Hodgkin lymphoma has added to the efficacy of such regimens outside of the CNS and is now hoped to do the same in the CNS variant. The use of hyperfractionation is used to further improve the therapeutic ratio and decrease the likelihood of neurotoxicity. Results of this trial, particularly the neurocognitive endpoints, may help to define the role of reduced-dose hyperfractionated radiotherapy in primary CNS lymphoma. Table 3 summarizes modern prospective trials for the treatment of primary CNS lymphoma.

MENINGIOMA
Current Treatment Paradigms for Meningioma

Because meningiomas are generally benign and indolent tumors, treatment is generally indicated only in scenarios of symptomatic or radiographically progressive tumors. A corollary to this concept is that meningiomas do need to undergo a period of close observation after diagnosis to rule out the rare tumor that is more rapidly progressive. The optimal treatment regimen for meningioma depends on the location of the tumor. Meningiomas in a vertex location can generally be managed with surgery alone, if and when treatment is indicated. Meningiomas located at the skull base can pose a more difficult management dilemma because the surgical morbidity associated with these locations is significant. As such, surgical debulking followed by radiation therapy, radiosurgery, or fractionated radiation therapy alone are all reasonable treatment options. The need for surgical debulking in the skull base region depends on the degree of symptoms and whether the patient may benefit from an immediate decompression.

Postoperative management of meningioma depends on the adequacy of resection and the histologic grade of the tumor. In the 1950s, Simpson[33] documented the recurrence rates after various grades of resection and developed the Simpson Grade as a measure of adequacy of resection. Although the Simpson Grade was developed before the advent of better imaging and newer surgical techniques, recent data have confirmed that the adequacy of resection as predicted by the Simpson Grade still predicts recurrence risk.[34] The dominant prognostic factor for meningioma is the World Health Organization (WHO) grade. WHO grade II and III meningioma represent atypical meningioma and malignant meningioma, respectively. Patients with atypical meningioma should be considered for adjuvant radiotherapy, whereas patients with malignant meningioma should almost always receive it.

Radiosurgery is an alternative to surgery and external beam radiotherapy in the treatment of meningioma. Radiosurgery involves the delivery of a single large fraction of radiation therapy to the tumor and requires significantly better precision and patient immobilization than external beam radiotherapy. Radiosurgery has an excellent control rate for meningioma, but the time course for a radiographic response is in the order of several years.[35] The advantage of radiosurgery is the convenience of a single-day, outpatient procedure as well as the ability to avoid the higher integral doses to normal tissues delivered by external beam radiotherapy. The limits of radiosurgery include a size limitation of approximately 3 cm and a close proximity to the optic nerve or optic chiasm.

Table 3
Contemporary prospective trials on primary therapy for primary CNS lymphoma

Trial	Number of Patients	Treatment Regimen	2-y PFS (%)	2-y OS (%)
RTOG 9310	98	MVP + IT MTX + 45 Gy	50	64
EORTC 20962	52	MBVP + 40 Gy		69
MSKCC	30	R-MPV + 23.4 Gy (if CR) or 45 Gy (if PR)	67	57
NABTT 9607	25	MTX	68	35
Univ Bonn	65	MTX + ara-C + IV MTX, prednisolone, ara-C		69
RTOG 0227	Currently open	Rituxan, MTX, TMZ + 36 Gy (1.2 Gy bid)		

Abbreviations: ara-C, arabinofuranosyl cytidine; CR, complete response; IT MTX, intrethecal methotrexate; IV, intraventricular; MBVP, methotrexate, teniposide, carmustine, methylprednisolone given before radiation; MSKCC, Memorial Sloan-Kettering Cancer Center; MTX, methotrexate; MVP, methotrexate, vincristine, procarbazine; PR, partial response; R-MPV, Rituxan, methotrexate, procarbazine, vincristine given before radiation; TMZ, temozolomide.

Current Trials

Randomized trials are lacking in the determination of the optimal postoperative treatment for meningioma. The EORTC 26021 trial was designed as a randomized phase III trial evaluating the role of adjuvant radiotherapy in the setting of subtotally resected benign meningioma. It was designed as a 3-arm trial that randomized patients to adjuvant external beam radiotherapy, adjuvant radiosurgery, or observation. However, the trial was closed early due to poor accrual. The question that the trial sought to answer, however, remains a controversy in the management of meningioma. Although subtotally resected low-grade meningiomas do have a high recurrence rate, the patients with these tumors still have an excellent prognosis. As such, the up-front adjuvant treatment with external beam radiotherapy is of unknown relative significance. Moreover, focal treatment with radiosurgery to the residual disease remains an attractive option, given its more limited toxicity profile with less amount of parenchymal brain exposed to high doses of radiotherapy.

At present, the EORTC has an open phase II trial evaluating the outcomes and toxicities of high-dose postoperative radiotherapy in the treatment of atypical meningioma. Although this is not a randomized trial, it attempts to assess the post-treatment global cognitive function of treated patients. This trial addresses a crucial issue of neurocognitive function in this patient population that has a lengthy expected survival despite a high recurrence risk.

SUMMARY

The role of radiotherapy in brain tumors continues to evolve. Clinical trials provide the cornerstone to this evolutionary process. The current focus of clinical trials is no longer purely on the control of tumor but has shifted to also include the avoidance of normal tissue toxicity. Patients with longer life expectancies are more likely to experience significant toxicity in the late setting, because radiation-induced toxicity is an actuarial event. The integration of newer technologies and novel drug therapies allows for higher doses of radiotherapy to be safely delivered to tumors that require higher doses. The better elucidation of risk factors for tumor recurrence may help to spare patients who have a lesser relative gain of radiotherapy from unnecessary treatment.

REFERENCES

1. Walker MD, Strike TA, Sheline GE. An analysis of dose-effect relationship in the radiotherapy of malignant gliomas. Int J Radiat Oncol Biol Phys 1979;5:1725–31.

2. Walker MD, Green SB, Byar DP, et al. Randomized comparisons of radiotherapy and nitrosoureas for the treatment of malignant glioma after surgery. N Engl J Med 1980;303:1323–9.

3. Kristiansen K, Hagen S, Kollevold T, et al. Combined modality therapy of operated astrocytomas grade III and IV. Confirmation of the value of postoperative irradiation and lack of potentiation of bleomycin on survival time: a prospective multicenter trial of the Scandinavian Glioblastoma Study Group. Cancer 1981;47:649–52.

4. Shapiro WR, Green SB, Burger PC, et al. Randomized trial of three chemotherapy regimens and two radiotherapy regimens and two radiotherapy regimens in postoperative treatment of malignant glioma. Brain Tumor Cooperative Group Trial 8001. J Neurosurg 1989;71:1–9.

5. Garden AS, Maor MH, Yung WK, et al. Outcome and patterns of failure following limited-volume irradiation for malignant astrocytomas. Radiother Oncol 1991;20:99–110.

6. Halperin EC, Bentel G, Heinz ER, et al. Radiation therapy treatment planning in supratentorial glioblastoma multiforme: an analysis based on post mortem topographic anatomy with CT correlations. Int J Radiat Oncol Biol Phys 1989;17:1347–50.

7. Coughlin C, Scott C, Langer C, et al. Phase II, two-arm RTOG trial (94-11) of bischloroethyl-nitrosourea plus accelerated hyperfractionated radiotherapy (64.0 or 70.4 Gy) based on tumor volume (> 20 or < or = 20 cm(2), respectively) in the treatment of newly-diagnosed radiosurgery-ineligible glioblastoma multiforme patients. Int J Radiat Oncol Biol Phys 2000;48:1351–8.

8. Deutsch M, Green SB, Strike TA, et al. Results of a randomized trial comparing BCNU plus radiotherapy, streptozotocin plus radiotherapy, BCNU plus hyperfractionated radiotherapy, and BCNU following misonidazole plus radiotherapy in the postoperative treatment of malignant glioma. Int J Radiat Oncol Biol Phys 1989;16:1389–96.

9. Werner-Wasik M, Scott CB, Nelson DF, et al. Final report of a phase I/II trial of hyperfractionated and accelerated hyperfractionated radiation therapy with carmustine for adults with supratentorial malignant gliomas. Radiation Therapy Oncology Group Study 83-02. Cancer 1996;77:1535–43.

10. Nelson DF, Diener-West M, Horton J, et al. Combined modality approach to treatment of malignant gliomas–re-evaluation of RTOG 7401/ECOG 1374 with long-term follow-up: a joint study of the Radiation Therapy Oncology Group and the Eastern Cooperative Oncology Group. NCI Monogr 1988;6:279–84.

11. Fitzek MM, Thornton AF, Harsh GT, et al. Dose-escalation with proton/photon irradiation for Daumas-

Duport lower-grade glioma: results of an institutional phase I/II trial. Int J Radiat Oncol Biol Phys 2001;51: 131–7.

12. Stupp R, Mason WP, van den Bent MJ, et al. Radiotherapy plus concomitant and adjuvant temozolomide for glioblastoma. N Engl J Med 2005;352: 987–96.

13. Wallner KE, Galicich JH, Krol G, et al. Patterns of failure following treatment for glioblastoma multiforme and anaplastic astrocytoma. Int J Radiat Oncol Biol Phys 1989;16:1405–9.

14. Hess CF, Schaaf JC, Kortmann RD, et al. Malignant glioma: patterns of failure following individually tailored limited volume irradiation. Radiother Oncol 1994;30:146–9.

15. Grosu AL, Weber WA, Riedel E, et al. L-(methyl-11C) methionine positron emission tomography for target delineation in resected high-grade gliomas before radiotherapy. Int J Radiat Oncol Biol Phys 2005;63: 64–74.

16. Pirzkall A, McKnight TR, Graves EE, et al. MR-spectroscopy guided target delineation for high-grade gliomas. Int J Radiat Oncol Biol Phys 2001;50: 915–28.

17. Gonzalez J, Kumar AJ, Conrad CA, et al. Effect of bevacizumab on radiation necrosis of the brain. Int J Radiat Oncol Biol Phys 2007;67:323–6.

18. Torcuator R, Zuniga R, Mohan YS, et al. Initial experience with bevacizumab treatment for biopsy confirmed cerebral radiation necrosis. J Neurooncol 2009;94(1):63–8.

19. Vredenburgh JJ, Desjardins A, Herndon JE 2nd, et al. Bevacizumab plus irinotecan in recurrent glioblastoma multiforme. J Clin Oncol 2007;25:4722–9.

20. Reardon DA, Nabors LB, Stupp R, et al. Cilengitide: an integrin-targeting arginine-glycine-aspartic acid peptide with promising activity for glioblastoma multiforme. Expert Opin Investig Drugs 2008;17:1225–35.

21. van den Bent MJ, Afra D, de Witte O, et al. Long-term efficacy of early versus delayed radiotherapy for low-grade astrocytoma and oligodendroglioma in adults: the EORTC 22845 randomised trial. Lancet 2005;366:985–90.

22. Karim AB, Maat B, Hatlevoll R, et al. A randomized trial on dose-response in radiation therapy of low-grade cerebral glioma: European Organization for Research and Treatment of Cancer (EORTC) Study 22844. Int J Radiat Oncol Biol Phys 1996;36:549–56.

23. Shaw E, Arusell R, Scheithauer B, et al. Prospective randomized trial of low- versus high-dose radiation therapy in adults with supratentorial low-grade glioma: initial report of a North Central Cancer Treatment Group/Radiation Therapy Oncology Group/

24. Pignatti F, van den Bent M, Curran D, et al. Prognostic factors for survival in adult patients with cerebral low-grade glioma. J Clin Oncol 2002;20:2076–84.

25. Keles GE, Lamborn KR, Berger MS. Low-grade hemispheric gliomas in adults: a critical review of extent of resection as a factor influencing outcome. J Neurosurg 2001;95:735–45.

26. Nelson DF, Martz KL, Bonner H, et al. Non-Hodgkin's lymphoma of the brain: can high dose, large volume radiation therapy improve survival? Report on a prospective trial by the Radiation Therapy Oncology Group (RTOG): RTOG 8315. Int J Radiat Oncol Biol Phys 1992;23:9–17.

27. DeAngelis LM, Seiferheld W, Schold SC, et al. Combination chemotherapy and radiotherapy for primary central nervous system lymphoma: Radiation Therapy Oncology Group Study 93-10. J Clin Oncol 2002;20:4643–8.

28. Abrey LE, Yahalom J, DeAngelis LM. Treatment for primary CNS lymphoma: the next step. J Clin Oncol 2000;18:3144–50.

29. Poortmans PM, Kluin-Nelemans HC, Haaxma-Reiche H, et al. High-dose methotrexate-based chemotherapy followed by consolidating radiotherapy in non-AIDS-related primary central nervous system lymphoma: European Organization for Research and Treatment of Cancer Lymphoma Group Phase II Trial 20962. J Clin Oncol 2003;21:4483–8.

30. Batchelor T, Carson K, O'Neill A, et al. Treatment of primary CNS lymphoma with methotrexate and deferred radiotherapy: a report of NABTT 96-07. J Clin Oncol 2003;21:1044–9.

31. Shah GD, Yahalom J, Correa DD, et al. Combined immunochemotherapy with reduced whole-brain radiotherapy for newly diagnosed primary CNS lymphoma. J Clin Oncol 2007;25:4730–5.

32. Gavrilovic IT, Hormigo A, Yahalom J, et al. Long-term follow-up of high-dose methotrexate-based therapy with and without whole brain irradiation for newly diagnosed primary CNS lymphoma. J Clin Oncol 2006;24:4570–4.

33. Simpson D. The recurrence of intracranial meningiomas after surgical treatment. J Neurol Neurosurg Psychiatry 1957;20:22–39.

34. Pollock BE, Stafford SL, Utter A, et al. Stereotactic radiosurgery provides equivalent tumor control to Simpson grade 1 resection for patients with small- to medium-size meningiomas. Int J Radiat Oncol Biol Phys 2003;55:1000–5.

35. Kondziolka D, Mathieu D, Lunsford LD, et al. Radiosurgery as definitive management of intracranial meningiomas. Neurosurgery 2008;62:53–8 [discussion: 58–60].

Clinical Trials in Brain Tumor Surgery

Jason M. Hoover, MD[a], Susan M. Chang, MD[b],
Ian F. Parney, MD, PhD[a],*

KEYWORDS

- Brain tumor • Gliomas • Central nervous system
- Cytoreductive surgery

Central nervous system tumors represent a continued medical and surgical challenge. Primary intra-axial brain tumors, more specifically gliomas, have an annual incidence of approximately 14 per 100,000.[1,2] Glioblastoma is the most frequent and malignant histologic subtype (World Health Organization [WHO] grade IV). Surgery has an established role in the diagnosis and treatment of brain tumors and forms a key part of standard therapy along with radiation and chemotherapy. Outcomes for most brain tumor patients, however, remain humbling and continued efforts to improve and refine brain tumor treatment (including surgery) are needed. This article focuses on clinical trials in primary intra-axial brain tumor surgery, including a review of outcome data with standard surgical maneuvers, techniques to maximize safe surgical resection, and trials of surgically delivered therapeutics.

STANDARD NEUROSURGICAL TECHNIQUES

Standard neurosurgical techniques in brain tumor management can be divided into those primarily directed at diagnosis (ie, techniques for biopsy) and those directed at tumor debulking (ie, techniques for craniotomy and resection). This section reviews clinical trials of these standard techniques, including outcome studies.

Frame-Based Stereotactic Biopsy

Stereotactic biopsy can be defined as biopsy of intracranial lesions through a burr hole using stereotactic target coordinates determined on prebiopsy imaging. Stereotactic biopsy techniques were first developed using rigid frames attached to a patient's skull.[3] A rigid fiducial marker box is attached to the frame base before imaging (CT or MR imaging), thus defining the stereotactic space to determine the target, entry point, depth, and trajectory based on X, Y, and Z coordinates and a Cartesian system. The fiducial marker box is replaced by a stereotactic guide system attached to the frame that directs a biopsy needle from the entry point to the target along the selected trajectory to the depth calculated by the system (Fig. 1). Frame-based stereotactic needle biopsy can be performed with local or general anesthetic. The technique is generally safe and has a high chance of obtaining diagnostic material. Diagnostic yields are 91% to 98.4% with transient morbidity of 2.9% to 9%, permanent morbidity of 1.5% to 5%, and mortality of approximately 1% in modern series.[4–6] Small, deep lesions in eloquent brain are associated with higher rates of morbidity and nondiagnosis. In addition, the number of separate trajectories needed to obtain diagnostic material has been associated with increased morbidity.[5] Finally, there remains the potential for sampling error with stereotactic biopsy. In a series of patients at the MD Anderson Cancer Center who underwent craniotomy and tumor resection after previously undergoing stereotactic biopsy for glioma, the final pathologic diagnosis changed in 38% once further tissue was available.[7] This was largely accounted for by differences in tumor grade.

[a] Department of Neurologic Surgery, Mayo Clinic, 200 First Street SW, Rochester, MN 55905, USA
[b] Department of Neurologic Surgery, University of California, 505 Parnassus Avenue, San Francisco, CA 94143, USA
* Corresponding author.
E-mail address: parney.ian@mayo.edu

neuroimaging.theclinics.com

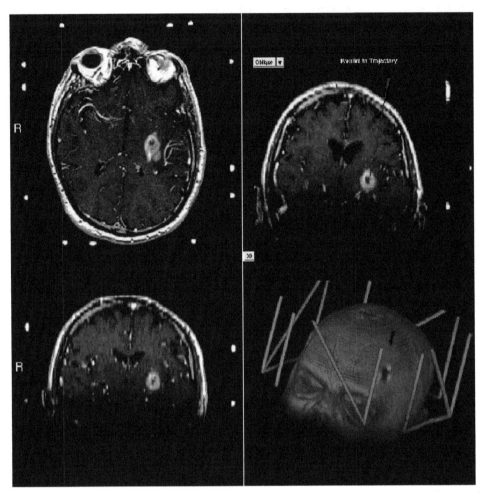

Fig. 1. Postcontrast T1-weighted MR imaging and reconstructions of a 73-year-old right-handed man who presented with a right hemiparesis secondary to an enhancing mass in his left insular cortex and basal ganglia. The hyperintense fiducial markers from the Compass stereotactic frame can be seen surrounding his head. The entry point, trajectory, and target are shown in the upper and lower right images. The final pathology was GBM.

Frameless Stereotactic Needle Biopsy

Frameless stereotactic biopsy performed using an intraoperative neuronavigation system, such as Stealth, BrainLab, or ISG Wand, is increasingly common.[8] Preoperative imaging (MR imaging or CT) is obtained after placing multiple adhesive fiducial markers on the patient's scalp. This information is transferred to an intraoperative computer connected to a binocular sensing device (eg, infrared camera) that can register the preoperative imaging in stereotactic space using the fiducial markers (Fig. 2). Alternatively, some systems register preoperative imaging using bony landmarks. Once the imaging and patient are registered, a viewing wand or other tool can be used to demonstrate the underlying anatomy in 3-D. An entry point, trajectory, depth, and target can then be determined for the biopsy. A guide system

attached to the skull or head holder keeps the biopsy instrument steady, allowing careful depth measurement and strict adherence to the proposed trajectory. Frameless stereotactic needle biopsy is often performed under general anesthetic.

Frameless stereotactic biopsy has been extensively reported in recent years, with diagnostic yields of 85% to 91% and permanent morbidity rates of 3% to 6%.[8–10] Studies with imaging phantoms have suggested that frameless and frame-based stereotactic biopsy accuracy are comparable.[11] Fiducial markers or surface landmarks used to register images for frameless systems may shift, however, during positioning for surgery. This is not an issue for rigid frame-based systems. Thus, some investigators advocate continued reliance on frame-based biopsy

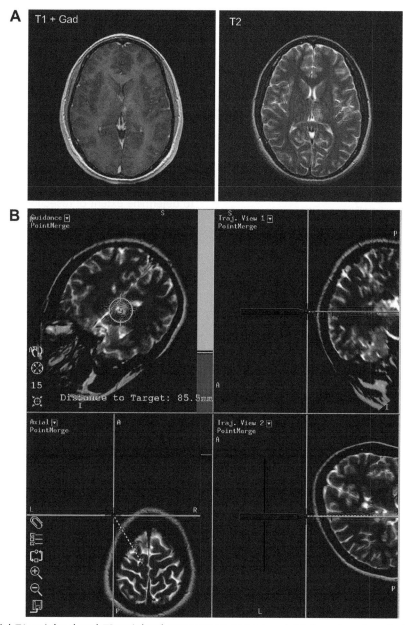

Fig. 2. (A) Axial T1-weighted and T2-weighted postcontrast images and (B) frameless stereotaxic biopsy plan (using the Stealth system) for an 18-year-old right-handed woman presenting with diplopia secondary to a partially enhancing mass in the left medial thalamus and midbrain tectum. The final pathology was primitive neuroectodermal tumor.

for small or deep lesions. Furthermore, there are potential advantages to frame-based biopsies in terms of reduced use of anesthesia, operating room, and hospital resources,[10] although this may vary with individual practice patterns. In contrast, some investigators have concluded that frameless stereotactic biopsy is comparable with frame bases with regard to diagnostic yield and complications but has distinct advantages. Although a recent series from the Johns Hopkins Hospital found no significant differences in diagnostic yield or complications, more than one needle trajectory was required more frequently to obtain diagnostic tissue from cortical lesions with frame-based compared with frameless stereotaxy.[8] In other studies, increased number of needle trajectories has been strongly associated with increased morbidity.[5] The Johns Hopkins investigators concluded that frameless stereotaxy may represent a more efficient means of obtaining biopsy specimens of cortical lesions but is otherwise similar to the frame-based technique.

Craniotomy for Surgical Resection

Craniotomy and resection has an established role in managing intra-axial primary central nervous system tumors to establish diagnosis and reduce mass effect. Resection is also often used for cytoreduction. Its value in this case, however, remains controversial. This section reviews outcome data for patients undergoing craniotomy and resection of diffuse intra-axial gliomas.

Cytoreductive Surgery for Malignant Gliomas

Malignant gliomas (WHO grade III or IV) include anaplastic (grade III) astrocytomas (AAs), oligodendrogliomas, and mixed oligoastrocytomas as well as glioblastoma multiforme (GBM) (grade IV). Craniotomy and resection of tumor is clearly indicated as a lifesaving measure in patients with raised intracranial pressure and impending herniation. Similarly, smaller tumors centered in deep gray matter (basal ganglia or thalamus) are often biopsied without resection due to the high morbidity associated with attempted surgical resection. Most malignant glioma patients fall in-between these extremes. For these patients, most neurosurgeons generally advocate maximal safe resection. There remains controversy, however, regarding this due to the lack of class I evidence demonstrating a survival advantage for patients under going resection for cytoreduction.[12]

The authors reviewed the literature on surgery for malignant gliomas published between 1987 and 2007. A PubMed search was performed using combinations of the key words, "malignant", "anaplastic", "high-grade", "glioma", "astrocytoma", "oligodendroglioma", glioblastoma multiforme, "surgery", and "outcome." In addition, further key publications were identified by cross-references in the resulting articles. Studies were excluded if they did not contain information on outcome with varying degrees of resection, did not determine extent of resection on the basis of postoperative imaging, or did not include formal statistical evaluation. Similarly, studies including children or patients with grade I or II tumors were excluded unless these populations were analyzed separately. Forty-two articles were identified that met the criteria for inclusion.[13–38] Twenty-eight studies, involving 5874 patients, were identified that found that more extensive resection of malignant gliomas was associated with significantly prolonged survival. Fourteen studies, involving

2122 patients, did not find any significant association.

It is not possible to pool data meaningfully from these disparate studies. Nevertheless, a trend to prolonged survival with more extensive resection is seen when the available data are collated. Several important sources of bias need to be considered, however. The majority of these studies are retrospective and, among prospective studies, only 2 were randomized. One of these was a limited study of 23 patients. Actual survival times often not recorded. Only 4 studies used formal computer-based volumetric assessment to determine extent of resection.[15,17,39,40] Finally, postsurgical treatment (radiation therapy and chemotherapy) varied widely in these studies.

Over the past decade, several investigators have addressed these concerns with varying degrees of success. In 2001, Sawaya and colleagues[17] reported results from their single-institution prospective series, demonstrating that survival was correlated with extent of resection. In 2003, Laws and colleagues[19] reported the landmark findings of the Glioma Outcomes Project (a prospective outcome study in 788 malignant glioma patients from 55 centers across North America). In this study, mean survival for newly diagnosed GBM patients undergoing craniotomy and resection was 49 weeks compared with 21 weeks for those undergoing biopsy. In 2006, Stummer and colleagues[22] published some of the most compelling data supporting cytoreductive surgery to date. In a multicenter randomized controlled trial, patients receiving fluorescence-guided surgery with 5-aminolevulinic acid (5-ALA) (discussed later) had an increased likelihood of gross total resection of enhancing tumor (65% vs 36%, $P<.0001$). These patients also had a prolonged 6-month progression-free survival when compared with those patients who had their tumor resected using white light (40% vs 21%, $P = .0003$).[22] Although this study was not powered to detect significant differences in overall survival, a trend was seen in this direction.

Cytoreductive Surgery for WHO Grade II Gliomas

WHO grade II gliomas (diffuse infiltrating astrocytomas, oligodendrogliomas, and mixed oligoastrocytomas) are related to and often progress to become malignant gliomas.[41] Managing patients with grade II gliomas has been controversial.[42,43] As with malignant gliomas, most neurosurgeons advocate maximal safe resection,[44] based in part on several nonrandomized studies that show trends to improved survival and improved response to adjuvant therapy with more extensive resection. The definition of maximal safe resection, however, differs widely among neurosurgeons.

The authors reviewed the literature from the past 20 years using a similar strategy to that described previously for malignant gliomas. A PubMed search was performed using combinations of the key words, "low-grade", "grade I", "diffuse", "glioma", "astrocytoma", "oligodendroglioma", "oligoastrocytoma", "surgery", and "outcome". In addition, further key publications were identified by cross-references in the resulting articles. Studies without information on outcome with varying degrees of resection, where extent of resection was not determined on the basis of post-operative imaging or where formal statistical evaluation was lacking, were excluded. Similarly, studies including children or patients with grade I, III, or IV tumors were excluded unless these populations were analyzed separately. In addition, studies with short median follow-up (<3 years) were excluded in recognition of the longer median survival seen in most patients with grade II gliomas. The authors identified 10 articles meeting criteria for inclusion.[45–54] Eight studies, involving 1115 patients, found a significantly positive association between extent of resection and survival. Two studies, involving 1075 patients, did not demonstrate any significant association.

As with high-grade gliomas, the lack of randomized controlled trials precludes meta-analysis of data from these studies. Nevertheless, collated data from these studies suggest a trend to prolonged survival with greater extent of resection. Furthermore, the magnitude of this effect is much greater than that seen with malignant gliomas. Five-year survival for grade II glioma patients is improved from 40% to 71% with simple biopsy to 80% to 98% with gross total resection, suggesting that resection could be associated with prolonged survival of several years compared with biopsy. This is in contrast to GBM patients where median survival after biopsy was 15 to 33 weeks and after gross total resection was 45 to 167 weeks, suggesting resection was often associated with prolonged survival of several months compared with biopsy. Two recent articles are particularly valuable. Smith and colleagues[54] used true computer-assisted volumetric analysis to evaluate the prognostic effect of extent of resection in a retrospective study of 216 adult patients undergoing initial resection of hemispheric low-grade gliomas. Patients with at least 90% extent of resection had 5- and 8-year overall survival rates of 97% and 91%, respectively, whereas patients with less than 90% extent of resection had 5- and 8-year overall survival rates

of 76% and 60%, respectively. They concluded that improved outcome among adult patients with hemispheric low-grade glioma is predicted by greater extent of resection.[54] Similarly, Shaw and colleagues examined recurrence in 111 adults less than 40 years of age with cerebral low-grade glioma who underwent a neurosurgeon-determined gross total resection. Overall survival rates at 2 and 5 years were 99% and 93% and progression-free survival rates at 2 and 5 years were 82% and 48%. Three prognostic factors predicted significantly poorer progression-free survival: (1) preoperative tumor diameter greater than or equal to 4 cm; (2) astrocytoma/oligoastrocytoma, histologic type; and (3) residual tumor greater than or equal to 1 cm according to MR imaging. They concluded that young adult patients with low-grade glioma who undergo a neurosurgeon-determined gross total resection still have a greater than 50% risk of tumor progression 5 years postoperatively and should be closely followed and considered for adjuvant treatment.[55]

The grade II glioma studies were subject to the same biases as the high-grade glioma studies. All the studies reported a statistical analysis of association between extent of resection and survival but only 78% actually reported specific 5-year survival percentages. Five-year survival statistics were missing from 1 of the 2 studies that failed to show an association between survival and extent of resection.[46] Coincidentally, this was the largest study that met criteria for inclusion (n = 993). Only 3 studies used volumetric assessments of residual tumor[45,52,54] whereas the remainder relied on 2-D estimates. All the studies were retrospective or based on post hoc analysis of data collected prospectively in trials designed to answer questions other than the influence of resection on survival. Postsurgical treatment varied between and within studies. Finally, all the studies were non-randomized, making them subject to considerable selection bias. Despite these potential biases, most studies demonstrate a compelling association between greater extent of resection and prolonged quality survival for many years.[45,47–49,51,52,54,56] As a result, it is reasonable to strongly advocate early maximal safe resection for patients with newly diagnosed grade II gliomas.

TECHNIQUES TO MAXIMIZE SAFE SURGICAL RESECTION
Advanced Imaging in Brain Tumor Surgery

Imaging studies going beyond purely anatomic data are increasingly incorporated into planning for brain tumor surgery. This imaging generally falls into 2 categories: (1) physiologic imaging (magnetic resonance spectroscopy [MRS], cerebral perfusion, and positron emission tomography [PET]), which can be used to provide information about the nature and extent of the tumor itself; and (2) functional imaging (functional MR imaging, diffusion tensor imaging, PET, and magnetoencephalography), which can provide information about adjacent eloquent brain. This section reviews recent clinical studies about physiologic and functional imaging in brain tumor surgery.

Physiologic imaging

Several imaging modalities have been used to elucidate information about tumor physiology that can be beneficial in surgical planning by highlighting more aggressive areas or further delineating the extent of tumor beyond enhancing margins.[57] For example, proton-based MRS can distinguish tumor (increased choline to N-acetylaspartate [NAA] ratio) from normal tissue (choline: NAA ratio <1) and necrosis (globally decreased metabolites). MRS can identify more malignant areas (greater choline:NAA ratios) within nonenhancing lesions and tumor extension within non-enhancing T2-weighted/fluid-attenuated inversion recovery signal abnormality around an enhancing mass. This information has been used successfully to target stereotactic biopsies and guide extent of resection.[58] Similar information can be obtained from fluorodeoxyglucose PET that demonstrates increased metabolic activity in tumor tissue and decreased metabolic activity in necrosis. Finally, cerebral perfusion studies have been used extensively to identify areas of increased blood flow within tumors.[59] Not only has this been beneficial in identifying more malignant areas within otherwise nonenhancing tumors but also it has been helpful in surgical preparation by identifying areas likely to be more vascular. (See **Fig. 3** for examples of physiologic imaging).

Functional imaging

Imaging eloquent areas of brain preoperatively so that their relationships to tumor can be appreciated and they can be avoided at surgery has definite advantages in surgical planning. PET has been used for many years to map eloquent areas of the brain and can be helpful in surgical planning. Functional PET often requires isotopes beyond fluorodeoxyglucose, however, such as ^{15}O-H_2O, that are not widely available. As a result, functional MR imaging has recently received more attention. This relies on changes in regional blood flow during task performance to generate a blood oxygenation level–dependent signal, which is an indirect measure of neuronal activity.[60] Similarly, diffusion tensor imaging (DTI) with MR imaging can map subcortical white matter tracts based on local water diffusion characteristics.[61] Functional MR imaging and DTI can be incorporated into preoperative image-guidance systems (discussed later) and have been widely used in clinical neurosurgery for preoperative planning in brain tumor patients.[62-65] (See **Fig. 4** for examples of functional MR imaging and DTI). Ongoing concerns about their sensitivity and specificity,[66,67] however, suggest that other functional mapping techniques may be necessary. Magnetoencephalography is one such promising technique, based on direct detection of neuronal activity. Small studies using magnetoencephalography in surgical planning for brain tumors have been reported and seem to show a good correlation with intraoperative electrophysiologic mapping.[68,69] This technology requires significant infrastructure and is not yet widely available.

Image Guidance

Gliomas are diffusely infiltrating by their nature and determining their boundaries at surgery can be difficult. Image guidance using frameless stereotaxy (as described previously for stereotactic biopsies) can be helpful for localizing tumor and for determining extent of resection. This has been described extensively in the past decade.[70] Image-guided resection was associated with improved outcome in 486 newly diagnosed malignant glioma patients in the Glioma Outcomes Project.[71] It was unclear, however, if these improved outcomes were due to the selection of a more favorable patient population (younger and good performance status) or to the image-guidance techniques themselves.

Intraoperative MR Imaging

As most neuronavigation systems are based on preoperative MR imaging, there is potential for significant shift in the surrounding brain as a tumor is debulked.[72] Thus, image-guidance systems may become increasingly inaccurate as tumor resection proceeds. Intraoperative MR imaging is one of the most robust methods to address brain shift during frameless stereotactic-guided tumor resection.[73,74] Early-generation intraoperative MR imaging scanners tended to be low field strength (eg, 0.2 tesla).[75] Although some investigators maintain that the images produced by such low-field magnets are adequate,[45,76,77] many prefer high-field (1.5 tesla or greater) magnets for intraoperative imaging.[64,78,79] These systems typically require significant infrastructure with nonferromagnetic instruments but produce images comparable with standard clinical 1.5-tesla MR

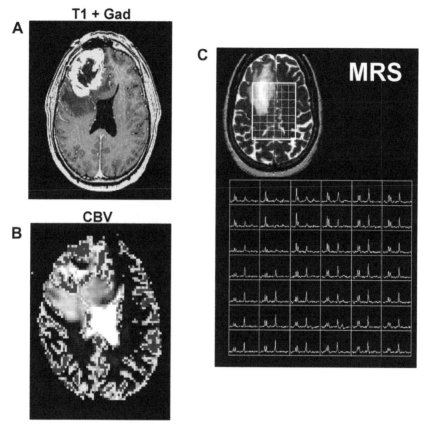

Fig. 3. (A) Standard axial T1-weighted postcontrast MR imaging of the head demonstrating a right frontal glioblastoma. (B) Cerebral blood volume/perfusion MR imaging demonstrating increased blood flow (red) in enhancing areas of same glioblastoma. (C) Multivoxel 3-D MRS of the same patient demonstrating increased choline:NAA ratio in tumor and surrounding T2 hyperintensity.

imaging scanners. Furthermore, they can be used to reregister image-guidance systems. A recent study from the University of California in Los Angeles reported a series documenting extent of resection with varying image guidance and intraoperative MR imaging systems.[80] As expected, extent of resection was generally larger with image guidance than without. Low-field intraoperative or high-field intraoperative MR imaging alone did not improve on this but high-field intraoperative MR imaging with reregistration of a neuronavigation system resulted in the highest degree of resection of any combination of image guidance and intraoperative imaging systems. (See Fig. 5 for an example of imaging obtained with high-field intraoperative MR imaging.)

Electrophysiologic Mapping

Although preoperative functional imaging can be incorporated into many neuronavigation systems, intraoperative electrophysiologic mapping remains the gold standard for identifying functional cortex

and subcortical fiber tracts. This is not a new technique, having been originally developed by Penfield and Boldrey in the 1930s to facilitate epilepsy surgery.[81] It has since been adapted to a variety of neurosurgical indications, including intra-axial tumor resection.[82,83] It has been suggested that, as long as the resection remains exclusively within the tumor itself, the risk of neurologic injury is low. This is not always possible, however, and data from large prospective series suggest that functional neurons occur within tumors adjacent to functional cortex in up to 8% of cases.[84] Mapping motor cortex and subcortical fibers can be done while patients are awake or asleep (with appropriate anesthetic management)[85] but speech mapping requires awake craniotomy and patient cooperation. As experience has grown with speech mapping in tumor surgery, it has become evident that this can allow aggressive tumor resection in brain areas traditionally felt to be inoperable due to their proximity to critical areas for speech. In a recent prospective series of 250 patients with gliomas,

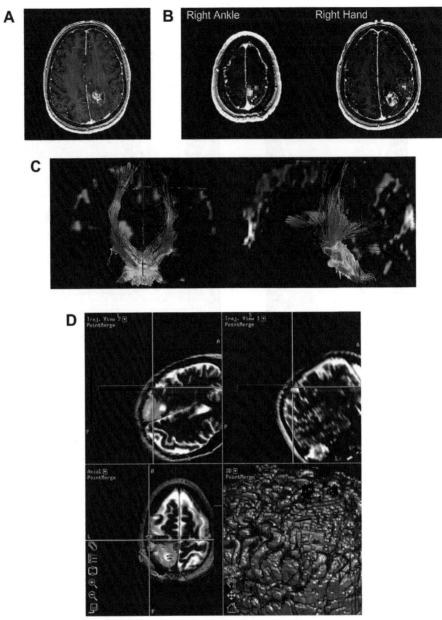

Fig. 4. (A) Standard axial T1-weighted postcontrast MR imaging of the head demonstrating a left parietal glioblastoma. (B) Functional MR imaging demonstrating areas of activation (*red and yellow*) with right ankle and hand motor tasks anterior and superior to the tumor. (C) DTI demonstrating displacement of white matter tracts by the tumor. (D) Frameless stereotactic images of the same patient with motor areas for right hand (*green*) and ankle (*pink*) superimposed. The viewing wand (*blue*) has been placed at a critical motor area for right hand function identified by intraoperative electrical stimulation mapping with a bipolar electrode. Note that this corresponds to only a portion of the larger area identified by functional MR imaging, suggesting that functional MR imaging was sensitive but not specific for motor function in this case.

Berger and colleagues[86] reported that critical speech areas were identified in 58%. One week after surgery, speech function was worsened in 22%; it resolved in most patients, however, and only 1.6% of surviving patients at 6 months continued to have increased speech deficits.[86]

Surface cortical electrophysiologic mapping is useful for identifying appropriate safe entry points for surgical resection. It does not identify subcortical fibers, however, that may deviate from their surface origin as they pass. For this, subcortical electrophysiologic mapping is critical, particularly

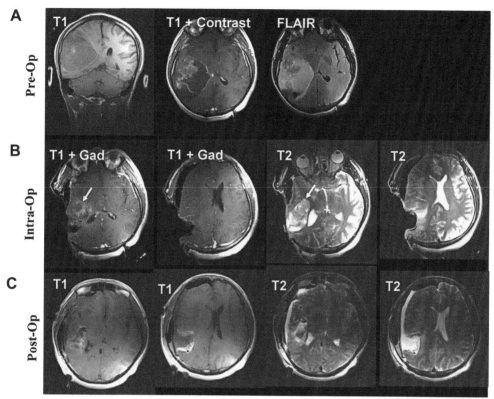

Fig. 5. (A) Preoperative, (B) intraoperative, and (C) postoperative MR imaging obtained in a 23-year-old man with a malignant glioneuronal tumor undergoing resection in a high-field (1.5-tesla) intraoperative MR imaging scanner. Note the significant residual tumor (*arrows*) seen on the intraoperative images. The image-guidance system was reregistered at this point and further tumor removal was performed, leading to a gross total resection (C). Gad, gadolinium.

for motor mapping,[85] and uses techniques similar to surface mapping and can be used intermittently as resection proceeds.

Fluorescence-Guided Resection

Fluorescence-guided resection relies on administration of a pharmacologic agent that localizes to tumor but not surrounding brain and fluoresces when exposed to light of the appropriate wavelength. Tumor resection can be guided by the fluorescence seen at surgery, potentially allowing a surgeon to identify tumor tissue that otherwise might not be obvious at craniotomy. Fluorescence-guided surgery for brain tumors has been used most commonly with 5-ALA. 5-ALA is orally available and accumulates in glioma tissue where it is metabolized to protoporphyrin IX and fluoresces pink when exposed to light at 375 to 440 nm.[87] Stummer and colleagues[22] have published results of a multicenter randomized controlled trial comparing 5-ALA fluorescence-guided resection with standard white light resection in 322 newly diagnosed GBM patients.

Patients undergoing fluorescence-guided resection were more likely to have a gross total resection (65% vs 36%, $P<.0001$). They were also more likely to be progression-free at 6 months (40% vs 21%, $P = .0003$). This was not associated with any significant difference in performance status. Although this study was not powered to detect differences in overall survival, it remains a source of some of the most compelling data supporting cytoreductive surgery in glioblastomas.[88]

LOCAL DELIVERY OF THERAPEUTIC AGENTS

As time and technology progress, surgeons become more skilled at operating on difficult brain tumors with increasingly minimal complications. Although there will always continue to be improvements, an era may be approaching where the biggest advances in neurosurgical oncology do not come about from enhancements in technique but from advances in surgically delivered anti-tumor agents.

Brachytherapy

Brachytherapy can be defined as implanting interstitial radioactive sources directly into the tumor at surgery to allow delivery of local high-dose irradiation while leaving surrounding tissues relatively spared. Iodine 125 and iridium 132 are commonly used sources. At least two forms have been investigated in malignant glioma treatment: temporary/high-dose brachytherapy and permanent/low-dose brachytherapy.[89,90] Although initial studies with high-dose temporary brachytherapy were promising, they failed to show benefit in a randomized controlled trial.[88] Single-arm studies of radical resection of recurrent malignant gliomas followed by permanent low-dose brachytherapy have shown modest efficacy.[91,92] GliaSite, another method for delivering temporary brachytherapy, has also been investigated. In this method, an inflatable balloon catheter is placed in the resection cavity at craniotomy for a recurrent malignant glioma.[93] An aqueous solution of organically bound ^{125}I is delivered to the balloon via a subcutaneous port 1 to 2 weeks after craniotomy and removed after 3 to 6 days. Gliasite has been safe and relatively promising in single-arm studies.[93–95] These results remain to be evaluated, however, in randomized studies.

Chemotherapy with Biodegradable Wafers

Several strategies have been used to deliver chemotherapeutic agents surgically to patients with malignant gliomas. Initial efforts focused on direct injection into tumor or surrounding parenchyma had limited efficacy but relatively high toxicity.[96] As an alternative to bolus injection, Brem and colleagues[97] developed methods to line malignant glioma resection cavities with biodegradable wafers impregnated with chemotherapeutic agents. In randomized controlled trials, recurrent malignant glioma patients receiving carmustine (BCNU)-impregnated polymer wafers had modest but significantly prolonged median survival compared with patients who underwent simple resection (31 weeks vs 23 weeks).[96–98] In the largest study, a statistical survival benefit persisted for up to 3 years.[99] In a recent institutional review, 1013 patients undergoing craniotomy for malignant astrocytomas over a 10-year period at Johns Hopkins Hospital were reviewed. Perioperative morbidity (within 3 months) and overall survival were assessed. Of 1013 patients who had craniotomies for malignant astrocytoma, 288 (28%) received Gliadel wafers (250 patients had GBM and 38 patients had AA/anaplastic oligodendroglioma [AA/AO]). Patients receiving Gliadel were older and more frequently underwent gross total resection (75% vs 36%). The patients in Gliadel versus non-Gliadel cohorts had similar perioperative morbidity. For patients receiving Gliadel for GBM, median survival was 13.5 months after primary resection (20% alive at 2 years) and 11.3 months after revision resection (13% alive at 2 years). For patients receiving Gliadel for AA/AO, median survival was 57 months after primary resection (66% alive at 2 years) and 23.6 months after revision resection (47% alive at 2 years).[100]

Convection-Enhanced Delivery

There remains concern as to whether or not chemotherapy-impregnated wafers are the most effective way to deliver therapeutic agents locally to patients with malignant gliomas at surgery. Just like bolus injection, chemotherapy wafers rely on diffusion to carry their agents into the surrounding brain parenchyma. Concerns have been raised that delivery via chemotherapy wafers may be too limited. As an alternative, Oldfield and colleagues[101,102] at the National Institutes of Health pioneered an approach, termed, *convection-enhanced delivery (CED)*. Between 1 and 3 small-diameter sialastic tubes are placed stereotactically in the tumor itself or in brain parenchyma surrounding a resection cavity and tunneled subcutaneously through the scalp. Therapeutic agents are then delivered via slow constant infusion (eg, 0.2 mL/h) through these catheters over 3 to 5 days postoperatively. The pressure from the slow infusion sets up a local convection current within the brain from the catheter tip (convection-enhanced) that results in a large volume of distribution for the agent in question. In ideal circumstances, an entire lobe can be perfused from a single catheter.

Most CED clinical trials to date have focused on small fusion proteins that have linked an intracellular toxin (eg, pseudomonas exotoxin or diphtheria toxin) to a ligand for surface receptors that are overexpressed on malignant glioma cells (eg, interleukin-13 or transferrin). Promising results from several phase I and II studies have been reported in newly diagnosed and recurrent malignant gliomas.[103,104] These therapies have potential for local inflammatory reactions that can be followed on post-treatment MR imaging scans and occasionally require treatment.[105] Two large multicenter randomized controlled trials have been completed in patients with recurrent glioblastomas (PRECISE and TransMID). These trials demonstrated that CED of these agents was safe and well tolerated. Unfortunately, they did not show any survival benefit. To date, these results have only been reported as press releases. Experimental efforts are ongoing to track and improve delivery by CED[106] and to expand the types of agents that can be delivered using this approach.[107]

Oncolytic Viral Vectors and Suicide Gene Therapy

Oncolytic virus therapy is a novel treatment option for GBM patients. These viruses are naturally occurring or genetically engineered viruses with a predilection to infect and kill tumor cells while leaving normal cells unharmed. They are derived from a variety of viruses, including herpes simplex virus (HSV-1), adenovirus, reovirus, measles, and Newcastle disease virus. The mechanisms underlying their relative tumor specificity are not always clear. Although work is ongoing to develop oncolytic viruses that can be systemically delivered, clinical trials so far in malignant gliomas have been limited to viruses that are delivered locally at surgery.[108–110] Oncolytic measles virus strains derived from the Edmonston vaccine lineage serve as a good example of the types viruses used in this manner. They have been effective in preclinical studies when delivered to intracranial tumors.[111,112] This strain was engineered to express the marker peptide measles virus–carcinoembryonic antigen (MV-CEA) and MV-CEA levels can serve as a correlate of viral gene expression. In support of a phase I clinical trial of intratumoral and resection cavity administration of MV-CEA to patients with recurrent gliomas, safety was demonstrated in rhesus macaques. The investigators found that more than 36 months from study initiation there had been no clinical or biochemical evidence of toxicity, including lack of neurologic symptoms, fever, or other systemic symptoms and lack of immunosuppression.[113] This approach is currently in phase I clinical trials.

Finally, Ram and colleagues[114] have evaluated the use of sitimagene ceradenovec (Cerepro) and ganciclovir gene therapy in the treatment of primary high-grade gliomas. This differs from a true oncolytic virus approach in that the virus has no inherent anticancer properties. Instead, a genetically engineered adenovirus delivers a suicide gene (HSV thymidine kinase) that kills tumor cells only when they are exposed to ganciclovir. The primary outcome measures for this randomized controlled trial are time from surgery to reintervention or death. Although data analyses are not complete, preliminary results suggest that patients in the Cerepro arm have a statistically significant improvement in outcome. Further data will be reported as they become available.[114]

SUMMARY

Brain tumor surgery, specifically glioma surgery, spans a broad range of pathologies and techniques. There is a continued need to improve the therapies available for treating these devastating tumors. As reviewed in this article, many clinical studies have examined new surgical techniques to perform and guide brain tumor biopsy and resection, the value of cytoreductive surgery, and the potential to introduce novel therapeutic agents locally at surgery. These studies have expanded the breadth of knowledge regarding optimal surgical approaches and have opened the door to new technologies that will hopefully have an impact on survival for patients with gliomas in the future.

REFERENCES

1. Davis FG, Kupelian V, Freels S, et al. Prevalence estimates for primary brain tumors in the United States by behavior and major histology groups. Neuro Oncol 2001;3(3):152–8.
2. Wrensch M, Minn Y, Chew T, et al. Epidemiology of primary brain tumors: current concepts and review of the literature. Neuro Oncol 2002;4(4):278–99.
3. Bernstein M, Parent AG. Complications of CT-guided stereotactic biopsy of intra-axial brain lesions. J Neurosurg 1994;81(2):165–8.
4. Kongkham PN, Knifed E, Tamber MS, et al. Complications in 622 cases of frame-based stereotactic biopsy, a decreasing procedure. Can J Neurol Sci 2008;35(1):79–84.
5. McGirt MJ, Woodworth GF, Coon AL, et al. Independent predictors of morbidity after image-guided stereotactic brain biopsy: a risk assessment of 270 cases. J Neurosurg 2005;102(5): 897–901.
6. Owen CM, Linskey ME. Frame-based stereotaxy in a frameless era: current capabilities, relative role, and the positive- and negative predictive values of blood through the needle. J Neurooncol 2009; 93(1):139–49.
7. Jackson RJ, Fuller GN, Abi-Said D, et al. Limitations of stereotactic biopsy in the initial management of gliomas. Neuro Oncol 2001;3(3):193–200.
8. Woodworth GF, McGirt MJ, Samdani A, et al. Frameless image-guided stereotactic brain biopsy procedure: diagnostic yield, surgical morbidity, and comparison with the frame-based technique. J Neurosurg 2006;104(2):233–7.
9. Air EL, Leach JL, Warnick RE, et al. Comparing the risks of frameless stereotactic biopsy in eloquent and noneloquent regions of the brain: a retrospective review of 284 cases. J Neurosurg 2009;111(4): 820–4.

10. Smith JS, Quinones-Hinojosa A, Barbaro NM, et al. Frame-based stereotactic biopsy remains an important diagnostic tool with distinct advantages over frameless stereotactic biopsy. J Neurooncol 2005;73(2):173–9.

11. Quinones-Hinojosa A, Ware ML, Sanai N, et al. Assessment of image guided accuracy in a skull model: comparison of frameless stereotaxy techniques vs. frame-based localization. J Neurooncol 2006;76(1):65–70.

12. Kreth FW, Warnke PC, Ostertag CB. Progress in malignant glioma. J Neurosurg 2004;100:1132–3.

13. Brown PD, Maurer MJ, Rummans TA, et al. A prospective study of quality of life in adults with newly diagnosed high-grade gliomas: the impact of the extent of resection on quality of life and survival. Neurosurgery 2005;57(3):495–504 [discussion: 495–504].

14. Buckner JC, Schomberg PJ, McGinnis WL, et al. A phase III study of radiation therapy plus carmustine with or without recombinant interferon-alpha in the treatment of patients with newly diagnosed high-grade glioma. Cancer 2001;92(2):420–33.

15. Keles GE, Anderson B, Berger MS. The effect of extent of resection on time to tumor progression and survival in patients with glioblastoma multiforme of the cerebral hemisphere. Surg Neurol 1999;52(4):371–9.

16. Kiwit JC, Floeth FW, Bock WJ. Survival in malignant glioma: analysis of prognostic factors with special regard to cytoreductive surgery. Zentralbl Neurochir 1996;57(2):76–88.

17. Lacroix M, Abi-Said D, Fourney DR, et al. A multivariate analysis of 416 patients with glioblastoma multiforme: prognosis, extent of resection, and survival. J Neurosurg 2001;95(2):190–8.

18. Lamborn K, Chang S, Prados M. Prognostic factors for survival of patients with glioblastoma: recursive partitioning analysis. Neuro Oncol 2004;6:227–35.

19. Laws ER, Parney IF, Huang W, et al. Survival following surgery and prognostic factors for recently diagnosed malignant glioma: data from the Glioma Outcomes Project. J Neurosurg 2003; 99(3):467–73.

20. Mohan DS, Suh JH, Phan JL, et al. Outcome in elderly patients undergoing definitive surgery and radiation therapy for supratentorial glioblastoma multiforme at a tertiary care institution. Int J Radiat Oncol Biol Phys 1998;42(5):981–7.

21. Nitta T, Sato K. Prognostic implications of the extent of surgical resection in patients with intracranial malignant gliomas. Cancer 1995;75:2727–31.

22. Stummer W, Pichlmeier U, Meinel T, et al. Fluorescence-guided surgery with 5-aminolevulinic acid for resection of malignant glioma: a randomised controlled multicentre phase III trial. Lancet Oncol 2006;7(5):392–401.

23. Nomiya T, Nemoto K, Kumabe T, et al. Prognostic significance of surgery and radiation therapy in cases of anaplastic astrocytoma: retrospective analysis of 170 cases. J Neurosurg 2007;106(4): 575–81.

24. Quigley MR, Flores N, Maroon JC, et al. Value of surgical intervention in the treatment of glioma. Stereotact Funct Neurosurg 1995;65(1–4):171–5.

25. Slotman BJ, Kralendonk JH, van Alphen HA, et al. Hypofractionated radiation therapy in patients with glioblastoma multiforme: results of treatment and impact of prognostic factors. Int J Radiat Oncol Biol Phys 1996;34(4):895–8.

26. Stark AM, Nabavi A, Mehdorn HM, et al. Glioblastoma multiforme-report of 267 cases treated at a single institution. Surg Neurol 2005;63(2):162–9 [discussion: 169].

27. Albert FK, Forsting M, Sartor K, et al. Early postoperative magnetic resonance imaging after resection of malignant glioma: objective evaluation of residual tumor and its influence on regrowth and prognosis. Neurosurgery 1994;34(1):45–60 [discussion: 1].

28. Ammirati M, Vick N, Liao YL, et al. Effect of the extent of surgical resection on survival and quality of life in patients with supratentorial glioblastomas and anaplastic astrocytomas. Neurosurgery 1987; 21(2):201–6.

29. Devaux BC, O'Fallon JR, Kelly PJ. Resection, biopsy, and survival in malignant glial neoplasms. A retrospective study of clinical parameters, therapy, and outcome. J Neurosurg 1993;78(5): 767–75.

30. Jeremic B, Grujicic D, Antunovic V, et al. Hyperfractionated radiation therapy followed by multiagent chemotherapy in patients with malignant glioma: a phase II study. Int J Radiat Oncol Biol Phys 1994;30:1179–85.

31. Kelly PJ, Hunt C. The limited value of cytoreductive surgery in elderly patients with malignant gliomas. Neurosurgery 1994;34(1):62–6 [discussion: 66–7].

32. Ushio Y, Kochi M, Hamada J, et al. Effect of surgical removal on survival and quality of life in patients with supratentorial glioblastoma. Neurol Med Chir (Tokyo) 2005;45(9):454–60 [discussion: 460–1].

33. Vuorinen V, Hinkka S, Farkkila M, et al. Debulking or biopsy of malignant glioma in elderly people - a randomised study. Acta Neurochir (Wien) 2003; 145(1):5–10.

34. Shibamoto Y, Yamashita J, Takahashi M, et al. Supratentorial malignant glioma: an analysis of radiation therapy in 178 cases. Radiother Oncol 1990;18(1):9–17.

35. Simpson JR, Horton J, Scott C, et al. Influence of location and extent of surgical resection on survival of patients with glioblastoma multiforme: results of three consecutive Radiation Therapy Oncology

Group (RTOG) clinical trials. Int J Radiat Oncol Biol Phys 1993;26(2):239–44.

36. Vecht CJ, Avezaat CJ, van Putten WL, et al. The influence of the extent of surgery on the neurological function and survival in malignant glioma. A retrospective analysis in 243 patients. J Neurol Neurosurg Psychiatry 1990;53(6):466–71.

37. Winger MJ, Macdonald DR, Cairncross JG. Supratentorial anaplastic gliomas in adults. The prognostic importance of extent of resection and prior low-grade glioma. J Neurosurg 1989;71(4):487–93.

38. Shinoda J, Sakai N, Murase S, et al. Selection of eligible patients with supratentorial glioblastoma multiforme for gross total resection. J Neurooncol 2001;52(2):161–71.

39. Keles GE, Chang EF, Lamborn KR, et al. Volumetric extent of resection and residual contrast enhancement on initial surgery as predictors of outcome in adult patients with hemispheric anaplastic astrocytoma. J Neurosurg 2006;105(1):34–40.

40. Pope WB, Sayre J, Perlina A, et al. MR imaging correlates of survival in patients with high-grade gliomas. AJNR Am J Neuroradiol 2005;26(10): 2466–74.

41. Schmidt M, Berger M, Lamborn K, et al. Repeated operations for infiltrative low-grade gliomas without intervening therapy. J Neurosurg 2003; 98:1165–9.

42. Frappaz D, Chinot O, Bataillard A, et al. Summary version of the standards, options and recommendations for the management of adult patients with intracranial glioma (2002). Br J Cancer 2003; 89(Suppl 1):S73–83.

43. Team L-GGG. Practice parameters in adults with suspected or known supratentorial nonoptic pathway low-grade glioma. Neurosurg Focus 1998;4:e10.

44. Keles G, Lamborn K, Berger M. Low-grade hemispheric gliomas in adults: a critical review of extent of resection as a factor influencing outcome. J Neurosurg 2001;95:735–45.

45. Claus E, Horlacher A, Hsu L, et al. Survival rates in patients with low-grade glioma after intraoperative magnetic resonance image guidance. Cancer 2005;103:1227–33.

46. Johannesen T, Langmark F, Lote K. Progress in long-term survival in adult patients with supratentorial low-grade gliomas: a population-based study of 993 patients in whom tumors were diagnosed between 1970 and 1993. J Neurosurg 2003;99: 854–62.

47. Leighton C, Fisher B, Bauman G, et al. Supratentorial low-grade glioma in adults: an analysis of prognostic factors and timing of radiation. J Clin Oncol 1997;15(4):1294–301.

48. Nakamura M, Konishi N, Tsunoda S, et al. Analysis of prognostic and survival factors related to treatment of low-grade astrocytomas in adults. Oncology 2000;58(2):108–16.

49. Philippon JH, Clemenceau SH, Fauchon FH, et al. Supratentorial low-grade astrocytomas in adults. Neurosurgery 1993;32(4):554–9.

50. Rajan B, Pickuth D, Ashley S, et al. The management of histologically unverified presumed cerebral gliomas with radiotherapy. Int J Radiat Oncol Biol Phys 1994;28(2):405–13.

51. Shaw E, Arusell R, Scheithauer B, et al. Prospective randomized trial of low- versus high-dose radiation therapy in adults with supratentorial low-grade glioma: initial report of a North Central Cancer Treatment Group/Radiation Therapy Oncology Group/Eastern Cooperative Oncology Group study. J Clin Oncol 2002; 20(9):2267–76.

52. van Veelen M, Avezaat C, Kros J, et al. Supratentorial low grade astrocytoma: prognostic factors, dedifferentiation, and the issue of early versus late surgery. J Neurol Neurosurg Psychiatry 1998; 64:581–7.

53. Yeh SA, Ho JT, Lui CC, et al. Treatment outcomes and prognostic factors in patients with supratentorial low-grade gliomas. Br J Radiol 2005;78(927): 230–5.

54. Smith JS, Chang EF, Lamborn KR, et al. Role of extent of resection in the long-term outcome of low-grade hemispheric gliomas. J Clin Oncol 2008;26(8):1338–45.

55. Shaw EG, Berkey B, Coons SW, et al. Recurrence following neurosurgeon-determined gross-total resection of adult supratentorial low-grade-glioma: results of a prospective clinical trial. J Neurosurg 2008;109(5):835–41.

56. Yeh DD, Warnick RE, Ernst RJ. Management strategy for adult patients with dorsal midbrain gliomas. Neurosurgery 2002;50(4):735–8 [discussion: 738–40].

57. Chang SM, Nelson S, Vandenberg S, et al. Integration of preoperative anatomic and metabolic physiologic imaging of newly diagnosed glioma. J Neurooncol 2009;92(3):401–15.

58. Dowling C, Bollen AW, Noworolski SM, et al. Preoperative proton MR spectroscopic imaging of brain tumors: correlation with histopathologic analysis of resection specimens. AJNR Am J Neuroradiol 2001;22(4):604–12.

59. Lupo JM, Cha S, Chang SM, et al. Dynamic susceptibility-weighted perfusion imaging of high-grade gliomas: characterization of spatial heterogeneity. AJNR Am J Neuroradiol 2005;26(6): 1446–54.

60. Kwong K, Belliveau J, Chesler D, et al. Dynamic magnetic resonance imaging of human brain activity during primary sensory stimulation. Proc Natl Acad Sci U S A 1992;89:5675–9.

61. Basser P, Jones D. Diffusion-tensor MRI: theory, experimental design and data analysis - a technical review. NMR Biomed 2002;15:456–67.

62. Binder J, Rao S, Hammeke T, et al. Lateralized human brain language systems demonstrated by task subtraction functional magnetic resonance imaging. Arch Neurol 1995;52:593–601.

63. Bittar R, Olivier A, Sadikot A, et al. Presurgical motor and somatosensory cortex mapping with functional magnetic resonance imaging and positron emission tomography. J Neurosurg 1999;91:915–21.

64. Nimsky C, Ganslandt O, Fahlbusch R. Comparing 0.2 tesla with 1.5 tesla intraoperative magnetic resonance imaging analysis of setup, workflow, and efficiency. Acad Radiol 2005;12(9):1065–79.

65. Berman J, Berger M, Mukherjee P, et al. Diffusion-tensor imaging-guided tracking of fibers of the pyramidal tract combined with intraoperative cortical stimulation mapping in patients with gliomas. J Neurosurg 2004;101:66–72.

66. Roberts T, Disbrow E, Roberts H, et al. Quantification and reproducibility of tracking cortical extent of activation by use of functional MR imaging and magnetoencephalography. AJNR Am J Neuroradiol 2000;21:1377–87.

67. Nimsky C, Ganslandt O, Hastreiter P, et al. Preoperative and intraoperative diffusion tensor imaging-based fiber tracking in glioma surgery. Neurosurgery 2007;61(Suppl 1):178–85 [discussion: 86].

68. Nagarajan S, Kirsch H, Lin P, et al. Preoperative localization of hand motor cortex by adaptive spatial filtering of magnetoencephalography data. J Neurosurg 2008;109(2):228–37.

69. Gaetz W, Cheyne D, Rutka JT, et al. Presurgical localization of primary motor cortex in pediatric patients with brain lesions by the use of spatially filtered magnetoencephalography. Neurosurgery 2009;64(Suppl 3):177–85 [discussion: 186].

70. Berger MS, Hadjipanayis CG. Surgery of intrinsic cerebral tumors. Neurosurgery 2007;61(Suppl 1):279–304 [discussion: 305].

71. Litofsky NS, Bauer AM, Kasper RS, et al. Image-guided resection of high-grade glioma: patient selection factors and outcome. Neurosurg Focus 2006;20(4):E16.

72. Keles G, Lamborn K, Berger M. Coregistration accuracy and detection of brain shift using intraoperative sononavigation during resection of hemispheric tumors. Neurosurgery 2003;53:556–62.

73. Ram Z, Hadani M. Intraoperative imaging—MRI. Acta Neurochir Suppl 2003;88:1–4.

74. Benveniste R, Germano IM. Evaluation of factors predicting accurate resection of high-grade gliomas by using frameless image-guided stereotactic guidance. Neurosurg Focus 2003;14(2):e5.

75. Nimsky C, Ganslandt O, Tomandl B, et al. Low-field magnetic resonance imaging for intraoperative use in neurosurgery: a 5-year experience. Eur Radiol 2002;12(11):2690–703.

76. Senft C, Seifert V, Hermann E, et al. Usefulness of intraoperative ultra low-field magnetic resonance imaging in glioma surgery. Neurosurgery 2008;63(4 Suppl 2):257–66 [discussion: 266–7].

77. Schneider JP, Trantakis C, Rubach M, et al. Intraoperative MRI to guide the resection of primary supratentorial glioblastoma multiforme—a quantitative radiological analysis. Neuroradiology 2005;47(7):489–500.

78. Kaibara T, Saunders JK, Sutherland GR. Advances in mobile intraoperative magnetic resonance imaging. Neurosurgery 2000;47(1):131–7 [discussion: 137–8].

79. Hatiboglu MA, Weinberg JS, Suki D, et al. Impact of intraoperative high-field magnetic resonance imaging guidance on glioma surgery: a prospective volumetric analysis. Neurosurgery 2009;64(6):1073–81 [discussion: 1081].

80. Bergsneider M, Sehati N, Villablanca P, et al. Mahaley Clinical Research Award: extent of glioma resection using low-field (0.2 T) versus high-field (1.5 T) intraoperative MRI and image-guided frameless neuronavigation. Clin Neurosurg 2005;52:389–99.

81. Penfield W, Boldrey E. Somatic motor and sensory representation in the cerebral cortex of man as studied by electrical stimulation. Brain 1937;60:389–443.

82. Berger M, Cohen W, Ojemann G. Correlation of motor cortex brain mapping data with magnetic resonance imaging. J Neurosurg 1990;72:383–7.

83. Ojemann G, Ojemann J, Lettich E, et al. Cortical language localization in left, dominant hemisphere. An electrical stimulation mapping investigation in 117 patients. J Neurosurg 1989;71(3):316–26.

84. Skirboll S, Ojemann G, Berger M, et al. Functional cortex and subcortical white matter located within gliomas. Neurosurgery 1996;38:678–84.

85. Keles G, Lundin D, Lamborn K, et al. Intraoperative subcortical stimulation mapping for hemispherical perirolandic gliomas located within or adjacent to the descending motor pathways: evaluation of morbidity and assessment of functional outcome in 294 patients. J Neurosurg 2004;100:369–75.

86. Sanai N, Mirzadeh Z, Berger MS. Functional outcome after language mapping for glioma resection. N Engl J Med 2008;358(1):18–27.

87. Stummer W, Novotny A, Stepp H, et al. Fluorescence-guided resection of glioblastoma multiforme by using 5-aminolevulinic acid-induced porphyrins: a prospective study in 52 consecutive patients. J Neurosurg 2000;93(6):1003–13.

88. Stummer W, Reulen HJ, Meinel T, et al. Extent of resection and survival in glioblastoma multiforme: identification of and adjustment for bias. Neurosurgery 2008;62(3):564–76 [discussion: 576].

89. McDermott M, Berger M, Kunwar S, et al. Stereotactic radiosurgery and interstitial brachytherapy for glial neoplasms. J Neurooncol 2004;69:83–100.

90. Laperriere NJ, Leung PM, McKenzie S, et al. Randomized study of brachytherapy in the initial management of patients with malignant astrocytoma. Int J Radiat Oncol Biol Phys 1998;41(5): 1005–11.

91. Larson D, Suplica J, Chang S, et al. Permanent iodine 125 brachytherapy in patients with progressive or recurrent glioblastoma multiforme. Neuro Oncol 2004;6:119–26.

92. Patel S, Breneman J, Warnick R, et al. Permanent iodine-125 interstitial implants for the treatment of recurrent glioblastoma multiforme. Neurosurgery 2000;46:1123–8.

93. Tatter S, Shaw E, Rosenblum M, et al. An inflatable balloon catheter and liquid 125I radiation source (GliaSite Radiation Therapy System) for treatment of recurrent malignant glioma: multicenter safety and feasibility trial. J Neurosurg 2003;99:297–303.

94. Chan TA, Weingart JD, Parisi M, et al. Treatment of recurrent glioblastoma multiforme with GliaSite brachytherapy. Int J Radiat Oncol Biol Phys 2005; 62(4):1133–9.

95. Gabayan AJ, Green SB, Sanan A, et al. GliaSite brachytherapy for treatment of recurrent malignant gliomas: a retrospective multi-institutional analysis. Neurosurgery 2006;58(4):701–9 [discussion: 9].

96. Walter KA, Tamargo RJ, Olivi A, et al. Intratumoral chemotherapy. Neurosurgery 1995;37(6):1128–45.

97. Brem H, Mahaley MS Jr, Vick NA, et al. Interstitial chemotherapy with drug polymer implants for the treatment of recurrent gliomas. J Neurosurg 1991; 74(3):441–6.

98. Westphal M, Hilt D, Bortey E, et al. A phase 3 trial of local chemotherapy with biodegradable carmustine (BCNU) wafers (Gliadel wafers) in patients with primary malignant glioma. Neuro Oncol 2003;5:79–88.

99. Westphal M, Ram Z, Riddle V, et al. Gliadel wafer in initial surgery for malignant glioma: long-term follow-up of a multicenter controlled trial. Acta Neurochir (Wien) 2006;148:269–75.

100. Attenello FJ, Mukherjee D, Datoo G, et al. Use of Gliadel (BCNU) wafer in the surgical treatment of malignant glioma: a 10-year institutional experience. Ann Surg Oncol 2008;15(10):2887–93.

101. Bobo RH, Laske DW, Akbasak A, et al. Convection-enhanced delivery of macromolecules in the brain. Proc Natl Acad Sci U S A 1994;91(6):2076–80.

102. Lieberman DM, Laske DW, Morrison PF, et al. Convection-enhanced distribution of large molecules in gray matter during interstitial drug infusion. J Neurosurg 1995;82(6):1021–9.

103. Vogelbaum MA, Sampson JH, Kunwar S, et al. Convection-enhanced delivery of cintredekin besudotox (Interleukin-13-Pe38qqr) followed by radiation therapy with and without temozolomide in newly diagnosed malignant gliomas: phase 1 study of final safety results. Neurosurgery 2007;61(5): 1031–7.

104. Kunwar S, Prados MD, Chang SM, et al. Direct intracerebral delivery of cintredekin besudotox (IL13-PE38QQR) in recurrent malignant glioma: a report by the Cintredekin Besudotox Intraparenchymal Study Group. J Clin Oncol 2007;25(7):837–44.

105. Parney IF, Kunwar S, McDermott M, et al. Neuroradiographic changes following convection-enhanced delivery of the recombinant cytotoxin interleukin 13-PE38QQR for recurrent malignant glioma. J Neurosurg 2005;102(2):267–75.

106. Sampson J, Brady M, Petry N, et al. Intracerebral infusate distribution by convection-enhanced delivery in humans with malignant gliomas: descriptive effects of target anatomy and catheter positioning. Neurosurgery 2007;60(2 Suppl 1): ONS89–98.

107. Kaiser MG, Parsa AT, Fine RL, et al. Tissue distribution and antitumor activity of topotecan delivered by intracerebral clysis in a rat glioma model. Neurosurgery 2000;47(6):1391–8 [discussion: 1398–9].

108. Forsyth P, Roldan G, George D, et al. A phase I trial of intratumoral administration of reovirus in patients with histologically confirmed recurrent malignant gliomas. Mol Ther 2008;16(3):627–32.

109. Chiocca EA, Abbed KM, Tatter S, et al. A phase I open-label, dose-escalation, multi-institutional trial of injection with an E1B-Attenuated adenovirus, ONYX-015, into the peritumoral region of recurrent malignant gliomas, in the adjuvant setting. Mol Ther 2004;10(5):958–66.

110. Liu TC, Galanis E, Kirn D. Clinical trial results with oncolytic virotherapy: a century of promise, a decade of progress. Nat Clin Pract 2007;4(2): 101–17.

111. Liu C, Sarkaria JN, Petell CA, et al. Combination of measles virus virotherapy and radiation therapy has synergistic activity in the treatment of glioblastoma multiforme. Clin Cancer Res 2007;13(23): 7155–65.

112. Phuong LK, Allen C, Peng KW, et al. Use of a vaccine strain of measles virus genetically engineered to produce carcinoembryonic antigen as a novel therapeutic agent against glioblastoma multiforme. Cancer Res 2003;63(10):2462–9.

113. Myers R, Harvey M, Kaufmann TJ, et al. Toxicology study of repeat intracerebral administration of a measles virus derivative producing carcinoembryonic antigen in rhesus macaques

in support of a phase I/II clinical trial for patients with recurrent gliomas. Hum Gene Ther 2008; 19(7):690–8.

114. Ram Z, Westphal M, Warnke P, et al. Treatment of primary high-grade glioma with sitimagene ceradenovec (Cerepro) and ganciclovir gene medicine: update of phase III results. Abstract presentation at the 2009 Joint Meeting of the Society for Neuro-Oncology and the AANS/CNS Section on Tumors.

Novel Medical Therapeutics in Glioblastomas, Including Targeted Molecular Therapies, Current and Future Clinical Trials

Eudocia C. Quant, MD, Patrick Y. Wen, MD*

KEYWORDS

- Targeted therapy • Glioblastoma
- Tyrosine kinase inhibitors • Clinical trials

Glioblastoma multiforme (GBM) is the most common type of malignant primary brain tumor in adults. More than 10,000 new cases are diagnosed every year in the United States.[1] Despite surgery, radiation, and chemotherapy, median survival is only 12 to 18 months.[2] The demand for better therapies is high. In recent years, there has been significant progress in understanding the molecular pathways involved gliomagenesis and disease progression.[3–6] Malignant transformation in gliomas is the result of sequential accumulation of genetic aberrations and deregulation of growth factor signaling pathways (**Fig. 1**).[7] Targeted therapies have been developed against these pathways.

GLIOBLASTOMA MULTIFORME

The incidence of GBM has increased over the past two decades primarily as a result of improved imaging.[7] The diagnostic imaging modality of choice is magnetic resonance imaging (MRI) with gadolinium administration, which typically demonstrates an irregular ring-enhancing lesion with central necrosis and surrounding vasogenic edema. Definitive diagnosis is based on histology. GBM is a highly cellular tumor marked by mitoses, vascular proliferation, and pseudopallisading necrosis.[8]

Glioblastomas can be separated into primary and secondary GBMs based on biologic and genetic differences.[6,7] Primary GBMs occur typically in older patients and are characterized by epidermal growth factor receptor (EGFR) amplification and mutations, loss of heterozygosity of chromosome 10q, deletion of phosphatase and tensin homologue on chromosome 10 (PTEN), and p16 deletion. Secondary GBMs arise from lower grade gliomas over several years; these are much less common than primary GBMs and usually occur in younger patients. Secondary GBMs are characterized by p53 mutations, overexpression of platelet-derived growth factor receptor (PDGFR), abnormalities in the p16 and retinoblastoma pathways, loss of heterozygosity of chromosome 10q, and mutations of the isocitrate dehydrogenase 1 and 2 genes.[6] Despite their genetic differences, primary and secondary GBMs

Division of Cancer Neurology, Department of Neurology, Brigham and Women's Hospital and Center for Neuro-Oncology, Dana-Farber/Brigham and Women's Cancer Center, Harvard Medical School, 44 Binney Street, SW 430D, Boston, MA 02115, USA
* Corresponding author.
E-mail address: pwen@partners.org

Neuroimag Clin N Am 20 (2010) 425–448
doi:10.1016/j.nic.2010.04.007

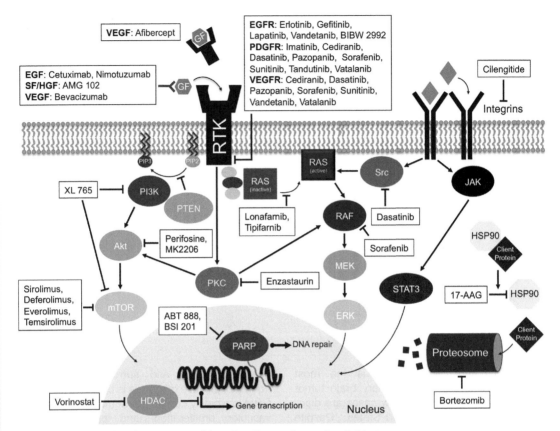

Fig. 1. Important molecular targets and key signaling pathways in glioblastoma.

are morphologically similar and likely share similar responses to conventional cytotoxic agents. On the other hand, these GBM subtypes may respond differently to targeted agents.

The standard of care for newly diagnosed GBM is based on results from a multicenter randomized trial.[2] Although the addition of temozolomide (TMZ) to radiation therapy (RT) significantly prolonged survival in this study, the benefit was modest (median overall survival 12.1 months for RT alone versus 14.6 months for RT combined with TMZ).[2] Most tumors eventually develop resistance to TMZ (median time to tumor progression is 6.9 months),[2] and there is no standard chemotherapy for recurrent or progressive GBM because of unfavorable outcomes with currently available cytotoxic therapies.

Knowledge of GBM biology has revealed new potential therapeutic targets. Several novel agents against these molecular targets are now in clinical trials (**Table 1**). Targeted therapy may provide greater specificity toward tumor cells with potentially less toxicity than conventional chemotherapy. The success of these agents in other systemic cancers[9] demonstrates their potential in

tumors with well-defined molecular targets. Even though the complexity of the molecular abnormalities in GBMs and the redundancy of the signaling pathways make it unlikely that single agents will achieve great success, there has been significant interest in this approach.

CELLULAR SIGNAL TRANSDUCTION PATHWAY
Tyrosine Kinase Inhibitors

Tyrosine kinases are a group of protein kinases that are critical to many signal transduction pathways involved in cell proliferation, growth, survival, adhesion, motility, and differentiation.[10] This group includes receptor tyrosine kinases (RTKs), which are transmembrane proteins containing an extracellular binding domain that binds ligands and an intracellular kinase domain that activates intracellular signaling pathways.

Epidermal growth factor
The EGFR pathway is an attractive target because it is frequently dysregulated in GBMs through overexpression, amplification, or activating mutations.[11–13] EGFR dysregulation results in aberrant

Table 1
Selected targeted agents in clinical trials for glioblastoma

Target	Mechanism of Action	Molecular Agent	Other Targets
Growth factors and growth factor receptors			
EGFR	Reversible small-molecule inhibitor	Erlotinib (OSI-774, Tarceva)	
		Gefitinib (ZD1839, Iressa)	
		Lapatinib (GW-572016, Tykerb)	HER2
		Vandetanib (ZD-6474, Zactima)	VEGFR
	Irreversible small-molecule inhibitor	BIBW-2992	HER2
		PF-00299804	HER2, HER4
	Monoclonal antibody	Cetuximab (Erbitux)	
		Nimotuzumab (h-R3, TheraCIM, TheraLOC)	
		EMD 55 900	
		Iodine-125 labeled monoclonal antibody-425	
EGFRvIII	Peptide based vaccine	CDX-110	
	Monoclonal antibody	mAb 806	
SF/HGF	Monoclonal antibody	AMG-102	
PDGFR	Small-molecule inhibitor	Cediranib (AZD-2171, Recentin)	VEGFR, c-Kit
		Dasatinib (BMS-354825, Sprycel)	Src, Abl, VEGFR, Flt-3
		Imatinib mesylate (STI-571, Gleevec)	Bcr-Abl, c-Fms, c-Kit
		Pazopanib (GW-786034)	VEGFR, c-Kit
		Sorafenib (BAY-439006, Nexavar)	VEGFR, Raf, c-Kit
		Sunitinib (SU-11248, Sutent)	VEGFR, c-Kit, Flt-3
		Tandutinib (MLN-518)	Flt-3, c-Kit
		Vatalanib (PTK-787/AK-222584)	VEGFR, c-Kit, c-Fms
PDGFR-α	Monoclonal antibody	IMC-3G3	
Intracellular signaling			
Ras	Farnesyl transferase inhibitor	Lonafarnib (SCH-66336, Sarasar)	
		Tipifarnib (R115777, Zanestra)	
Raf	Small-molecule inhibitor	Sorafenib (BAY-439006, Nexavar)	VEGFR, PDGFR, Flt-3, c-Kit, FGFR
mTOR	Small-molecule inhibitor	Ridaforolimus (AP-23573)	
		Everolimus (RAD-001, Afinitor)	
		Sirolimus (Rapamycin, Rapamune)	
		Temsirolimus (CCI-779, Torisel)	
		XL-765	PI3K
PI3K	Small-molecule inhibitor	XL-765	mTOR
		XL147	
		BKM 120	
Akt	Alkylphospholipid	Perifosine (KRX-0401)	
	Small-molecule inhibitor	MK2206	
PKC	Small-molecule inhibitor	Enzastaurin (LY-317615)	
Tumor vasculature			
VEGF	Soluble decoy receptor	Afibercept (VEGF-Trap)	
	Monoclonal antibody	Bevacizumab (Avastin)	
VEGFR	Small-molecule inhibitor	Cediranib (AZD-2171, Recentin)	PDGFR, c-Kit
		Dasatinib (BMS-354825, Sprycel)	Src, Abl, PDGFR, Flt-3
		Pazopanib (GW-786034)	PDGFR, c-Kit
		Sorafenib (BAY-439006, Nexavar)	PDGFR, Raf, c-Kit
		Sunitinib (SU-11248, Sutent)	PDGFR, c-Kit, Flt-3
		Vandetanib (ZD-6474, Zactima)	EGFR
		Vatalanib (PTK-787/AK-222584)	PDGFR, c-Kit, c-Fms
		XL184	Met
		Foretinib	Met, PDGFR
	Adnectin	CT-332 (Angiocept)	
	Monoclonal antibody	IMC-1121B	

(continued on next page)

Table 1
(continued)

Target	Mechanism of Action	Molecular Agent	Other Targets
Met	Small-molecule inhibitor	XL184	VEGFR
Integrins	Small-molecule inhibitor	Cilengitide (EMD-121974) ATN-161	
Cytokines			
TGF-β	Antisense oligonucleotide	AP 12009	
Protein turnover			
	Proteasome inhibitor	Bortezomib (MLN-341, Velcade)	
Chromatin remodeling			
	HDAC inhibitor	Vorinostat (SAHA, Zolinza) Panobinostat (LBH589)	
Heat shock proteins			
	HSP90 inhibitor	Tanespimycin (17-AAG, KOS-953)	
DNA repair			
	PARP inhibitor	ABT-888 BSI-201	

Abbreviations: EGFR, epidermal growth factor receptor; FGFR, fibroblast growth factor receptor; HDAC, histone deacetylase; HER, human epidermal growth factor receptor; mTOR, mammalian target of rapamycin; PARP, poly(ADP-ribose) polymerase; PDGFR, platelet-derived growth factor receptor; PKC, protein kinase C; SF/HGF, scatter factor/hepatic growth factor; TGF-β, transforming growth factor β; VEGF, vascular endothelial growth factor; VEGFR, vascular endothelial growth factor receptor.

signaling which, in turn, is associated with increased proliferation, motility, and survival of tumor cells in vitro.[14–18] The most common EGFR mutation, found in 20% to 30% of GBMs, is EGFRvIII, which causes constitutive activation and phosphorylation of the receptor without ligand binding.[19–21] Several approaches exist for targeting EGFR including small-molecule tyrosine kinase inhibitors (TKIs), monoclonal antibodies (mAbs), and vaccines.

The most extensively studied TKIs in GBM are erlotinib and gefitinib. Both are oral, low molecular weight, reversible inhibitors of tyrosine kinase activity associated with EGFR. When combined with RT in newly diagnosed GBM patients, the addition of these agents did not prolong 6-month progression-free survival (6M-PFS) or overall survival (OS) in multicenter trials as compared with standard therapy.[22,23] In several phase 2 clinical trials of recurrent high-grade gliomas, neither gefitinb[24–26] nor erlotinib[27–30] monotherapy demonstrated any significant survival benefit as compared with historical controls. Clinical activity was modest in the GBM subset, with radiographic responses (RR) ranging from 0% to 13% for gefitinib and 0% to 26% for erlotinib, and with 6M-PFS ranging from 9% to 13% for gefitinib and 0% to 26% for erlotinib. Small subgroups of patients had durable responses. Both TKIs were generally well tolerated with rash, diarrhea, and fatigue as the most common side effects. The combination of EGFR inhibitors with other therapies is discussed later in this article.

Lapatinib, which inhibits ErbB2/HER2 (human epidermal growth factor receptor 2) as well as EGFR, has also been evaluated in recurrent glioblastomas. This agent achieves therapeutic concentrations in gliomas[31] but has limited activity.[32,33]

Although subsets of GBM patients have sustained responses to reversible TKIs that target EGFR, the studies to date have been largely disappointing. Potential reasons for lack of response include poor blood-brain barrier penetration, insufficient local tumor concentrations, coactivation of multiple TKIs,[34] redundant signaling pathways, and resistance. Irreversible EGFR inhibitors, such as BIBW 2992 and PF-00299804, could have better efficacy in GBM than gefitinib or elotinib due to increased potency and in the case of PF-00299804, better brain concentration. This newer class of EGFR inhibitors has been shown to circumvent mechanisms of response to gefitinib or erlotinib in non–small cell lung cancer cells.[35–40]

Attempts to define subsets of erlotinib or gefitinib responders have also been met with limited success. The activating mutations found in EGFR in non–small cell lung cancer that increase response to EGFR inhibitors are not present in GBM.[41,42] Initial molecular studies suggested that gefitinib and erlotinib were more effective in tumors with EGFRvIII mutations and intact PTEN.[43] However, recent studies failed to validate these results.[23,30]

Monoclonal antibodies (mAb) as well as vaccines that target EGFR are currently under investigation in GBM. These therapies have been well tolerated in early clinical trials. Results from a phase 1/2 study combining nimotuzumab (a humanized anti-EGFR mAb) with radiotherapy in patients were favorable (**Table 2**).[44] Both nimo-tuzumab and cetuximab, a chimeric anti-EGFR human-mouse mAb, are now being studied in combination with radiation and temozolomide as upfront GBM therapies. Preliminary results from a phase 2 clinical trial suggest that the addition of CDX-110, a peptide based EGFRvIII vaccine, to standard therapy prolongs survival in patients with newly diagnosed GBM (see **Table 2**).[45] However, patients were required to have gross total resections as well as EGFRvIII positivity by immunohistochemistry in order to be eligible for this trial.

Scatter factor/hepatocyte growth factor

Scatter factor/hepatocyte growth factor (SF/HGF) and its tyrosine kinase receptor c-Met play a role in cell growth, cell motility, morphogenesis, and angiogenesis.[46] HGF and c-Met are overexpressed in gliomas, and expression levels correlate with grade and the degree of malignancy.[47–51] AMG-102 is a fully human monoclonal antibody that selectively targets SF/HGF. A phase 2 study of AMG-102 in recurrent GBM was recently completed but failed to produce any benefit.[52] It is unclear whether the lack of activity was related to the inability of AMG-102 to pass through the blood-tumor barrier or whether inhibiting HGF alone was insufficient. A recent study suggests that the combination of EGFR inhibitors and Met inhibitors may be more effective than either agent alone in PTEN-null GBM tumors.[53] Met TKIs such as XL184 are in clinical trial in GBM.[53]

Platelet-derived growth factor

Platelet-derived growth factors (PDGFs) are a pleiotropic family of peptides that signal through PDGFR to stimulate cellular functions including growth, proliferation, and differentiation.[54] PDGF and PDGFR are overexpressed in gliomas and are associated with more malignant tumors.[55–57] Blocking PDGF-mediated phosphorylation causes either apoptosis or growth inhibition in glioma cell lines.[58,59] PDGF-C also induces angiogenic activity via activation of PDGFR-α and -β

receptors[60] as well as upregulation of vascular endothelial growth factor (VEGF).[61,62]

Imatinib mesylate, an inhibitor of PDGFR-α, PDGFR-β, Bcr-Abl, c-Fms, and c-Kit tyrosine kinases, demonstrated activity in preclinical models of glioma.[63] However, in two multicenter phase 2 clinical trials, imatinib monotherapy was not associated with clinically useful activity in GBM, with RR of 3% to 13% and 6M-PFS of 3% to 16%.[64,65] Results were also disappointing in a multicenter phase 3 trial of imatinib plus hydroxy-urea (a ribonucleoside diphosphate reductase inhibitor) versus hydroxyurea monotherapy in progressive GBM.[66] Radiographic response rates by central review and 6M-PFS were similar in both arms. One explanation for the lack of efficacy is that imatinib is a substrate for the P-glycoprotein efflux pump, which limits its passage over an intact blood-brain barrier.[67] Two second-generation PDGFR inhibitors with improved central nervous system penetration, tandutinib and dasatinib, are in clinical trials for recurrent high-grade glioma, as is IMC-3G3, an antibody against PDGFR-α.

INTRACELLULAR SIGNALING KINASES
Serine-Threonine Kinases

The serine-threonine kinases are a family of enzymes that phosphorylate serine and threonine residues. Many of these kinases serve as interme-diates in important signaling pathways.

PI3K/Akt pathway inhibitors

Phosphatidylinositol 3-kinase/AKT (PI3K/Akt) is a signaling pathway important for cell growth and survival.[68] The pathway is activated by several RTKs, including EGFR and PDGFR, and is in-hibited by PTEN. Activation of the PI3K-Akt pathway is associated with poor prognosis in glioma patients and with more aggressive tumors.[69] In vivo studies suggest that PI3K inhibi-tors sensitize GBM cells to apoptosis.[70] Several PI3K and Akt inhibitors are in development or early clinical trials. XL765, an inhibitor of PI3K and mTOR, is currently in a phase 1 clinical trial in combination with temozolomide for patients with high-grade glioma. Akt inhibitors undergoing eval-uation in high-grade glioma include perifosine and MK2206.

PI3K/Akt signaling leads to downstream acti-vation of several targets including the mamma-lian target of rapamycin (mTOR). The mTOR inhibitor sirolimus (rapamycin) and its analogues temsirolimus, everolimus, and ridaforolimus are the most clinically advanced PI3K/Akt pathway inhibitors. Despite promising results from preclin-ical studies, temsirolimus monotherapy was not

Table 2
Selected clinical trials of combination therapy in newly diagnosed glioblastoma

Therapy	Trial Phase	Patient Population	Trial Number and Sponsor	Status
ABT-888, RT, TMZ	Multicenter phase 1/2 study	GBM	NCT00770471, ABTC	Ongoing
Aflibercept, RT, TMZ	Multicenter phase 1/2 study	High-grade glioma	NCT00650923, ABTC	Ongoing
Bevacizumab, irinotecan, RT vs bevacizumab, TMZ, RT	Multicenter randomized phase 2 study	GBM	NCT00817284, Rigshospitalet	Ongoing
Bevacizumab, RT, TMZ vs RT, TMZ	Multicenter randomized phase 3 study	GBM, gliosarcoma	NCT00884741, RTOG	Ongoing
Bevacizumab, RT, TMZ vs RT, TMZ	Multicenter randomized phase 3 study	GBM	NCT00943826 Roche	Ongoing
Bevacizumab, erlotinib, TMZ	Single-center phase 2 study	GBM with stable disease following concurrent RT and TMZ	NCT00525525, University of California at San Francisco	Ongoing
BSI-201, RT, TMZ	Multicenter Phase 1/2 study	High-grade glioma	NCT00687765, ABTC	Ongoing
Cediranib, RT, TMZ	Multicenter phase 1/2 study	GBM	NCT00662506, Massachusetts General Hospital	Ongoing
Cetuximab, RT, TMZ	Single-center phase 1/2 study	GBM	NCT00311857, University of Heidelberg	Ongoing
CDX-110, RT, TMZ	Multicenter phase 2 study	GBM with gross total resection and EGFRvIII positivity by IHC	NCT00458601, Pfizer	Preliminary results[45]: median OS 33.3 months, median PFS 16.6 months
Cilengitide, RT, TMZ vs RT, TMZ	Multicenter randomized phase 3 study	GBM with methylated MGMT	NCT00689221, EORTC	Ongoing
Cilengitide, RT, TMZ	Single-center phase 2 study	GBM with unmethylated MGMT	NCT00813943, Merck Serono	Ongoing
Cilengitide, RT, TMZ	Multicenter phase 1/2 study	GBM	NCT00085254, Merck Serono	Ongoing
CT-322, RT, TMZ	Multicenter phase 1 study	GBM	NCT00768911, Adnexus	Ongoing
Dasatinib, RT, TMZ	Mutlicenter NCCTG phase 1/2 study	GBM	NCT00869401, NCCTG	Not yet recruiting

Drug, therapy	Study type	Condition	Identifier, sponsor	Status/results
Enzastaurin, RT	Multicenter phase 2 study	GBM with unmethylated MGMT	NCT00509821, Eli Lilly and Company	Ongoing
Enzastaurin, RT, TMZ	Single-center phase 1/2 study	GBM, gliosarcoma	NCT00402116, Eli Lilly and Company, University of California at San Francisco	Ongoing
Erlotinib, RT, TMZ	Multicenter phase 1/2 study	GBM	NCT00039494, NCCTG	Results[23]: median OS 15.3 mo, median PFS 7.2 mo
Erlotinib, RT, TMZ	Single-center phase 2 study	GBM, gliosarcoma	NCT00187486, University of California at San Francisco	Results[181]: median OS 19.3 mo, median PFS 8.2 mo
Erlotinib, RT, TMZ	Single-center phase 2 study	GBM	NCT00274833, Case Comprehensive Cancer Center	Ongoing
Everolimus, RT, TMZ	Multicenter phase 1/2 study	GBM	NCT00553150, NCCTG	Ongoing
Everolimus, TMZ	Multicenter phase 1 study	GBM with stable disease following concurrent RT and TMZ	NCT00387400, National Cancer Institute of Canada	Ongoing
Gefitinib, RT	Multicenter phase 1/2 study	GBM	NCT00052208, RTOG	Preliminary results[22]: median OS 11.0 mo, median PFS 5.1 mo
Nimotuzumab, RT	Multicenter phase 1/2 study	High-grade glioma	National Center for Clinical Trials (Cuba)	Results[44]: median OS 17.47 mo for GBM subset, RR 31.3% for GBM subset
Nimotuzumab, RT, TMZ	Multicenter randomized phase 3 study	GBM	NCT00753246, Oncoscience AG	Ongoing
Sorafenib, RT, TMZ	Single-center phase 1/2 study in GBM	GBM, gliosarcoma	NCT00734526, MD Anderson Cancer Center	Ongoing
Sorafenib, TMZ following RT and TMZ	Multicenter phase 2 study	GBM	NCT00544817, SCRI Oncology Research Consortium	Ongoing
Temsirolimus, RT, TMZ	Multicenter phase 1 study	GBM	NCT00316849, NCCTG	Ongoing
Tipifarnib, RT	Multicenter phase 1/2 study	GBM	NCT00209989, Institut Claudius Regaud	Ongoing

(continued on next page)

Table 2
(continued)

Therapy	Trial Phase	Patient Population	Trial Number and Sponsor	Status
Tipifarnib (prior to RT)	Multicenter phase 2 study	GBM with residual enhancing disease	NCT00058097, NABTT CNS Consortium	Results[81] median OS 7.7 mo, RR 0, study stopped early due to progression of disease in 48%
Tipifarnib, RT, TMZ	Multicenter NABTC phase 1 study in GBM	GBM, Gliosarcoma	NCT00049387, NABTC	Ongoing
Vandetanib, RT, TMZ	Multicenter phase 1/2 study in GBM	GBM, gliosarcoma	NCT00441142, Dana Farber Cancer Institute	Ongoing
Vatalanib, RT, TMZ vs RT, TMZ	Multicenter randomized phase 1/2 study	GBM	NCT00128700, EORTC	Phase 1 study completed,[182] phase 2 study ongoing
Vatalanib, RT, TMZ	Multicenter phase 1 study	GBM on enzyme-inducing antiepiletics	NCT00385853, Massachusetts General Hospital	Ongoing
Vorinostat, RT, TMZ	Multicenter phase 1/2 study	GBM	NCT00731731, NCCTG and ABTC	Ongoing

Abbreviations: ABTC, Adult Brain Tumor Consortium; EORTC, European Organization for Research and Treatment of Cancer; IHC, immunohistochemistry; MGMT, O^6-methylguanine methyltransferase; NABTC, North American Brain Tumor Coalition; NABTT, New Approaches to Brain Tumor Therapy; NCCTG, North Central Cancer Treatment Group; OS, overall survival; PFS, progression-free survival; RR, radiographic response rate; RT, radiation therapy; RTOG, Radiation Therapy Oncology Group; SCRI, Sarah Cannon Research Institute; TMZ, temozolomide.

Data from National Institutes of Health. Available at: http://www.clinicaltrials.gov.

clinically active in recurrent GBM in two multi-center phase 2 clinical trials.[71,72] Radiographic response rates were 0% and 5% while 6M-PFS rates were 2% and 8%. One possible explanation for the lack of efficacy is that rapamycin inhibition of TOR complex 1 (TORC1) disrupts the negative feedback loop on the Akt pathway, which may lead paradoxically to Akt activation.[73–75] An Akt inhibitor, such as perifosine or MK2206, or a combined PI3K/mTOR inhibitor, such as XL765, may ultimately prove more favorable. Studies combining mTOR inhibitors with other targeted agents are discussed later in this article.

Ras-mitogen activated protein kinase pathway inhibitors

The mitogen-activated protein kinase (MAPK) pathway is involved in important signaling cascades that regulate normal cell proliferation, survival, and differentiation.[76] The pathway is triggered by several RTKs, including EGFR and vascular endothelial growth factor receptor (VEGFR), and results in downstream activation of Ras, a guanine nucleotide triphosphatase. Ras then transmits signals to MAPK, PI3K, and other signaling pathways.

Several posttranslational modifications of Ras are necessary for proper functioning. One of these modifications is the addition of a farnesyl group, which enables Ras to translocate from the cytoplasm to the cell membrane. Farnesyl transferase inhibitors (FTIs), such as tipifarnib and lonafarnib, are designed to block farnesylation and ultimately prevent proper functioning of Ras. These agents demonstrated activity in human glioma cell lines,[77–79] but results from clinical trials have been disappointing.[80,81] Both tipifarnib and lonafarnib are now being studied in combination with TMZ for high-grade gliomas.

The Raf serine/threonine kinases are the main downstream effectors of Ras in the MAPK pathway. Inhibiting at the level of Raf may be more efficacious because it is a key element situated at the convergence of several redundant signaling pathways.[82] Activating Raf mutations have been found in several malignancies, including GBM. Sorafenib is a potent inhibitor of Raf kinase but also inhibits proangiogenic RTKs including VEGFR-2, VGFRR-3, PDGFR-β, Flt-3, c-Kit, and fibroblast growth factor receptor 1. Several trials of sorafenib in high-grade glioma are underway.

Protein kinase C inhibitors

Protein kinase C (PKC) is a family of serine/threonine kinases that are involved in cell proliferation, differentiation, angiogenesis, and apoptosis. PKCs are activated by RTKs and G-protein–coupled receptors and help regulate several signaling pathways including PI3K/Akt and MAPK. Several PKC isoforms are overexpressed in glioma cell lines.[83,84] Enzastaurin is an oral serine/threonine kinase inhibitor that targets the PKC and Akt pathways. In a multi-center phase 2 open-label trial, patients with recurrent GBM were randomized to either enzastaurin or lomustine.[85] Unfortunately, enrollment was stopped after interim futility analysis due to a lack of difference in PFS between the 2 arms. Other studies of enzastaurin in combination with radiation and/or chemotherapeutic agents are in progress.[86]

MULTITARGETED INHIBITORS AND COMBINED THERAPIES

In an attempt to improve the effectiveness of targeted molecular therapy, there is growing interest in using multitargeted agents that inhibit several kinases (see **Table 1**) or combinations of targeted agents with other therapies (see **Table 2; Table 3**). For example, the EGFR inhibitor erlotinib has been studied in combination with mTOR inhibitors such as sirolimus[87] and temsirolimus.[88] Preliminary results from these erlotinib combination studies suggest only modest efficacy, and some combinations are poorly tolerated.[89–91] However, other combinations of agents may be better tolerated and several trials are underway. Because antiangiogenic agents can potentially have synergistic effects with RT, two randomized multicenter trials combining bevacizumab with radiation and temozolomide are underway. In addition, several multitargeted agents are in clinical trials for GBM including vandetanib (which targets EGFR and VEGFR), sunitinib (which targets VEGFR-2, PDGFR, c-Kit and Flt-3), and tandutinib (which targets c-Kit and Flt-3).

TUMOR VASCULATURE

Angiogenesis, the process of new blood vessel formation, is critical for the growth of many solid tumors including gliomas.[92,93] GBM cells produce various proangiogenic factors including VEGF, basic fibroblast growth factor (bFGF), PDGF, and SF/HGF. Integrins also play a role in angiogenesis regulation.[94]

Vascular Endothelial Growth Factor

The best characterized of the proangiogenic growth factors is the VEGF family. Members include VEGF-B, VEGF-C, VEGF-D, and placental

Table 3
Selected clinical trials of combination therapy in progressive or recurrent glioblastoma

Therapy	Trial Phase	Patient Population	Trial # and Sponsor	Status
ATN-161, Carboplatin	Single-center phase 1/2 study	High-grade glioma	NCT00352313, NCI Neuro-Oncology Branch	Completed but results not available
Bevacizumab, bortezomib	Single-center phase 1 study	High-grade glioma	NCT00611325, Duke University	Ongoing
Bevacizumab, carmustine	Single-center phase 2 study	High-grade glioma	NCT00795665, University of California at Davis	Ongoing
Bevacizumab, cediranib	Single-center phase in brain tumors (including GBM)	Advanced malignancies including GBM, gliosarcoma, anaplastic astrocytoma	NCT00458731, MD Anderson Cancer Center	Ongoing
Bevacizumab, etoposide	Single-center phase 2 study	GBM	NCT00612430, Duke University	Preliminary results[183]: PFS 18 wk, 6M-PFS 44%
Bevacizumab, metronomic TMZ	Single-center phase 2 study	High-grade Glioma	NCT00501891, Duke University	Ongoing
Bevacizumab, panobinostat	Multicenter phase 1/2 study	High-grade glioma	NCT00859222, Dana Farber Cancer Institute	Ongoing
Bevacizumab, RT	Single-center phase 1 study	High-grade glioma	NCT00595322, Memorial Sloan Kettering Cancer Center	Ongoing
Bevacizumab, sorafenib	Multicenter phase 2 study	GBM	NCT00621686, NCCTG	Ongoing
Bevacizumab, temsirolimus	Single-center phase 2 in recurrent GBM		NCT00800917, Rigshospitalet	Ongoing
BIBW 2992, TMZ	Multicenter phase 1/2 in recurrent high-grade glioma	High-grade glioma	NCT00727506, Boehringer Ingelheim Pharmaceuticals	Ongoing
Bortezomib, tamoxifen	Single-center phase 2 study	High-grade glioma	NCT00112762, NCI Neuro-Oncology Branch	Ongoing
Cediranib, lomustine vs lomustine	Multicenter randomized phase 3 study	GBM	NCT00777153, AstraZeneca	Ongoing
Cetuximab, bevacizumab, irinotecan	Multicenter phase 2 study	GBM	NCT00463073, Rigshospitalet	Preliminary results[184]: median PFS 24 wk, RR 33%
CT-322, irinotecan	Multicenter phase 2 study	GBM	NCT00562419, Adnexus	Ongoing

Drug combination	Study type	Disease	Identifier, Institution	Status/Results
CYT997, carboplatin, etoposide	Single-center phase 1b/2 study	GBM	NCT00650949, Cytopia Research Pty Ltd	Ongoing
Dasatinib, erlotinib	Single-center phase 1 study	High-grade glioma	NCT00609999, Duke University	Ongoing
Enzastaurin, bevacizumab	Single-center phase 2 study	High-grade glioma	NCT00559923, NCI Neuro-Oncology Branch	Ongoing
Enzastaurin, carboplatin	Single-center phase 1 study	Gliomas	NCT00438997, NCI Neuro-Oncology Branch	Ongoing
Erlotinib, bevacizumab	Single-center phase 2 study	High-grade glioma	NCT00671970, Duke University	Preliminary results[185,186]: 6M-PFS 24%, RR 50%
Erlotinib, carboplatin	Single-center phase 2 study	GBM	MD Anderson Cancer Center	Results[187]: median PFS 9 weeks, 6M-PFS 14%, RR 2%
Erlotinib, sirolimus	Single-center phase 2 study	GBM	NCT00672243, Duke University	Preliminary results[87]: RR 0
Erlotinib, sirolimus	Single-center phase 1/2 study	High-grade glioma	NCT00509431, University of California at Los Angeles	Ongoing
Erlotinib, sorafenib	Multicenter phase 2 study	GBM	NCT00445588, NABTT CNS Consortium	Ongoing
Erlotinib, temsirolimus	Multicenter phase 1/2 study	High-grade glioma	NCT00112736, NABTC	Preliminary results[91]: for GBM patients, no PR, 6M-PFS 12.5%. Phase 2 study ongoing
Everolimus, TMZ	Multicenter phase 1 study	GBM	NCT00387400, National Cancer Institute of Canada	Ongoing
Gefitinib, everolimus	Multicenter phase 1/2 study	GBM	NCT00085566, Memorial Sloan Kettering Cancer Center	Preliminary results[188]: median PFS 2.6 mo, 6M-PFS 4.5%
Gefitinib, sirolimus	Single-center phase 1 study	GBM	Cedars-Sinai Medical Center	Phase 1 study completed[189]
Gefitinib, TMZ	Multicenter phase 1 study	High-grade Glioma	NCT00027625, NABTC	Phase 1 study completed[190]
Imatinib mesylate, hydroxyurea, everolimus	Single-center phase 1 study	High-grade glioma	NCT00613132, Duke University	Ongoing, preliminary phase 1 results[191]
Imatinib mesylate, hydroxyurea, vatalanib	Single-center phase 1 study	High-grade glioma	NCT00387933, Duke University	Phase 1 study completed[192]
Lonafarnib, TMZ	Single-center phase 1/1b study	GBM	NCT00102648, MD Anderson Cancer Center	Ongoing
Lonafarnib, TMZ	Single-center phase 1 study	High-grade gliomas	NCT00612651, Duke University	Ongoing
Lonafarnib, TMZ	Multicenter phase 1 study	Supratentorial gliomas	NCT00083096, EORTC	Ongoing

(continued on next page)

Table 3
(continued)

Therapy	Trial Phase	Patient Population	Trial # and Sponsor	Status
Pazopanib, lapatinib	Multicenter phase 1/2 study	High-grade glioma on enzyme-inducing antiepiletics	NCT00350727, GlaxoSmithKline	Ongoing
Sorafenib combined with erotinib, tipifarnib, or temsirolimus	Multicenter phase 1/2	GBM, gliosarcoma	NCT00335764, NABTC	Ongoing
Sorafenib, temsirolimus	Multicenter phase 1/2 study	GBM	NCT00329719, NCCTG	Ongoing
Sunitinib, irinotecan	Single-center phase 1 study	High-grade glioma	NCT00611728, Duke University	Ongoing
Tandutinib, bevacizumab	Single-center phase 2 study	High-grade glioma	NCT00667394, NCI Neuro-Oncology Branch	Ongoing
Vandetanib, etoposide	Single-center phase 1 study	High-grade glioma	NCT00613223, Duke University	Ongoing
Vandetanib, imatinib, hydroxyurea	Single-center phase 1 study	High-grade glioma	NCT00613054, Duke University	Ongoing
Vandetanib, sirolimus	Multicenter phase 1 study	GBM	NCT00821080, Massachusetts General Hospital	Ongoing
Vatalanib, imatinib, hydroxyurea	Single-center phase 1 study	High-grade glioma	NCT00387933, Duke University	Phase 1 study completed[193]
Vorinostat, bortezomib	Multicenter phase 2 study	GBM	NCT00641706, NCCTG	Ongoing
Vorinostat, isotretinoin, carboplatin	Single-center phase 1/2 study	GBM	NCT00555399, MD Anderson Cancer Center	Ongoing
Vorinostat, TMZ	Multicenter phase 1 study	High-grade glioma	NCT00268385, NABTC	Ongoing
XL765, TMZ	Multicenter phase 1 study	High-grade glioma	NCT00704080, Exelixis	Ongoing

Abbreviations: EORTC, European Organization for Research and Treatment of Cancer; NABTC, North American Brain Tumor Coalition; NABTT, New Approaches to Brain Tumor Therapy; NCCTG, North Central Cancer Treatment Group; NCI, National Cancer Institute; OS, overall survival; PFS, progression-free survival; RR, radiographic response rate; RT, radiation therapy; RTOG, Radiation Therapy Oncology Group; SCRI, Sarah Cannon Research Institute; TMZ, temozolomide; 6M-PFS, 6-month progression-free survival.

Data from National Institutes of Health. Available at: http://www.clinicaltrials.gov.

growth factor (PIGF), but only VEGF-A has an established role in pathologic angiogenesis.[95] VEGF-A levels correlate with the degree of malignancy in gliomas.[51] This angiogenic factor acts on endothelial cell receptors VEGF receptor 2 (VEGFR-2) via a paracrine loop to stimulate endothelial cell growth and division.[96] VEGF is also a potent inducer of increased permeability, which contributes to vasogenic edema.[92]

Bevacizumab, a humanized monoclonal antibody against VEGF-A, was the first VEGF inhibitor to be studied in patients with GBM (**Fig. 2**). Bevacizumab has now been tested in several phase 2 clinical trials as a single agent[97,98] or in combination with irinotecan[97,99,100] for recurrent high-grade glioma. Response rates for the GBM subsets based on the criteria of MacDonald and colleagues[101] for single-agent bevacizumab range from 28% to 35% and for bevacizumab plus irinotecan from 38% to 61%. Six-month PFS for bevacizumab monotherapy ranges from 29% to 43% and for combination 30% to 50%. Treatment

with bevacizumab seems to reduce the need for corticosteroids and the drug is well tolerated. The risk of hemorrhage appears to be low even in patients who require anticoagulation.[102,103] Based on these results, single-agent bevacizumab received accelerated approval by the Food and Drug Administration on May 5, 2009 for the treatment of recurrent glioblastomas.

Another class of antiangiogenic agents is small-molecule TKIs. A large number of agents directed against VEGFR are undergoing evaluation including cediranib, sorafenib, sunitinib, pazopanib, XL184, and CT-322.[93] Cediranib is an oral tyrosine kinase inhibitor that targets all subtypes of VEGFR in addition to PDGFR and c-Kit. A phase 2 clinical trial of cediranib in recurrent GBM yielded a favorable RR of 27% and a 6M-PFS of 25.8%.[104,105] Hypertension was a common adverse effect, as is seen with most antiangiogenesis drugs. MRI scans were also obtained at frequent intervals throughout the study and provided evidence for "normalization" of

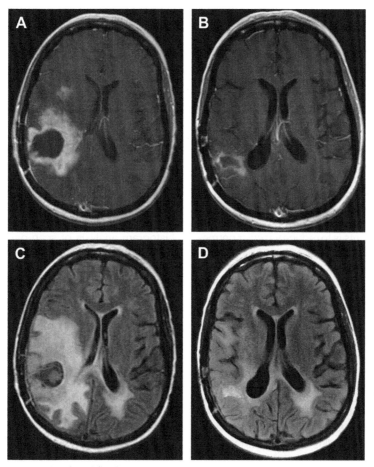

Fig. 2. Postcontrast T1-weighted and fluid-attenuation inversion recovery images of a patient with glioblastoma before (*A, C*) and during (*B, D*) treatment with bevacizumab.

tumor vasculature. In other words, antiangiogenic agents may transiently normalize the abnormal structure and function of tumor vasculature, potentially improving oxygen and drug delivery.[106,107] Using MRI methods discussed below, relative tumor vessel size decreased as early as 1 day after onset of cediranib treatment, reversed toward abnormal values at day 56 on continuous cediranib treatment, and increased when cediranib was held, suggesting a window period for normalization during treatment and the reversibility of normalization during drug holiday. In addition, MRI demonstrated a significant reduction in vascular permeability and vasogenic edema. These data combined with a reduction of steroid usage suggests that cediranib has a steroid-sparing effect.

Newer agents that target the VEGF pathway are in the pipeline. Aflibercept is a soluble decoy VEGF receptor fused with an immunoglobulin constant region and binds to VEGF-A with several hundred times more affinity than bevacizumab.[108,109] Preliminary response rates from a single-arm phase 2 clinical trial of aflibercept in recurrent high-grade glioma are comparable to those of bevacizumab.[110]

Despite the apparent clinical efficacy of anti-VEGF/VEGFR agents, their biologic effects on humans remain unknown. Thus far, radiographic response and progression have been defined by the criteria of MacDonald and colleagues,[101] which measures changes in tumor size based on T1-weighted post-gadolinium images. Because anti-VEGF therapy reduces vascular permeability, it may also decrease gadolinium enhancement without changing tumor size. Changes in vascular permeability can occur as early as 24 hours following a single dose of anti-VEGF therapy.[105,111] Some have proposed that the primary effect of antiangiogenic agents is to reduce vascular permeability and vasogenic edema without killing tumor cells.[112] Indeed, Kamoun and colleagues[113] showed that reductions in vascular permeability, vessel diameter, and vasogenic cerebral edema by cediranib prolonged OS in orthotopic GBM models despite continued tumor growth. These findings are particularly compelling because some tumors may adapt a more invasive, infiltrating phenotype on continued anti-VEGF therapy. Retrospective studies suggest that a subset of patients treated with bevacizumab develop enlarging regions of abnormal hyperintensity on T2-weighted or fluid-attenuation inversion recovery images without concordant findings on post-gadolinium sequences.[103,114–116] Although not pathologically proven in humans, these areas of T2 hyperintensity may represent nonenhancing tumor infiltration with

decreased tumor vascularity. This hypothesis is supported by data from orthotopic GBM models in which blockade of VEGF-mediated angiogenesis facilitated growth along normal vasculature (a process known as co-option) and promoted tumor invasion.[117,118] As a result of these radiographic controversies and other challenges[119] with the current response criteria, new radiographic response criteria for high-grade gliomas are being developed by an international Response Assessment in Neuro-Oncology Working Group.[120,121]

There is also active research in developing new neuroimaging techniques to assess tumor growth, response to treatment, and angiogenesis.[122] Dynamic susceptibility contrast (DSC) and dynamic contrast enhanced (DCE) MRI can measure vascular parameters, such as cerebral blood flow, cerebral blood volume, mean transit time, and vessel size and permeability. As seen with cediranib, these surrogate MRI markers of angiogenesis could be used to assess tumor vasculature during treatment. Recently, the same group defined a "vascular normalization index" based on K^{trans} (a surrogate marker of vascular permeability obtained from DCE MRI), cerebral blood volume (an indicator of microvessel size obtained from MRI), and serum collagen IV levels (a putative measure of vascular basement membrane thickness), which was highly correlated with both progression-free and overall survival.[123]

Diffusion-weighted imaging may provide information regarding tumor density because increased cell numbers restrict diffusion. Apparent diffusion coefficient (ADC) maps can be used to estimate tumor cellularity; histologic studies in mice and humans have correlated low ADC values with increased cell density and proliferation.[124,125] In a preliminary retrospective study of 41 bevacizumab-treated patients with recurrent GBM, ADC histogram analysis of scan data obtained before treatment was a better independent predictor of PFS6 than conventional MRI parameters. Similar findings were not detected in analyzing ADC data from control patients.[126]

Other imaging advances include diffusion tensor imaging and the development of new radiolabeled positron emission tomography (PET) tracers. Fractional anisotropy maps (diffusion tensor imaging) can be used to assess phenomena that perturb white mater tracks such as vasogenic edema and tumor infiltration. ^{18}F-fluoromisonidazole (FMISO) is a nitroimidazole derivative developed as a PET agent to image hypoxia,[127] a potent stimulator of angiogenesis. FMISO PET may play a role in directing and monitoring targeted hypoxic therapy. 3'-Deoxy-3'-^{18}F-fluorothymidine (FLT) is a thymidine analogue whose uptake correlates with activity of thymidine kinase-1, an enzyme expressed during DNA synthesis. In gliomas, elevated FLT uptake is associated with higher mitotic activity.[128,129] Thus, FLT PET has the potential to monitor treatment response.

Integrins

Integrins are heterodimeric cell surface adhesion receptors that cluster with other receptors and adaptor proteins to regulate tumor cell invasion, migration, proliferation, survival, and angiogenesis.[94] Integrins αvβ3 and αvβ5 are particularly important in angiogenesis.[130–133] Cilengitide is a synthetic cyclic pentapeptide small-molecule inhibitor of αvβ3 and αvβ5 integrins. In a phase 2 study of patients with recurrent GBM, cilengitide was well tolerated and exhibited modest antitumor activity with a 6M-PFS of 15% and a median OS of 9.9 months.[134] A trial combining cilengitide with RT and TMZ in patients with newly diagnosed GBM is underway.[135]

NEW MOLECULAR TARGETS
Histone Deacetylases

Protein acetylation by histone acetyltransferases and deacetylation by histone deacetylases (HDACs) affect the regulation of gene expression through chromatin remodeling and acetylation of transcription factors.[136] HDAC inhibitors cause the growth arrest, differentiation, or apoptosis of many transformed cells by altering transcription of various genes, including those involved in regulation of cell survival, proliferation, tumor cell differentiation, cell cycle arrest, and apoptosis.[137] Vorinostat (suberoylanilide hydroxamic acid, SAHA) is a small-molecule inhibitor of most human class I and class II histone deacetylases. This HDAC inhibitor demonstrated moderate clinical activity in a phase 2 study of patients with recurrent GBMs. 6M-PFS was 15.2%.[138] The Adult Brain Tumor Consortium and the North Central Cancer Treatment Group are now jointly conducting a trial of vorinostat with RT and temozlomide in patients with newly diagnosed high-grade glioma. Clinical trials combining HDAC inhibitors with other agents such as bortezomib, a proteasome inhibitor, or bevacizumab are currently underway for recurrent GBM.

UBIQUITIN-PROTEASOME SYSTEM

The ubiquitin/proteasome pathway plays a critical role in the regulated degradation of proteins involved in cell cycle control, apoptosis, and tumor growth.[139] The pathway is initiated by the addition of multiple ubiquitin monomers; this targets proteins for degradation by the 26S proteasome. Several in vitro studies demonstrate that proteasome inhibitors have activity in GBM cell lines, resulting in cell growth arrest and induction of apoptosis.[140–142] Bortezomib, a proteasome inhibitor, is well tolerated when administered as a single agent[143] and in combination TMZ and RT[144] in patients with high-grade glioma. Bortezomib is now in clinical trials in high-grade gliomas.

HEAT SHOCK PROTEINS

Heat shock protein 90 (HSP90) is a chaperone protein that assists in proper folding and functioning of client proteins.[145] Several proteins and signaling pathways implicated in GBM are stabilized by HSP90 function, including Akt[146] and EGFRvIII.[147] Tanespimycin (17-allylamino-geldanamycin, 17-AAG), a benzoquinone antibiotic derived from geldanamycin, was the first HSP90 inhibitor to enter clinical trials. HSP90 inhibitors act by binding to HSP90 and inducing proteasomal degradation of HSP90 client proteins.[148–153] HSP90 binds with 100-fold higher affinity to 17-AAG in tumor cells than in normal cells.[154] Preclinical data demonstrate that tanespimycin significantly inhibits growth of glioma cell lines in vitro[155,156] and intracranial tumors in orthotopic models.[155,157] HSP90 inhibitors are entering clinical trials in GBM.

CYTOKINES

Transforming growth factor β (TGF-β) is a cytokine involved in maintaining tissue homeostasis by controlling proliferation and apoptosis of various cell types.[158] TGF-β binding activates several downstream signaling cascades including Smad, MAPK, and PI3K.[159,160] Tumors use different mechanisms to evade immune surveillance including production of TGF-β. This cytokine is overexpressed in high-grade glioma.[161,162] Trabedersen (AP12009), an antisense oligonucleotide that targets TGF-β, is delivered using convection-enhanced delivery directly into the tumor tissue. Preliminary results from a phase 2b study that randomizes patients with recurrent high-grade gliomas to low-dose AP 12009, high-dose AP 12009, or standard therapy (TMZ or procarbazine/lomustine/vincristine) suggests improved outcome in the low-dose AP12009 arm compared to standard chemotherapy.[163]

DNA REPAIR

Poly(ADP-ribose) polymerase (PARP) is a nuclear enzyme that signals the presence of DNA breaks and facilitates DNA repair by engaging mechanisms such as base excision repair (BER).[164] Because PARP inhibitors disrupt BER, an important mediator of TMZ resistance, these agents may enhance temozolomide's antitumor effects against gliomas. Two PARP inhibitors, BSI-201 and ABT-888, are currently being tested in combination with radiation and temozolomide for newly diagnosed high-grade gliomas.

GLIOMA STEM CELLS

Glioma stem cells are believed to represent a subpopulation of cells in the tumor with the ability to self-renew, proliferate, and give rise to progeny of multiple neuroepithelial lineages.[165] Several years ago, the discovery of stemlike cells embedded within fresh surgical isolates of malignant gliomas lent support to this hypothesis.[166] Evidence from in vivo and in vitro studies suggest that these cells may be important for glioma-genesis[166,167] and mediating resistance to therapy.[168,169] As a result, there is significant interest in molecular therapies targeting stem cell pathways, such as notch (eg, MRK0752 and R4929097) and sonic hedgehog (GDC4409),[165,166,168] as well as hypoxia-inducible factors 1 and 2α.[170]

OTHER THERAPEUTIC MODALITIES

A large number of other therapeutic modalities are being explored for high-grade gliomas. Examples include gene therapy,[171–173] stem cell therapies,[174] synthetic chlorotoxins (TM-601),[175] chemotherapeutic agents with enhanced ability to penetrate into tumor tissue, and convection-enhanced delivery (CED) of drugs and toxins.[176] Intracavitary TM-601, the synthetic version of a chlorotoxin found in the venom of the giant yellow Israeli scorpion, is under evaluation in a phase 2 study. Agents administered directly into high-grade gliomas via CED that have been studied in phase 3 clinical trials include IL13-*Pseudomonas aeruginosa* exotoxic (IL13-PE38, cintredekin besudotox) and transferrin-C diphtheriae toxin (Tf-CRM107, TransMID). Unfortunately, both trials were terminated for reasons of futility after interim analysis.[177] Nonetheless, CED may be a useful approach with more effective agents.

Gene therapy involves the insertion or modification of genes in a patient's cell to treat a disease.[173] Transfer of "suicidal" genes via viral vectors such as herpes simple virus thymidine kinase gene (HSV-tk) has demonstrated only limited survival benefit in several clinical trials for recurrent GBM.[173] However, gene transfer strategies continue to improve. Viral vectors can also deliver proapoptotic cytokines such as tumor necrosis factor–related apoptosis-inducing ligand (TRAIL) and p53 as well as cytokines such as interleukin-2 and interferon β. Other methods of delivery under investigation include cell-based transfer and synthetic vectors.

Antitumor vaccines based on peptide antigens, dendritic cells, or whole tumor cells represent another major avenue of investigation. Among the many promising vaccines are CDX-110,[178] a peptide vaccine directed against EGFRvIII; GVAX,[179] which involves administration of irradiated autologous tumor cells mixed with granulocyte macrophage colony-stimulating factor–producing cells; and vaccines against HSP90.[180] In small phase 2 studies, these vaccines appear to be well tolerated and show promising efficacy compared with historical controls. However, larger prospective controlled studies will be required to confirm any clinical benefit.

SUMMARY

Advances in our understanding of gliomagenesis and disease progression have led to a plethora of potential targets and novel anticancer drugs. The complexity of molecular abnormalities and the redundancy of signaling pathways in GBMs make it unlikely that single agents will achieve great success. However, multitargeted agents, combination therapies, and new treatment modalities are on the horizon. In addition, new agents continue to be developed against known as well as novel targets.

ACKNOWLEDGMENTS

We gratefully acknowledge the support of the Chris Elliott Fund for Glioblastoma Brain Cancer Research.

REFERENCES

1. Central Brain Tumor Registry of the United States. Statistical report: primary brain tumors in the United States, 2000-2004. Available at: http://www.cbtrus.org/reports//2007-2008/2007report.pdf. Accessed December 1, 2008.
2. Stupp R, Mason WP, van den Bent MJ, et al. Radiotherapy plus concomitant and adjuvant temozolomide for glioblastoma. N Engl J Med 2005; 352(10):987–96.
3. Network CGAR. Comprehensive genomic characterization defines human glioblastoma genes and core pathways. Nature 2008;455(7216):1061–8.
4. Furnari FB, Fenton T, Bachoo RM, et al. Malignant astrocytic glioma: genetics, biology, and paths to treatment. Genes Dev 2007;21(21):2683–710.

5. Parsons DW, Jones S, Zhang X, et al. An integrated genomic analysis of human glioblastoma multiforme. Science 2008;321(5897):1807–12.

6. Yan H, Parsons DW, Jin G, et al. IDH1 and IDH2 mutations in gliomas. N Engl J Med 2009;360(8): 765–73.

7. Wen PY, Kesari S. Malignant gliomas in adults. N Engl J Med 2008;359(5):492–507.

8. Kleihues P, Burger PC, Aldape KD, et al. Glioblastoma. In: Louis DN, Ohgaki H, Wiestler OD, et al, editors. WHO classification of tumours of the central nervous system. 4th edition. Lyon (France): International Agency for Research on Cancer; 2007. p. 33–46.

9. Druker BJ. Perspectives on the development of a molecularly targeted agent. Cancer Cell 2002; 1(1):31–6.

10. Futreal PA, Kasprzyk A, Birney E, et al. Cancer and genomics. Nature 2001;409(6822):850–2.

11. Agosti RM, Leuthold M, Gullick WJ, et al. Expression of the epidermal growth factor receptor in astrocytic tumours is specifically associated with glioblastoma multiforme. Virchows Arch A Pathol Anat Histopathol 1992;420(4):321–5.

12. Bigner SH, Humphrey PA, Wong AJ, et al. Characterization of the epidermal growth factor receptor in human glioma cell lines and xenografts. Cancer Res 1990;50(24):8017–22.

13. Humphrey PA, Wong AJ, Vogelstein B, et al. Amplification and expression of the epidermal growth factor receptor gene in human glioma xenografts. Cancer Res 1988;48(8):2231–8.

14. Berens ME, Rief MD, Shapiro JR, et al. Proliferation and motility responses of primary and recurrent gliomas related to changes in epidermal growth factor receptor expression. J Neurooncol 1996; 27(1):11–22.

15. Feldkamp MM, Lau N, Guha A. Signal transduction pathways and their relevance in human astrocytomas. J Neurooncol 1997;35(3):223–48.

16. Holland EC, Hively WP, DePinho RA, et al. A constitutively active epidermal growth factor receptor cooperates with disruption of G1 cell-cycle arrest pathways to induce glioma-like lesions in mice. Genes Dev 1998;12(23):3675–85.

17. Lund-Johansen M, Bjerkvig R, Humphrey PA, et al. Effect of epidermal growth factor on glioma cell growth, migration, and invasion in vitro. Cancer Res 1990;50(18):6039–44.

18. Sugawa N, Yamamoto K, Ueda S, et al. Function of aberrant EGFR in malignant gliomas. Brain Tumor Pathol 1998;15(1):53–7.

19. Batra SK, Castelino-Prabhu S, Wikstrand CJ, et al. Epidermal growth factor ligand-independent, unregulated, cell-transforming potential of a naturally occurring human mutant EGFRvIII gene. Cell Growth Differ 1995;6(10):1251–9.

20. Humphrey PA, Wong AJ, Vogelstein B, et al. Antisynthetic peptide antibody reacting at the fusion junction of deletion-mutant epidermal growth factor receptors in human glioblastoma. Proc Natl Acad Sci U S A 1990;87(11):4207–11.

21. Wong AJ, Ruppert JM, Bigner SH, et al. Structural alterations of the epidermal growth factor receptor gene in human gliomas. Proc Natl Acad Sci U S A 1992;89(7):2965–9.

22. Chakravarti A, Berkey B, Robins HI, et al. An update of phase II results from RTOG 0211: a phase I/II study of gefitinib with radiotherapy in newly diagnosed glioblastoma. In: Proceedings from the American Society of Clinical Oncology [abstract 1527]. Atlanta (GA), June 2–6, 2006.

23. Brown PD, Krishnan S, Sarkaria JN, et al. Phase I/II trial of erlotinib and temozolomide with radiation therapy in the treatment of newly diagnosed glioblastoma multiforme: north central cancer treatment group study N0177. J Clin Oncol 2008; 26(34):5603–9.

24. Franceschi E, Cavallo G, Lonardi S, et al. Gefitinib in patients with progressive high-grade gliomas: a multicentre phase II study by Gruppo Italiano Cooperativo di Neuro-Oncologia (GICNO). Br J Cancer 2007;96(7):1047–51.

25. Rich JN, Reardon DA, Peery T, et al. Phase II trial of gefitinib in recurrent glioblastoma. J Clin Oncol 2004;22(1):133–42.

26. Lieberman FS, Cloughesy T, Fine H, et al. NABTC phase I/II trial of ZD-1839 for recurrent malignant gliomas and unresectable meningiomas. In: Proceedings from the American Society of Clinical Oncology [abstract 1510]. New Orleans (LA), June 5–8, 2004.

27. Cloughesy T, Yung A, Vrendenberg J, et al. Phase II study of erlotinib in recurrent GBM: Molecular predictors of outcome. In: Proceedings from the American Society of Clinical Oncology [abstract 1507]. Orlando (FL), May 13–17, 2005.

28. Vogelbaum MA, Peereboom D, Stevens G, et al. Phase II study of erlotinib single agent therapy in recurrent glioblastoma multiforme. European Journal of Cancer Supplements 2005;3(2):135S.

29. Raizer JJ, Abrey LE, Lassman AB, et al. A phase II trial of Erlotinib in patients with non-progressive glioblastoma multiforme post radiation therapy, and recurrent malignant gliomas and meningiomas: a North American Brain Tumor Consortium Trial. Neuro Oncol 2010;12(1):95–103.

30. van den Bent MJ, Brandes AA, Rampling R, et al. Randomized phase II trial of erlotinib versus temozolomide or carmustine in recurrent glioblastoma: EORTC brain tumor group study 26034. J Clin Oncol 2009;27(8):1268–74.

31. Kuhn J, Robins I, Mehta M, et al. Tumor sequestration of lapatinib (NABTC 04-01). In: Proceedings

from the Thirteenth Annual Meeting of the Society for Neuro-Oncology [abstract ET-05]. Las Vegas (NV), November 20–23, 2008.

32. Reardon DA, Groves M, Wen P, et al. A phase II trial of lapatinib and pazopanib for patients with recurrent glioblastoma multiforme (GBM). In: Proceedings from the Twelfth Annual Meeting of the Society for Neuro-Oncology [abstract MA-07]. Dallas (TX), November 15–18, 2007.

33. Thiessen B, Stewart C, Tsao M, et al. A phase I/II trial of GW572016 (lapatinib) in recurrent glioblastoma multiforme: clinical outcomes, pharmacokinetics and molecular correlation. Cancer Chemother Pharmacol 2009. [Epub ahead of print].

34. Stommel JM, Kimmelman AC, Ying H, et al. Coactivation of receptor tyrosine kinases affects the response of tumor cells to targeted therapies. Science 2007;318(5848):287–90.

35. Greulich H, Chen TH, Feng W, et al. Oncogenic transformation by inhibitor-sensitive and -resistant EGFR mutants. PLoS Med 2005;2(11):e313.

36. Kobayashi S, Boggon TJ, Dayaram T, et al. EGFR mutation and resistance of non-small-cell lung cancer to gefitinib. N Engl J Med 2005;352(8):786–92.

37. Kobayashi S, Ji H, Yuza Y, et al. An alternative inhibitor overcomes resistance caused by a mutation of the epidermal growth factor receptor. Cancer Res 2005;65(16):7096–101.

38. Kwak EL, Sordella R, Bell DW, et al. Irreversible inhibitors of the EGF receptor may circumvent acquired resistance to gefitinib. Proc Natl Acad Sci U S A 2005;102(21):7665–70.

39. Li D, Ambrogio L, Shimamura T, et al. BIBW2992, an irreversible EGFR/HER2 inhibitor highly effective in preclinical lung cancer models. Oncogene 2008; 27(34):4702–11.

40. Shimamura T, Ji H, Minami Y, et al. Non-small-cell lung cancer and Ba/F3 transformed cells harboring the ERBB2 G776insV_G/C mutation are sensitive to the dual-specific epidermal growth factor receptor and ERBB2 inhibitor HKI-272. Cancer Res 2006; 66(13):6487–91.

41. Barber TD, Vogelstein B, Kinzler KW, et al. Somatic mutations of EGFR in colorectal cancers and glioblastomas. N Engl J Med 2004;351(27):2883.

42. Lassman AB, Rossi MR, Raizer JJ, et al. Molecular study of malignant gliomas treated with epidermal growth factor receptor inhibitors: tissue analysis from North American Brain Tumor Consortium Trials 01-03 and 00-01. Clin Cancer Res 2005;11(21):7841–50.

43. Mellinghoff IK, Wang MY, Vivanco I, et al. Molecular determinants of the response of glioblastomas to EGFR kinase inhibitors. [erratum appears in N Engl J Med 2006 Feb 23;354(8):884]. N Engl J Med 2005;353(19):2012–24.

44. Ramos TC, Figueredo J, Catala M, et al. Treatment of high-grade glioma patients with the humanized anti-epidermal growth factor receptor (EGFR) antibody h-R3: report from a phase I/II trial. Cancer Biol Ther 2006;5(4):375–9.

45. Sampson JH, Archer GE, Bigner DD, et al. Effect of EGFRvIII-targeted vaccine (CDX-110) on immune response and TTP when given with simultaneous standard and continuous temozolomide in patients with GBM. In: Proceedings from the American Society of Clinical Oncology [abstract 2011]. Chicago (IL), May 31–June 3, 2008.

46. Matsumoto K, Nakamura T. Emerging multipotent aspects of hepatocyte growth factor. J Biochem 1996;119(4):591–600.

47. Koochekpour S, Jeffers M, Rulong S, et al. Met and hepatocyte growth factor/scatter factor expression in human gliomas. Cancer Res 1997;57(23):5391–8.

48. Lamszus K, Laterra J, Westphal M, et al. Scatter factor/hepatocyte growth factor (SF/HGF) content and function in human gliomas. Int J Dev Neurosci 1999;17(5-6):517–30.

49. Moriyama T, Kataoka H, Kawano H, et al. Comparative analysis of expression of hepatocyte growth factor and its receptor, c-met, in gliomas, meningiomas and schwannomas in humans. Cancer Lett 1998;124(2):149–55.

50. Rosen EM, Laterra J, Joseph A, et al. Scatter factor expression and regulation in human glial tumors. Int J Cancer 1996;67(2):248–55.

51. Schmidt NO, Westphal M, Hagel C, et al. Levels of vascular endothelial growth factor, hepatocyte growth factor/scatter factor and basic fibroblast growth factor in human gliomas and their relation to angiogenesis. Int J Cancer 1999;84(1):10–8.

52. Reardon DA, Cloughsey TF, Raizer JJ, et al. Phase II study of AMG 102, a fully human neutralizing antibody against hepatocyte growth factor/scatter factor, in patients with recurrent glioblastoma multiforme. In: Proceedings from the American Society of Clinical Oncology [abstract 2051]. Chicago (IL), 2008.

53. Lal B, Goodwin CR, Sang Y, et al. EGFRvIII and c-Met pathway inhibitors synergize against PTEN-null/EGFRvIII+ glioblastoma xenografts. Mol Cancer Ther 2009;8(7):1751–60.

54. George D. Targeting PDGF receptors in cancer—rationales and proof of concept clinical trials. Adv Exp Med Biol 2003;532:141–51.

55. Di Rocco F, Carroll RS, Zhang J, et al. Platelet-derived growth factor and its receptor expression in human oligodendrogliomas. Neurosurgery 1998;42(2):341–6.

56. Hermanson M, Funa K, Hartman M, et al. Platelet-derived growth factor and its receptors in human glioma tissue: expression of messenger RNA and protein suggests the presence of autocrine

and paracrine loops. Cancer Res 1992;52(11): 3213–9.

57. Nister M, Libermann TA, Betsholtz C, et al. Expression of messenger RNAs for platelet-derived growth factor and transforming growth factor-alpha and their receptors in human malignant glioma cell lines. Cancer Res 1988;48(14):3910–8.

58. Chin LS, Murray SF, Zitnay KM, et al. K252a inhibits proliferation of glioma cells by blocking platelet-derived growth factor signal transduction. Clin Cancer Res 1997;3(5):771–6.

59. Vassbotn FS, Ostman A, Langeland N, et al. Activated platelet-derived growth factor autocrine pathway drives the transformed phenotype of a human glioblastoma cell line. J Cell Physiol 1994;158(2):381–9.

60. Cao R, Brakenhielm E, Li X, et al. Angiogenesis stimulated by PDGF-CC, a novel member in the PDGF family, involves activation of PDGFR-alphaalpha and -alphabeta receptors. FASEB J 2002; 16(12):1575–83.

61. Li X, Eriksson U. Novel PDGF family members: PDGF-C and PDGF-D. Cytokine Growth Factor Rev 2003;14(2):91–8.

62. Li X, Ponten A, Aase K, et al. PDGF-C is a new protease-activated ligand for the PDGF alpha-receptor. Nat Cell Biol 2000;2(5):302–9.

63. Kilic T, Alberta JA, Zdunek PR, et al. Intracranial inhibition of platelet-derived growth factor-mediated glioblastoma cell growth by an orally active kinase inhibitor of the 2-phenylaminopyrimidine class. Cancer Res 2000;60(18):5143–50.

64. Raymond E, Brandes AA, Dittrich C, et al. Phase II study of imatinib in patients with recurrent gliomas of various histologies: a European Organisation for Research and Treatment of Cancer Brain Tumor Group Study. J Clin Oncol 2008;26(28):4659–65.

65. Wen PY, Yung WK, Lamborn KR, et al. Phase I/II study of imatinib mesylate for recurrent malignant gliomas: North American Brain Tumor Consortium Study 99-08. Clin Cancer Res 2006;12(16): 4899–907.

66. Dresemann G, Weller M, Bogdahn U, et al. Imatinib plus hydroxyurea versus hydroxyurea monotherapy in progressive glioblastoma—an international multicenter, open-label, randomized phase III study (AMBROSIA-STUDY). In: Proceedings from the Thirteenth Annual Meeting of the Society for Neuro-Oncology [abstract MA-19]. Lake Las Vegas (NV), November 20–23, 2008.

67. Dai H, Marbach P, Lemaire M, et al. Distribution of STI-571 to the brain is limited by P-glycoprotein-mediated efflux. J Pharmacol Exp Ther 2003; 304(3):1085–92.

68. Hennessy BT, Smith DL, Ram PT, et al. Exploiting the PI3K/AKT pathway for cancer drug discovery. Nat Rev Drug Discov 2005;4(12):988–1004.

69. Chakravarti A, Zhai G, Suzuki Y, et al. The prognostic significance of phosphatidylinositol 3-kinase pathway activation in human gliomas. J Clin Oncol 2004;22(10):1926–33.

70. Opel D, Westhoff MA, Bender A, et al. Phosphatidylinositol 3-kinase inhibition broadly sensitizes glioblastoma cells to death receptor- and drug-induced apoptosis. Cancer Res 2008;68(15): 6271–80.

71. Chang SM, Wen P, Cloughesy T, et al. Phase II study of CCI-779 in patients with recurrent glioblastoma multiforme. Invest New Drugs 2005;23(4):357–61.

72. Galanis E, Buckner JC, Maurer MJ, et al. Phase II trial of temsirolimus (CCI-779) in recurrent glioblastoma multiforme: a North Central Cancer Treatment Group Study. J Clin Oncol 2005;23(23):5294–304.

73. Cloughesy TF, Yoshimoto K, Nghiemphu P, et al. Antitumor activity of rapamycin in a Phase I trial for patients with recurrent PTEN-deficient glioblastoma. PLoS Med 2008;5(1):e8.

74. Wan X, Harkavy B, Shen N, et al. Rapamycin induces feedback activation of Akt signaling through an IGF-1R-dependent mechanism. Oncogene 2007;26(13):1932–40.

75. O'Reilly KE, Rojo F, She QB, et al. mTOR inhibition induces upstream receptor tyrosine kinase signaling and activates Akt. Cancer Res 2006; 66(3):1500–8.

76. Sebolt-Leopold JS, Herrera R. Targeting the mitogen-activated protein kinase cascade to treat cancer. Nat Rev Cancer 2004;4(12):937–47.

77. Feldkamp MM, Lau N, Guha A. Growth inhibition of astrocytoma cells by farnesyl transferase inhibitors is mediated by a combination of anti-proliferative, pro-apoptotic and anti-angiogenic effects. Oncogene 1999;18(52):7514–26.

78. Glass TL, Liu TJ, Yung WK. Inhibition of cell growth in human glioblastoma cell lines by farnesyltransferase inhibitor SCH66336. Neuro Oncol 2000; 2(3):151–8.

79. Kurimoto M, Hirashima Y, Hamada H, et al. In vitro and in vivo growth inhibition of human malignant astrocytoma cells by the farnesyltransferase inhibitor B1620. J Neurooncol 2003;61(2):103–12.

80. Cloughesy TF, Wen PY, Robins HI, et al. Phase II trial of tipifarnib in patients with recurrent malignant glioma either receiving or not receiving enzyme-inducing antiepileptic drugs: a North American Brain Tumor Consortium Study. J Clin Oncol 2006; 24(22):3651–6.

81. Lustig R, Mikkelsen T, Lesser G, et al. Phase II pre-radiation R115777 (tipifarnib) in newly diagnosed GBM with residual enhancing disease. Neuro Oncol 2008;10(6):1004–9.

82. Beeram M, Patnaik A, Rowinsky EK. Raf: a strategic target for therapeutic development against cancer. J Clin Oncol 2005;23(27):6771–90.

83. Sharif TR, Sharif M. Overexpression of protein kinase C epsilon in astroglial brain tumor derived cell lines and primary tumor samples. Int J Oncol 1999;15(2):237–43.

84. Xiao H, Goldthwait DA, Mapstone T. The identification of four protein kinase C isoforms in human glioblastoma cell lines: PKC alpha, gamma, epsilon, and zeta. J Neurosurg 1994;81(5):734–40.

85. Wick W, Puduvalli VK, Chamberlain MC, et al. Phase III study of enzastaurin compared with lomustine in the treatment of recurrent intracranial glioblastoma. J Clin Oncol 2010;28(7):1168–74.

86. Butowski NA, Lamborn K, Chang S, et al. Phase I/II study of enzastaurin (ENZ) plus temozolomide (TMZ) and radiation therapy (XRT) in patients with glioblastoma multiforme (GBM) or gliosarcoma (GS). ASCO Meeting Abstracts 2008;26(Suppl 15):3559.

87. Friedman HS, Desjardins A, Vredenburgh JJ, et al. Phase II trial of erlotinib plus sirolimus for recurrent glioblastoma multiforme (GBM). In: Proceedings from the American Society of Clinical Oncology [abstract 2062]. Chicago (IL), May 30–June 3, 2008.

88. Wen P, Kuhn J, Chang S, et al. Phase I/II study of erlotinib and temsirolimus (CCI-779) for patients with recurrent malignant gliomas (NABTC 04-02). In: Thirteenth Annual Meeting of the Society for Neuro-Oncology. Dallas (TX), November 20–23, 2008.

89. Wen P, Cloughesy T, Kuhn J, et al. Phase I/II study of sorafenib and temsirolimus for patients with recurrent glioblastoma (GBM) (NABTC 05–02). In: Proceedings from the American Society of Clinical Oncology [abstract 2006]. Orlando (FL), May 29–June 2, 2009.

90. Prados M, Gilbert M, Kuhn J, et al. Phase I/II study of sorefenib and erlotinib for patients with recurrent glioblastoma (GBM) (NABTC 05-02). In: Proceedings from the American Society of Clinical Oncology [abstract 2005]. Orlando (FL), May 29–June 2, 2009.

91. Chang S, Kuhn J, Lamborn K, et al. Phase I/II study of erlotinib and temsirolimus for patients with recurrent malignant gliomas (MG) (NABTC 04-02). In: Proceedings from the American Society of Clinical Oncology [abstract 2004]. Orlando (FL), May 29–June 2, 2009.

92. Jain RK, di Tomaso E, Duda DG, et al. Angiogenesis in brain tumours. Nat Rev Neurosci 2007; 8(8):610–22.

93. Chi AS, Norden AD, Wen PY. Antiangiogenic strategies for treatment of malignant gliomas. Neurotherapeutics 2009;6(3):513–26.

94. Jin H, Varner J. Integrins: roles in cancer development and as treatment targets. Br J Cancer 2004; 90(3):561–5.

95. Norden AD, Drappatz J, Wen PY. Novel anti-angiogenic therapies for malignant gliomas. Lancet Neurol 2008;7(12):1152–60.

96. Millauer B, Shawver LK, Plate KH, et al. Glioblastoma growth inhibited in vivo by a dominant-negative Flk-1 mutant. Nature 1994;367(6463):576–9.

97. Friedman HS, Prados MD, Wen PY, et al. Bevacizumab alone and in combination with irinotecan in recurrent glioblastoma. J Clin Oncol 2009;27: 4733–40.

98. Kreisl TN, Kim L, Moore K, et al. Phase II trial of single-agent bevacizumab followed by bevacizumab plus irinotecan at tumor progression in recurrent glioblastoma. J Clin Oncol 2009;27(5):740–5.

99. Vredenburgh JJ, Desjardins A, Herndon JE 2nd, et al. Phase II trial of bevacizumab and irinotecan in recurrent malignant glioma. Clin Cancer Res 2007;13(4):1253–9.

100. Vredenburgh JJ, Desjardins A, Herndon JE 2nd, et al. Bevacizumab plus irinotecan in recurrent glioblastoma multiforme. J Clin Oncol 2007;25(30): 4722–9.

101. Macdonald DR, Cascino TL, Schold SC Jr, et al. Response criteria for phase II studies of supratentorial malignant glioma. J Clin Oncol 1990;8(7): 1277–80.

102. Nghiemphu P, Green RM, Pope WB, et al. Safety of anticoagulation use and bevacizumab in patients with glioma. Neuro Oncol 2008;10(3):355–60.

103. Norden AD, Young GS, Setayesh K, et al. Bevacizumab for recurrent malignant gliomas: efficacy, toxicity, and patterns of recurrence. Neurology 2008;70(10):779–87.

104. Batchelor TT, Duda DG, di Tomaso E, et al. Phase II study of cediranib, an oral pan-VEGF receptor tyrosine kinase inhibitor, in patients with recurrent glioblastoma. J Clin Oncol 2010. [Epub ahead of print].

105. Batchelor TT, Sorensen AG, di Tomaso E, et al. AZD2171, a pan-VEGF receptor tyrosine kinase inhibitor, normalizes tumor vasculature and alleviates edema in glioblastoma patients. Cancer Cell 2007;11(1):83–95.

106. Jain RK. Normalizing tumor vasculature with antiangiogenic therapy: a new paradigm for combination therapy. Nat Med 2001;7(9):987–9.

107. Jain RK. Normalization of tumor vasculature: an emerging concept in antiangiogenic therapy. Science 2005;307(5706):58–62.

108. Holash J, Davis S, Papadopoulos N, et al. VEGF-trap: a VEGF blocker with potent antitumor effects. Proc Natl Acad Sci U S A 2002;99(17): 11393–8.

109. Wachsberger PR, Burd R, Cardi C, et al. VEGF trap in combination with radiotherapy improves tumor control in u87 glioblastoma. Int J Radiat Oncol Biol Phys 2007;67(5):1526–37.

110. de Groot JF, Wen PY, Lamborn K, et al. Phase II single arm trial of aflibercept in patients with recurrent temozolomide-resistant glioblastoma: NABTC 0601. In: Proceedings from the American Society

of Clinical Oncology [abstract 2020]. Chicago (IL), May 30–June 3, 2008.

111. Desjardins A, Barboriak DP, Herndon JE, II, et al. Effect of bevacizumab (BEV) and irinotecan (CPT-11) on dynamic contrast-enhanced magnetic resonance imaging (DCE-MRI) in glioblastoma (GBM) patients. In: Proceedings from the American Society of Clinical Oncology [abstract 2026]. Chicago (IL), May 30–June 3, 2008.

112. Norden AD, Drappatz J, Muzikansky A, et al. An exploratory survival analysis of anti-angiogenic therapy for recurrent malignant glioma. J Neurooncol 2009;92(2):149–55.

113. Kamoun WS, Ley CD, Farrar CT, et al. Edema control by cediranib, a vascular endothelial growth factor receptor-targeted kinase inhibitor, prolongs survival despite persistent brain tumor growth in mice. J Clin Oncol 2009;27(15):2542–52.

114. Lassman AB, Iwamoto FM, Gutin PH, et al. Patterns of relapse and prognosis after bevacizumab (BEV) failure in recurrent glioblastoma (GBM). In: Proceedings from the American Society of Clinical Oncology [abstract 2028]. Chicago (IL), 2008.

115. Narayana A, Raza S, Golfinos JG, et al. Bevacizumab therapy in recurrent high grade glioma: Impact on local control and survival. In: Proceedings from the American Society of Clinical Oncology [abstract 13000]. Chicago (IL), 2008.

116. Zuniga RM, Torcuator R, Jain R, et al. Efficacy, safety and patterns of response and recurrence in patients with recurrent high-grade gliomas treated with bevacizumab plus irinotecan. J Neurooncol 2009;91(3):329–36.

117. Kunkel P, Ulbricht U, Bohlen P, et al. Inhibition of glioma angiogenesis and growth in vivo by systemic treatment with a monoclonal antibody against vascular endothelial growth factor receptor-2. Cancer Res 2001;61(18):6624–8.

118. Rubenstein JL, Kim J, Ozawa T, et al. Anti-VEGF antibody treatment of glioblastoma prolongs survival but results in increased vascular cooption. Neoplasia 2000;2(4):306–14.

119. Sorensen AG, Batchelor TT, Wen PY, et al. Response criteria for glioma. Nat Clin Pract Oncol 2008;5(11):634–44.

120. Wen PY, Macdonald DR, Reardon DA, et al. Updated response assessment criteria for high-grade gliomas: Response Assessment in Neuro-Oncology (RANO) Working Group. J Clin Oncol 2010;28(11):1963–72.

121. van den Bent MJ, Vogelbaum MA, Wen PY, et al. End point assessment in gliomas: novel treatments limit usefulness of classical Macdonald's criteria. J Clin Oncol 2009;27(18):2905–8.

122. Gerstner ER, Sorensen AG, Jain RK, et al. Advances in neuroimaging techniques for the evaluation of tumor growth, vascular permeability, and angiogenesis in gliomas. Curr Opin Neurol 2008; 21(6):728–35.

123. Sorensen AG, Batchelor TT, Zhang WT, et al. A "vascular normalization index" as potential mechanistic biomarker to predict survival after a single dose of cediranib in recurrent glioblastoma patients. Cancer Res 2009;69(13):5296–300.

124. Chenevert TL, Stegman LD, Taylor JM, et al. Diffusion magnetic resonance imaging: an early surrogate marker of therapeutic efficacy in brain tumors. J Natl Cancer Inst 2000;92(24):2029–36.

125. Higano S, Yun X, Kumabe T, et al. Malignant astrocytic tumors: clinical importance of apparent diffusion coefficient in prediction of grade and prognosis. Radiology 2006;241(3):839–46.

126. Pope WB, Kim HJ, Huo J, et al. Recurrent glioblastoma multiforme: ADC histogram analysis predicts response to bevacizumab treatment. Radiology 2009;252(1):182–9.

127. Rasey JS, Koh WJ, Evans ML, et al. Quantifying regional hypoxia in human tumors with positron emission tomography of [^{18}F]fluoromisonidazole: a pretherapy study of 37 patients. Int J Radiat Oncol Biol Phys 1996;36(2):417–28.

128. Chen W, Cloughesy T, Kamdar N, et al. Imaging proliferation in brain tumors with 18F-FLT PET: comparison with ^{18}F-FDG. J Nucl Med 2005; 46(6):945–52.

129. Ullrich R, Backes H, Li H, et al. Glioma proliferation as assessed by 3′-fluoro-3′-deoxy-L-thymidine positron emission tomography in patients with newly diagnosed high-grade glioma. Clin Cancer Res 2008;14(7):2049–55.

130. Brooks PC, Clark RA, Cheresh DA. Requirement of vascular integrin alpha v beta 3 for angiogenesis. Science 1994;264(5158):569–71.

131. Brooks PC, Montgomery AM, Rosenfeld M, et al. Integrin alpha v beta 3 antagonists promote tumor regression by inducing apoptosis of angiogenic blood vessels. Cell. 1994;79(7):1157–64.

132. Friedlander M, Brooks PC, Shaffer RW, et al. Definition of two angiogenic pathways by distinct alpha v integrins. Science 1995;270(5241):1500–2.

133. Trikha M, Zhou Z, Timar J, et al. Multiple roles for platelet GPIIb/IIIa and alphavbeta3 integrins in tumor growth, angiogenesis, and metastasis. Cancer Res 2002;62(10):2824–33.

134. Reardon DA, Fink KL, Mikkelsen T, et al. Randomized phase II study of cilengitide, an integrin-targeting arginine-glycine-aspartic acid peptide, in recurrent glioblastoma multiforme. J Clin Oncol 2008;26(34):5610–7.

135. Stupp R, Goldbrunner R, Neyns B, et al. Phase I/IIa trial of cilengitide (EMD121974) and temozolomide with concomitant radiotherapy, followed by temozolomide and cilengitide maintenance therapy in patients (pts) with newly diagnosed glioblastoma

(GBM). In: Proceedings from the American Society of Clinical Oncology [abstract 2000]. Chicago (IL), June 2–5, 2007.

136. Richon VM, Garcia-Vargas J, Hardwick JS. Development of vorinostat: Current applications and future perspectives for cancer therapy. Cancer Lett 2009;280(2):201–10.

137. Jones PA, Baylin SB. The fundamental role of epigenetic events in cancer. Nat Rev Genet 2002; 3(6):415–28.

138. Galanis E, Jaeckle KA, Maurer MJ, et al. Phase II trial of vorinostat in recurrent glioblastoma multiforme: a north central cancer treatment group study. J Clin Oncol 2009;27(12):2052–8.

139. Adams J, Palombella VJ, Sausville EA, et al. Proteasome inhibitors: a novel class of potent and effective antitumor agents. Cancer Res 1999; 59(11):2615–22.

140. Pedeboscq S, L'Azou B, Passagne I, et al. Cytotoxic and apoptotic effects of bortezomib and gefitinib compared to alkylating agents on human glioblastoma cells. J Exp Ther Oncol 2008;7(2): 99–111.

141. Laurent N, de Bouard S, Guillamo JS, et al. Effects of the proteasome inhibitor ritonavir on glioma growth in vitro and in vivo. Mol Cancer Ther 2004; 3(2):129–36.

142. Yin D, Zhou H, Kumagai T, et al. Proteasome inhibitor PS-341 causes cell growth arrest and apoptosis in human glioblastoma multiforme (GBM). Oncogene 2005;24(3):344–54.

143. Phuphanich S, Supko J, Carson KA, et al. Phase I trial of bortezomib in adults with recurrent malignant glioma. J Neurooncol 2010. [Epub ahead of print].

144. Kubicek GJ, Werner-Wasik M, Machtay M, et al. Phase I trial using proteasome inhibitor bortezomib and concurrent temozolomide and radiotherapy for central nervous system malignancies. Int J Radiat Oncol Biol Phys 2009;74(2):433–9.

145. Queitsch C, Sangster TA, Lindquist S. Hsp90 as a capacitor of phenotypic variation. Nature 2002; 417(6889):618–24.

146. Basso AD, Solit DB, Chiosis G, et al. Akt forms an intracellular complex with heat shock protein 90 (Hsp90) and Cdc37 and is destabilized by inhibitors of Hsp90 function. J Biol Chem 2002;277(42): 39858–66.

147. Lavictoire SJ, Parolin DA, Klimowicz AC, et al. Interaction of Hsp90 with the nascent form of the mutant epidermal growth factor receptor EGFRvIII. J Biol Chem 2003;278(7):5292–9.

148. An WG, Schulte TW, Neckers LM. The heat shock protein 90 antagonist geldanamycin alters chaperone association with p210bcr-abl and v-src proteins before their degradation by the proteasome. Cell Growth Differ 2000;11(7):355–60.

149. Miller P, Schnur RC, Barbacci E, et al. Binding of benzoquinoid ansamycins to p100 correlates with their ability to deplete the erbB2 gene product p185. Biochem Biophys Res Commun 1994; 201(3):1313–9.

150. Mimnaugh EG, Chavany C, Neckers L. Polyubiquitination and proteasomal degradation of the p185c-erbB-2 receptor protein-tyrosine kinase induced by geldanamycin. J Biol Chem 1996; 271(37):22796–801.

151. Schulte TW, An WG, Neckers LM. Geldanamycin-induced destabilization of Raf-1 involves the proteasome. Biochem Biophys Res Commun 1997; 239(3):655–9.

152. Schulte TW, Blagosklonny MV, Ingui C, et al. Disruption of the Raf-1-Hsp90 molecular complex results in destabilization of Raf-1 and loss of Raf-1-Ras association. J Biol Chem 1995;270(41):24585–8.

153. Whitesell L, Mimnaugh EG, De Costa B, et al. Inhibition of heat shock protein HSP90-pp60v-src heteroprotein complex formation by benzoquinone ansamycins: essential role for stress proteins in oncogenic transformation. Proc Natl Acad Sci U S A 1994;91(18):8324–8.

154. Kamal A, Thao L, Sensintaffar J, et al. A high-affinity conformation of Hsp90 confers tumour selectivity on Hsp90 inhibitors. Nature 2003; 425(6956):407–10.

155. Sauvageot CM, Weatherbee JL, Kesari S, et al. Efficacy of the HSP90 inhibitor 17-AAG in human glioma cell lines and tumorigenic glioma stem cells. Neuro Oncol 2009;11(2):109–21.

156. Garcia-Morales P, Carrasco-Garcia E, Ruiz-Rico P, et al. Inhibition of Hsp90 function by ansamycins causes downregulation of cdc2 and cdc25c and G(2)/M arrest in glioblastoma cell lines. Oncogene 2007;26(51):7185–93.

157. Xie Q, Thompson R, Hardy K, et al. A highly invasive human glioblastoma pre-clinical model for testing therapeutics. J Transl Med 2008;6:77.

158. Siegel PM, Massague J. Cytostatic and apoptotic actions of TGF-beta in homeostasis and cancer. Nat Rev Cancer 2003;3(11):807–21.

159. Javelaud D, Mauviel A. Crosstalk mechanisms between the mitogen-activated protein kinase pathways and Smad signaling downstream of TGF-beta: implications for carcinogenesis. Oncogene 2005;24(37):5742–50.

160. Moustakas A, Heldin CH. Non-Smad TGF-beta signals. J Cell Sci 2005;118(Pt 16):3573–84.

161. Jachimczak P, Hessdorfer B, Fabel-Schulte K, et al. Transforming growth factor-beta-mediated autocrine growth regulation of gliomas as detected with phosphorothioate antisense oligonucleotides. Int J Cancer 1996;65(3):332–7.

162. Kjellman C, Olofsson SP, Hansson O, et al. Expression of TGF-beta isoforms, TGF-beta receptors,

and SMAD molecules at different stages of human glioma. Int J Cancer 2000;89(3):251–8.

163. Hau P, Bogdahn U, Olyushin VE, et al. Results of a phase IIb study in recurrent or refractory glioblastoma patients with the TGF-beta-2 inhibitor AP 12009 [meeting abstracts]. J Clin Oncol 2007; 25(18 Suppl):12521.

164. Ma WW, Adjei AA. Novel agents on the horizon for cancer therapy. CA Cancer J Clin 2009;59(2):111–37.

165. Das S, Srikanth M, Kessler JA. Cancer stem cells and glioma. Nat Clin Pract Neurol 2008;4(8):427–35.

166. Stiles CD, Rowitch DH. Glioma stem cells: a midterm exam. Neuron 2008;58(6):832–46.

167. Li Z, Wang H, Eyler CE, et al. Turning cancer stem cells inside out: an exploration of glioma stem cell signaling pathways. J Biol Chem 2009;284(25): 16705–9.

168. Bao S, Wu Q, McLendon RE, et al. Glioma stem cells promote radioresistance by preferential activation of the DNA damage response. Nature 2006;444(7120):756–60.

169. Eyler CE, Rich JN. Survival of the fittest: cancer stem cells in therapeutic resistance and angiogenesis. J Clin Oncol 2008;26(17):2839–45.

170. Li Z, Bao S, Wu Q, et al. Hypoxia-inducible factors regulate tumorigenic capacity of glioma stem cells. Cancer Cell 2009;15(6):501–13.

171. Fulci G, Chiocca EA. The status of gene therapy for brain tumors. Expert Opin Biol Ther 2007;7(2): 197–208.

172. Aghi M, Rabkin S, Martuza RL. Effect of chemotherapy-induced DNA repair on oncolytic herpes simplex viral replication. J Natl Cancer Inst 2006; 98(1):38–50.

173. Germano IM, Binello E. Gene therapy as an adjuvant treatment for malignant gliomas: from bench to bedside. J Neurooncol 2009;93(1):79–87.

174. Nakamizo A, Marini F, Amano T, et al. Human bone marrow-derived mesenchymal stem cells in the treatment of gliomas. Cancer Res 2005;65(8): 3307–18.

175. Mamelak A, Rosenfeld S, Bucholz R, et al. Phase I single-dose study of intracavitary-administered iodine-131-TM-601 in adults with recurrent high-grade glioma. J Clin Oncol 2006; 24(22):3644–50.

176. Ferguson S, Lesniak MS. Convection enhanced drug delivery of novel therapeutic agents to malignant brain tumors. Curr Drug Deliv 2007;4(2): 169–80.

177. Celtic Pharma terminates TransMID trial KSB311R/CIII/001. Celtic Pharma; February 2, 2007. Available at: http://www.celticpharma.com/news/pr/transmid_020707.pdf. Accessed August 10, 2009.

178. Sampson JH, Archer GE, Bigner DD, et al. Effect of EGFRvIII-targeted vaccine (CDX-110) on immune response and TTP when given with simultaneous standard and continuous temozolomide in patients with GBM. J Clin Oncol 2008;26:2011.

179. Nemunaitis J, Jahan T, Ross H, et al. Phase 1/2 trial of autologous tumor mixed with an allogeneic GVAX vaccine in advanced-stage non-small-cell lung cancer. Cancer Gene Ther 2006;13(6): 555–62.

180. Parsa A, Crane C, Butkowski N, et al. Autologous heat shock protein vaccine for recurrent glioma: updated results of a phase I clinical trial. In: Proceedings from the Thirteenth Annual Meeting of the Society for Neuro-Oncology [abstract MA-91]. Lake Las Vegas (NV), November 20–23, 2008.

181. Prados MD, Chang SM, Butowski N, et al. Phase II study of erlotinib plus temozolomide during and after radiation therapy in patients with newly diagnosed glioblastoma multiforme or gliosarcoma. J Clin Oncol 2009;27(4):579–84.

182. Brandes AA, Stupp R, Hau P, et al. EORTC Study 26041–22041: Phase I/II study on concomitant and adjuvant temozolomide (TMZ) and radiotherapy (RT) with or without PTK787/ZK222584 (PTK/ZK) in newly diagnosed glioblastoma–results of a phase I trial. In: Proceedings from the American Society of Clinical Oncology [abstract 2026]. Chicago (IL), June 2–5, 2007.

183. Rich JN, Desjardins A, Sathornsumetee S, et al. Phase II study of bevacizumab and etoposide in patients with recurrent malignant glioma [meeting abstracts]. J Clin Oncol 2008;26(Suppl 15):2022.

184. Hasselbalch B, Lassen U, Soerensen M, et al. A phase II trial with cetuximab, bevacizumab and irinotecan for patients with primary glioblastoma and progression after radiation therapy and temozolomide. In: Proceedings from the Thirteenth Annual Meeting of the Society for Neuro-Oncology [abstract MA-44]. Lake Las Vegas (NV), November 20–23, 2008.

185. Sathornsumetee S, Desjardins A, Vredenburgh JJ, et al. Safety and efficacy of bevacizumab and erlotinib for recurrent glioblastoma patients in a phase II study. In: Proceedings from the Thirteenth Annual Meeting of the Society for Neuro-Oncology [abstract MA-41]. Lake Las Vegas (NV), November 20–23, 2008.

186. Sathornsumetee S, Vredenburgh JJ, Rich JN, et al. Phase II study of bevacizumab and erlotinib in patients with recurrent glioblastoma multiforme. In: Proceedings from the American Society of Clinical Oncology [abstract 13008]. Chicago (IL), May 30–June 3, 2008.

187. de Groot JF, Gilbert MR, Aldape K, et al. Phase II study of carboplatin and erlotinib (Tarceva, OSI-774) in patients with recurrent glioblastoma. J Neurooncol 2008;90(1):89–97.

188. Kreisl TN, Lassman AB, Mischel PS, et al. A pilot study of everolimus and gefitinib in the treatment

of recurrent glioblastoma (GBM). J Neurooncol 2009;92(1):99–105.

189. Phuphanich S, Rudnick J, Chu R, et al. A phase I trial of gefitinib and sirolimus in adults with recurrent glioblastoma multiforme (GBM). In: Proceedings from the American Society of Clinical Oncology [abstract 2088]. Chicago (IL), May 30–June 3, 2008.

190. Prados MD, Yung WK, Wen PY, et al. Phase-1 trial of gefitinib and temozolomide in patients with malignant glioma: a North American brain tumor consortium study. Cancer Chemother Pharmacol 2008;61(6):1059–67.

191. Reardon D, Quinn JA, Rich JN, et al. A phase I trial of imatinib, hydroxyurea and RAD001 for patients with recurrent malignant glioma. In: Proceedings from the American Society of Clinical Oncology [abstract 1580]. Atlanta (GA), June 2–6, 2006.

192. Kirkpatrick JP, Rich JN, Vredenburgh JJ, et al. Final report: phase I trial of imatinib mesylate, hydroxyurea, and vatalanib for patients with recurrent malignant glioma (MG). In: Proceedings from the American Society of Clinical Oncology [abstract 2057]. Chicago (IL), May 30–June 3, 2008.

193. Reardon DA, Egorin MJ, Desjardins A, et al. Phase I pharmacokinetic study of the vascular endothelial growth factor receptor tyrosine kinase inhibitor vatalanib (PTK787) plus imatinib and hydroxyurea for malignant glioma. Cancer 2009;115(10): 2188–98.

INDEX

Note: Page numbers of article titles are in **boldface** type